MEDICARE'S PROSPECTIVE PAYMENT SYSTEM

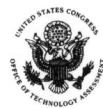

Office of Technology Assessment

The Office of Technology Assessment (OTA) was created in 1972 as an analytical arm of Congress. OTA's basic function is to help legislative policymakers anticipate and plan for the consequences of technological changes and to examine the many ways, expected and unexpected, in which technology affects people's lives. The assessment of technology calls for exploration of the physical, biological, economic, social, and political impacts that can result from applications of scientific knowledge. OTA provides Congress with independent and timely information about the potential effects—both beneficial and harmful—of technological applications.

Requests for studies are made by chairmen of standing committees of the House of Representatives or Senate; by the Technology Assessment Board, the governing body of OTA; or by the Director of OTA in consultation with the Board.

The Technology Assessment Board is composed of six members of the House, six members of the Senate, and the OTA Director, who is a nonvoting member.

OTA has studies under way in nine program areas: energy and materials; industry, technology, and employment; international security and commerce; biological applications; food and renewable resources; health; communication and information technologies; oceans and environment; and science, transportation, and innovation.

MEDICARE'S PROSPECTIVE PAYMENT SYSTEM

Office of Technology Assessment
Congress of the United States

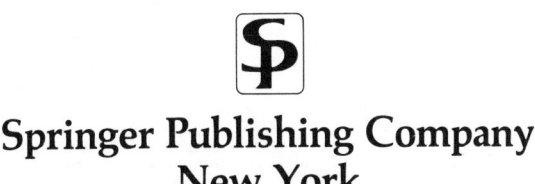

Springer Publishing Company
New York

Published in 1986 by:

Springer Publishing Company, Inc.
536 Broadway
New York, New York 10012

ISBN 0-8261-5720-3
Library of Congress Catalog Card Number 85-600604
Printed in the United States of America
All rights reserved.

OTA Reports are the principal documentation of formal assessment projects. These projects are approved in advance by the Technology Assessment Board. At the conclusion of a project, the Board has the opportunity to review the report, but its release does not necessarily imply endorsement of the results by the Board or its individual members.

Contents

Chapter   *Page*
Glossary of Acronyms and Terms ix

1. Introduction and Summary 3

Part One: A Framework for Evaluation 19
2. Predicted Effects of Medicare's Prospective Payment System 23
3. Preliminary Evidence of the Impacts of PPS 35
4. Issues in Designing an Evaluation of PPS 51

Part Two: Critical PPS Impact Areas 59
5. Expenditures and Costs 63
6. Quality of Care 77
7. Access to Health Care 95
8. Technological Change 113
9. Clinical Research 131

Part Three: Evaluation Strategies 139
10. Current PPS Evaluation Activities 143
11. Strategies for Evaluating PPS Impacts 165

Appendix   *Page*
A. Method of the Study 173
B. Acknowledgments and Health Program Advisory Committee 176
C. Major Population-Based Health Care Surveys 180
D. Major Databases Covering the Availability of Health Care Services 190
E. Medicare Part A Databases 195
F. Sources of Data on Aggregate Measures of Technological Change 200
G. PROs' Quality-of-Care Role in PPS 202
H. Alternative Patient Classification Systems 206

References 217

Office of Technology Assessment

Congressional Board of the 99th Congress

TED STEVENS, *Alaska, Chairman*

MORRIS K. UDALL, *Arizona, Vice Chairman*

Senate	House
ORRIN G. HATCH *Utah*	GEORGE E. BROWN, JR. *California*
CHARLES McC. MATHIAS, JR. *Maryland*	JOHN D. DINGELL *Michigan*
EDWARD M. KENNEDY *Massachusetts*	CLARENCE E. MILLER *Ohio*
ERNEST F. HOLLINGS *South Carolina*	COOPER EVANS *Iowa*
CLAIBORNE PELL *Rhode Island*	DON SUNDQUIST *Tennessee*

JOHN H. GIBBONS
(Nonvoting)

Advisory Council

WILLIAM J. PERRY, *Chairman* H&Q Technology Partners	CLAIRE T. DEDRICK *California Land Commission*	MICHEL T. HALBOUTY *Michel T. Halbouty Energy Co.*
DAVID S. POTTER, *Vice Chairman* General Motors Corp. (Ret.)	JAMES C. FLETCHER *University of Pittsburgh*	CARL N. HODGES *University of Arizona*
EARL BEISTLINE *Consultant*	S. DAVID FREEMAN *Consultant*	RACHEL McCULLOUCH *University of Wisconsin*
CHARLES A. BOWSHER *General Accounting Office*	GILBERT GUDE *Library of Congress*	LEWIS THOMAS *Memorial Sloan-Kettering Cancer Center*

Director

JOHN H. GIBBONS

The Technology Assessment Board approves the release of this report. The views expressed in this report are not necessarily those of the Board, OTA Advisory Council, or individual members thereof.

OTA Project Staff—Medicare's Prospective Payment System: Strategies for Evaluating Cost, Quality, and Medical Technology

Roger C. Herdman, *Assistant Director, OTA*
Health and Life Sciences Division

Clyde J. Behney, *Health Program Manager*

Judith L. Wagner, *Project Director*

Anne Kesselman Burns, *Analyst*
Mary Ann M. Hughes, *Research Assistant*
Cynthia P. King, *Analyst*
Elaine J. Power, *Research Analyst*
Kerry Britten Kemp, *Health and Life Sciences Division Editor*

Virginia Cwalina, *Administrative Assistant*
Beckie I. Erickson, *PC Specialist/Word Processor*[1]
Diann G. Hohenthaner, *PC Specialist/Word Processor*
Brenda L. Miller, *PC Specialist/Word Processor*[2]
Carol A. Guntow, *Secretary/Word Processor Specialist*

Contractors

Mary Ann Baily, *George Washington University*
Judith Barr, *Northeastern University*
Matthew Farber, *West Virginia University*
Marvin Feuerberg, *Washington, DC*
Stanley Finklestein, *MIT Sloane School of Management*
Bernard Friedman, *Northwestern University*
Kathleen Lohr, *Rand Corp.*
Peter McMenamin, *Washington, DC*
Ross Mullner, *American Hospital Association*
Jerri Perkins, *Perkins & Perkins Inc.*
Elliott Pickar, *Rockville, MD*
Neil Powe, *University of Pennsylvania*
Sankey Williams, *University of Pennsylvania*

---

[1]Until August 1985.
[2]Until January 1985.

Advisory Panel—Medicare's Prospective Payment System: Strategies for Evaluating Cost, Quality, and Medical Technology

John Eisenberg, *Panel Chair*
Associate Professor of Medicine
Hospital of the University of Pennsylvania

John R. Ball
Associate Executive Vice President for Health
 and Public Policy
American College of Physicians
Washington, DC

Morris Collen
Consultant
Department of Medical Methods Research
Kaiser-Permanente Medical Program
Oakland, CA

Helen Darling
Director
Human Resources Studies
Government Research Corp.
Washington, DC

Judith Feder
Center for Health Policy Studies
Georgetown University

Susan B. Foote
Assistant Professor
School of Business Administration
University of California at Berkeley

Anthony J. Gigliotti
President
Chief Operating Officer
United Hospitals, Inc.
Cheltenham, PA

Melvin Glasser
Director
Health Security Action Council
Washington, DC

Henry Grabowski
Department of Economics
Duke University

Rosalinda Haddon
Assistant Director
Newark Beth Israel Medical Center
Newark, NJ

Mark Hornbrook
Senior Investigator
Center for Health Research
Kaiser-Permanente, Northwest Region
Portland, OR

Ronald Hurst
Manager, Health Care Planning
Caterpillar Tractor
Peoria, IL

Judith Lave
Professor
Department of Health Economics
University of Pittsburgh

Barbara J. McNeil
Professor of Radiology and Clinical
 Epidemiology
Director, Center for Cost-Effective Care
Harvard Medical School
Brigham and Women's Hospital

Heather Palmer
Associate Dean for Students
Associate Professor of Health Services
Department of Health Policy and Management
Harvard School of Public Health

William Rial
Swarthmore, PA

Richard Riegelman
Associate Professor of Medicine and Health
 Care Sciences
George Washington University
School of Medicine

Leonard Saxe
Associate Professor of Psychology
Center for Applied Social Science
Boston University

Stephen Shortell
Professor of Hospital and Health Service
J.L. Kellogg Graduate School of Management
Northwestern University
Evanston, IL

Donald Sutherland
Director
Investor Affairs
E. I. du Pont de Nemours & Co.
Wilmington, DE

Bruce Vladeck
President
United Hospital Fund of New York

John E. Wennberg
Professor
Department of Community and Family
 Medicine
Dartmouth Medical School

James Young
Vice President and Medical Director
Blue Cross/Blue Shield of Massachusetts

Foreword

Twenty years ago, Congress made a major commitment to securing older Americans' access to acute medical care with the creation of Medicare. Subsequent legislation extended the Medicare program to disabled people and to victims of end-stage renal disease. Medicare has been an unquestioned success in reducing financial barriers to health care for its beneficiaries, but the program's costs have risen rapidly.

Medicare's payment methods have discouraged doctors, hospital managers, and patients from making cost-effective decisions regarding the use of medical technology. Retrospective cost-based hospital reimbursement was particularly troublesome and, most would agree, inflationary.

Congress ended cost-based reimbursement for inpatient hospital care for Medicare beneficiaries with the creation of Medicare's prospective payment system (PPS) in 1983. The new hospital payment system has reversed the financial incentives away from the provision of more care for hospitalized patients to the provision of less care. Now, the Nation needs to know what this radical change in financial incentives is doing to the quantity and quality of health care received by Medicare beneficiaries, and to the effectiveness of Medicare resources.

Early in 1984, two committees of Congress, the Senate Committee on Finance and the Senate Special Committee on Aging, asked OTA to conduct an assessment that would identify potential economic and health-related effects of PPS and develop a series of strategies for an evaluation of the most important effects.

In this report, OTA arrays the possible effects of PPS on the health care system and assesses the extent to which these effects can be measured. Potential PPS impacts are summarized, and critical evaluation questions are identified for each impact area. In addition to identifying specific studies that would address the critical evaluation questions, OTA also attempted to put the studies in a priority order, based on their cost and feasibility.

OTA was guided in the study by an advisory panel chaired by John Eisenberg. Drafts of the report and several working papers prepared as background were reviewed by members of the advisory panel, members of the OTA Health Program Advisory Committee, and other experts in the Federal and State governments and in health policy research. We are grateful for their assistance. Key OTA staff were Judith Wagner, Anne K. Burns, Mary Ann M. Hughes, Cynthia P. King, and Elaine J. Power.

JOHN H. GIBBONS
Director

Glossary of Acronyms and Terms

Glossary of Acronyms

ADAMHA	—Alcohol, Drug Abuse, and Mental Health Administration (PHS)
AHA	—American Hospital Association
ALOS	—average length of stay
APACHE	—Acute Physiology and Chronic Health Evaluation
ARF	—Area Resource File (HRSA)
ASPE	—Assistant Secretary for Planning and Evaluation (DHHS)
CBO	—Congressional Budget Office (U.S. Congress)
CDC	—Centers for Disease Control (PHS)
CHAS	—Center for Health Administration Studies (University of Chicago)
CON	—certificate of need
CPHA	—Commission on Professional and Hospital Activities
CPT-4	—Current Procedural Terminology, 4th Edition
CRS	—Congressional Research Service (U.S. Congress)
DHHS	—U.S. Department of Health and Human Services
DRG	—diagnosis-related group
ECOG	—Eastern Cooperative Oncology Group
ESRD	—end-stage renal disease
ESWL	—extracorporeal shock wave lithotripsy
FDA	—Food and Drug Administration (PHS)
FTE	—full-time equivalent
GAO	—General Accounting Office (U.S. Congress)
GCRC	—general clinical research center
HANES	—Health and Nutrition Examination Survey (NCHS)
HCFA	—Health Care Financing Administration (DHHS)
HCRIS	—Hospital Cost Report Information System (HCFA)
HCUP	—Hospital Cost and Utilization Project (NCHSR&HCTA)
NDS	—Hospital Discharge Survey (NCHS)
HES	—Health Examination Survey (NCHS)
HIM	—Health Insurance Master Enrollment Record (HCFA)
HIS	—Health Interview Survey (NCHS)
HRSA	—Health Resources and Services Administration (PHS)
HSQB	—Health Standards and Quality Bureau (HCFA)
ICD-9-CM	—International Classification of Diseases, 9th Revision, Clinical Modification
ICF	—intermediate care facility
ICU	—intensive care unit
IOLs	—intraocular lenses
IRS	—Internal Revenue Service
JCAH	—Joint Commission on the Accreditation of Hospitals
LOS	—length of stay
MADRS	—Medicare Automated Data Retrieval System (HCFA)
MEDISGRPS	—Medical Illness Severity Grouping System
MEDPAR	—Medicare Provider Analysis and Review (HCFA)
MFI	—Master Facility Inventory of Hospitals and Institutions (NCHS)
MHS	—Medicare History Sample
MMACS	—Medicare/Medicaid Automated Certification System (HCFA)
NAFAC	—National Association for Ambulatory Care Centers
NAMCS	—National Ambulatory Medical Care Survey (NCHS)
NCHS	—National Center for Health Statistics (PHS)
NCHSR	—National Center for Health Services Research (PHS)
NCHSR& HCTA	—National Center for Health Services Research and Health Care Technology Assessment (PHS)
NCI	—National Cancer Institute (NIH)
NIH	—National Institutes of Health (PHS)
NLTCS	—National Long-Term Care Survey (ASPE, HCFA)
NMCES	—National Medical Care Expenditure Survey (NCHSR)
NMCUES	—National Medical Care Utilization and Expenditure Survey (NCHS, HCFA)
NNHS	—National Nursing Home Survey (NCHS)
NSF	—National Science Foundation
NSPHPC	—National Survey of Personal Health Practices and Consequences (NCHS)
ODE	—Office of Demonstrations and Evaluation (ORD)

OHPE	—Office of Health Planning and Evaluation (PHS)
OHTA	—Office of Health Technology Assessment (NCHSR)
OR	—Office of Research (ORD)
ORD	—Office of Research and Demonstrations (HCFA)
OTA	—Office of Technology Assessment (U.S. Congress)
PATBILL	—Medicare's inpatient bills file
PHDDS	—PRO Hospital Discharge Data Set
PHS	—Public Health Service (DHHS)
PMAA	—premarket approval application
POS	—Provider of Services (MMACS)
PPO	—preferred provider organization
PPS	—prospective payment system (Medicare)
PRO	—utilization and quality control peer review organization
ProPAC	—Prospective Payment Assessment Commission
PSRO	—professional standards review organization
PTCA	—percutaneous transluminal coronary angioplasty
R&D	—research and development
SDW	—Survey of Disability and Work (SSA)
SIC	—Standard Industrial Classification
SIP	—Survey of Institutionalized Persons (Bureau of the Census)
SMSA	—Standard Metropolitan Statistical Area
SNF	—skilled nursing facility
SSA	—Social Security Administration (DHHS)
TDM	—therapeutic drug monitoring
TEFRA	—Tax Equity and Fiscal Responsibility Act of 1982
UHDDS	—Uniform Hospital Discharge Data Set
VA	—U.S. Veterans Administration
WHO	—World Health Organization

Glossary of Terms

Access: Potential and actual entry of a population into the health care delivery system.

Ambulatory care: Medical care provided to patients in physician offices, clinics, or outpatient facilities.

Ancillary services: Medical technologies used directly to support clinical care, such as diagnostic radiology, radiation therapy, clinical laboratory, and other special services.

Average length of stay (ALOS): The average length of hospital stay experienced by a group of patients.

Bad debt: Unpaid patient hospital bills.

Budget neutrality: A term used in the Social Security Amendments of 1983 (Public Law 98-21) to mean that the aggregate payments by Medicare for the operating costs of inpatient hospital services in fiscal years 1984 and 1985 will be neither more nor less than such payments would have been under the Tax Equity and Fiscal Responsibility Act (Public Law 97-248) for the costs of the same services.

Capital costs: Expenditures for capital plant and equipment used in providing a service. Under Medicare's prospective payment system (PPS) for hospitals, established by the Social Security Amendments of 1983 (Public Law 98-21), hospitals' capital costs (depreciation, interest, and return on equity to for-profit institutions) are treated as passthroughs (i.e., are not subject to the new system's controls).

Carriers: Organizations authorized by the Health Care Financing Administration to help administer the Part B benefits under Medicare. Carriers determine coverage and benefit amounts payable and make Part B payments to providers or beneficiaries.

Case mix: The relative frequency of admissions of various types of patients, reflecting different needs for hospital resources.

Clinical trial: A scientific research activity undertaken to define prospectively the effect and value of medical devices, agents, regimens, procedures, etc., applied to human subjects.

Conditions of participation (Medicare): Requirements that health care providers (including hospitals, skilled nursing homes, home health agencies, etc.) must meet in order to be eligible to receive payments for Medicare patients. An example is the requirement that hospitals conduct utilization review.

Copayment: A form of beneficiary cost-sharing whereby the insured pays a specific amount at the point of consumption of health services, e.g., $10 per visit.

Cost-based reimbursement: See *retrospective cost-based reimbursement*.

Current Procedure Terminology, 4th Edition (CPT-4): A coding system for procedures performed by physicians that is used in Medicare Part B billing.

Deductible: A form of beneficiary cost-sharing in which the insured incurs an initial expense of a specified amount within a given time period (e.g., $250 per year) before the insurer assumes liability for any additional costs of covered services.

Diagnosis-related groups (DRGs): Groupings of diagnostic categories that are the case-mix measure mandated by the Social Security Amendments of 1983 (Public Law 98-21) for Medicare's prospective payment system (PPS) for hospitals. DRG categories were drawn from the International Classification of Diseases, 9th Revision, Clinical Modification, and modified by the presence of a surgical procedure, patient age, presence or absence of significant comorbidities or complications, and other relevant criteria.

Discharge abstract: A shortened version of a discharged patient's medical record including items extracted from the medical record.

Discretionary adjustment factor: The component of the DRG update factor that accounts for cost increases or decreases that are not necessarily captured by inflation measures, e.g., quality of care. The discretionary adjustment factor was originally set at 1 percent per year but was later limited by Congress to 0.25 percent for fiscal years 1985 and 1986.

DRG weight: A weight assigned to a DRG that represents its assumed resource use relative to other DRGs. The higher the weight, the larger the Medicare payment.

Freestanding facilities: Health care facilities that are not physically, administratively, or financially connected to a hospital. An example is a freestanding ambulatory surgery center.

Full-time equivalent (FTE) employees: The number of full-time employees it would take to work the total number of hours worked by part-time, full-time, and over-time employees.

Hemodialysis: A process by which blood is pumped from a patient's body into a dialyzer and then returned to the body in a continuous extracorporeal blood loop. While in the dialyzer, the blood flows next to but separate from another fluid, a dialysate. The blood and the dialysate are separated from each other by a semipermeable membrane. Waste products and other molecules pass through the semipermeable membrane, and the blood takes on its appropriate properties.

Home health agency: An organization that is primarily engaged in providing skilled nursing services and other therapeutic services (e.g., physical, occupational, or speech therapy) in the patient's home.

Iatrogenic events: Infections, drug reactions, or other mishaps due to treatment in a hospital or by a physician.

Inpatient care: Medical care that includes an overnight stay in a medical facility. In this report, the term generally refers to overnight treatment in a hospital.

Intermediaries: Organizations authorized by the Health Care Financing Administration to make Medicare Part A payments to hospitals. Intermediaries also make payments for home health and outpatient hospital services covered under Part B.

International Classification of Diseases, 9th Revision, Clinical Modification (ICD-9-CM): A two-part system of coding patient medical information used in abstracting systems and for classifying patients into DRGs for Medicare. The first part is a comprehensive list of diseases with corresponding codes compatible with the World Health Organization's list of disease codes. The second part contains procedure codes, independent of the disease codes.

Length of stay (LOS): The number of days a patient remains in the hospital from admission to discharge.

Medical technology: The drugs, devices, and medical and surgical procedures used in medical care, and the organizational and supportive systems within which such care is provided.

Medicare: A nationwide, federally administered health insurance program authorized in 1965 to cover the cost of hospitalization, medical care, and some related services for most persons over age 65, persons receiving Social Security Disability Insurance payments for 2 years, and persons with end-stage renal disease. Medicare consists of two separate but coordinated programs—Part A (Hospital Insurance) and Part B (Supplementary Medical Insurance). Health insurance protection is available to Medicare beneficiaries without regard to income.

Medicare cost reports: Annual reports submitted by individual hospitals to Medicare intermediaries and used to calculate the amount of Medicare's obligation to the hospital under cost-based reimbursement.

Outliers: Cases with unusually high or low resource use. DRG outliers are defined by the Social Security Amendments of 1983 (Public Law 98-21) as atypical cases that have either an extremely long length of stay or extraordinarily high costs when compared to most discharges classified in the same DRG.

Outpatient care: Medical care that does not include an overnight stay in the facility in which care is provided.

Part A (Medicare): Medicare's Hospital Insurance program, which covers specified hospital inpatient services, posthospital extended care, and home health care services. Part A, which is an entitlement program for those who are eligible, is available without payment of a premium, although those not automatically eligible for Part A may enroll in the program by paying a monthly premium. The beneficiary is responsible for an initial deductible and/or copayment for some services.

Part B (Medicare): Medicare's Supplementary Medical Insurance program which covers physician services, hospital outpatient services, outpatient physical therapy and speech pathology services, and various other limited ambulatory services and supplies such as prosthetic devices and durable medical equipment. This program also covers home health services for Medicare beneficiaries who have Part B coverage only. Enrollment in Part B is optional and requires payment of a monthly premium. The beneficiary is also responsible for a deductible and a coinsurance payment for most covered services.

Passthroughs: Elements of hospital cost that are not covered by Medicare's prospective payment system (PPS) established by the Social Security Amendments of 1983 and continue to be paid for on the basis of cost-based reimbursement. Under Medicare's PPS, capital costs, direct teaching, and outpatient service expenses are passthroughs.

Per-case payment: A type of prospective payment for health care services in which the hospital (or other provider) is paid a specific amount for each patient treated, regardless of the number and types of services or number of days of care provided. Medicare's DRG-based prospective payment system (PPS) for inpatient services is a per-case payment system.

Procedure (medical or surgical): A medical technology involving any combination of drugs, devices, and provider skills and abilities. Appendectomy, for example, may involve at least drugs (for anesthesia), monitoring devices, surgical devices, and the skilled action of physicians, nurses, and support staff.

Professional standards review organizations (PSROs): Community-based, physician-directed, nonprofit agencies established under the Social Security Amendments of 1972 (Public Law 92-603) to review the quality and appropriateness of institutional health care provided to Medicare and Medicaid beneficiaries. PSROs have been replaced by utilization and quality control peer review organizations (PROs).

Prospective payment: A method of payment for health care services in which the amount of payment for services is set prior to the delivery of those services and the hospital (or other provider) is at least partially at risk for losses or stands to gain from surpluses that accrue in the payment period. Prospective payment rates may be per service, per capita, per diem, or per case rates.

Prospective Payment Assessment Commission (ProPAC): An independent commission established by the Social Security Amendments of 1983 (Public Law 98-21), the law that created Medicare's DRG-based prospective payment system (PPS), to advise the Secretary of Health and Human Services on the annual update factor and on adjustments of DRG classifications and weights.

Quality assessment: Measurement and evaluation of quality of care for individuals, groups, or populations.

Quality assurance: A term that refers to integrated programs that attempt to protect or raise quality of care by conducting assessments, taking action to correct problems found, and following up corrective interventions.

Quality of care: A term used in this report to refer to the kind of care that maximizes an inclusive measure of patient welfare after one has taken account of the balance of expected gains and losses that attend the process of care in all its parts.

Ratesetting: A method of payment for health care services in which a State (or other) regulatory body decides what prices a hospital, for example, may charge in a given year.

Recalibration: The periodic process of adjusting the prices of DRGs relative to each other, through changes in DRG weights.

Retrospective cost-based reimbursement: A method of payment for health care services in which hospitals (or other providers) are paid their incurred costs of treating patients after the treatment has occurred.

Reweighting: The adjustment of certain DRG weights to reflect changes in relative resource costs.

Short-stay hospitals: Hospitals in which the average length of stay is less than 30 days.

Skilled nursing facility (SNF): A specially qualified institution that has the staff and equipment to provide skilled nursing care or rehabilitation services and other related health services and that also meets specified regulatory certification requirements.

Standard Industrial Classification (SIC) codes: A categorization of data on products and companies that is used by the U.S. Department of Commerce. Establishments (plants) are assigned to SIC "industries" on the basis of their primary line of business. However, SIC data on shipments of a specific product include all shipments of the relevant product, regardless of the "industry" in which the producing establishment is classified.

Substantially equivalent device: A device first marketed after the 1976 Medical Device Amendments that the Food and Drug Administration has found to be similar to a device already being marketed. To be found substantially equivalent, a postamendments device need not be identical to a preamendments device, but must not differ markedly in materials, design, or energy source.

Technology diffusion: The diffusion or spread of a medical technology into the health care system. It is generally thought to be in two phases: the initial phase in which decisions are made to adopt or reject the technology, and a subsequent phase in which decisions are made to use the technology.

Updating: The annual process of increasing (or decreasing) all DRG prices by an "update factor" that determines the overall generosity of Medicare's prospective payment system for hospitals. The update factor used in this process has two components: 1) an inflation factor that reflects inflation in the hospital sector; and 2) a "discretionary adjustment factor" that reflects cost increases (or decreases) not captured by inflation measures.

Utilization and quality control peer review organizations (PROs): Physician organizations established by the Tax Equity and Fiscal Responsibility Act of

1982 (Public Law 97-248) to replace professional standards review organizations (PSROs). Hospitals are mandated by the Social Security Amendments of 1983 (Public Law 98-21) to contract with PROs to review quality of care and appropriateness of admissions and readmissions.

Waivered States: States holding waivers from the Health Care Financing Administration that allow them to participate in experimental payment programs as alternatives to Medicare's prospective payment system (PPS). Currently, they are Maryland, Massachusetts, New Jersey, and New York (New York will not have a waiver after Dec. 31, 1985). These States are required by their special contracts with the Federal Government to keep their aggregate Medicare expenditures below what they would be under the national PPS.

Chapter 1
Introduction and Summary

Contents

	Page
Introduction	3
Scope of the Report	4
Organization of the Report	4
Findings	5
Potential PPS Impacts	5
Potential for Evaluation	8
Options for Evaluating PPS	10
Options for Specific Studies	10
Options for Implementing PPS Evaluation	14

LIST OF TABLES

Table No.	Page
1-1. Summary of Potential PPS Impacts on Five Dimensions of Health System Performance	7
1-2. Studies and Data Sources Needed To Address Critical PPS Evaluation Questions	11

Chapter 1
Introduction and Summary

INTRODUCTION

In 1983, Congress passed a law that radically changed Medicare's method of payment for inpatient hospital services. The Social Security Amendments of 1983 (Public Law 98-21) mandated an end to cost-based reimbursement by Medicare and initiated a 3-year transition to a prospective payment system (PPS) for inpatient hospital services. The system mandated by this law is based on fixed per-case payment rates for patients in 468 diagnosis-related groups (DRGs).

The ultimate objective of Medicare's PPS is to reduce Medicare's outlays for inpatient hospital care while maintaining an acceptable level of quality and access for beneficiaries. This goal is to be sought through a fundamental restructuring of the financial incentives facing hospitals. Medicare's PPS is a striking change from the previous payment system, providing an entirely new set of incentives relating to medical technology[1] adoption and use by hospitals and other health care providers.

One incentive under PPS is for hospitals to reduce the cost of treating a patient over the course of a hospital stay, in some cases by reducing the length of that stay. PPS diminishes the financial incentives for hospitals managers and physicians to provide additional technologies (except where they lower per-case costs to the hospital), because it encourages such providers to weigh explicitly the benefits of those additional services against their added costs. Because payment is per admission, a second incentive is for hospitals to increase the number of admissions, particularly those that appear to be profitable. A third incentive under PPS is for hospitals to develop new sources of revenue by offering services not subject to DRG payment restrictions. All other incentives and resulting changes in the patterns of technology use arise from these three basic incentives.

Although the direction of the incentives under PPS and some of the resulting impacts were predicted by the designers of the new payment system, the assumptions behind them are largely untested. These uncertainties have not discouraged many observers from predicting serious undesirable results of PPS on patients' access to and quality of health care, on the rate of introduction of new technologies into the practice of medicine, and on the level of clinical research in this country. **The widespread concern that Medicare's PPS could pose a substantial threat to the health care system has made it a highly visible issue and argues for a deliberate strategy for development of valid and timely data on the actual impacts of PPS as they occur.**

Congressional awareness of potential problems with PPS was evident even as the law establishing the system was drafted, and some of the problems are explicitly addressed in the Social Security Amendments of 1983. For example, the PPS law mandated that the Secretary of the Department of Health and Human Services (DHHS) prepare annual reports on the impact of PPS through 1987.

Access to valid information on the impacts of Medicare's PPS is so vital, however, that two committees of Congress, the Senate Committee on Finance and the Senate Special Committee on Aging, asked OTA to conduct an assessment that would identify: 1) the *types* of economic and health-related effects, related to medical technology, that might result from implementation of Medicare's PPS; and 2) a series of strategies for congressional consideration that would provide an evaluation of the most important effects.

This report presents the results of OTA's assessment. It is not an evaluation of PPS; rather, its primary purpose is to identify the kinds of information that are required to give Congress and the American public an accurate and timely view of the impacts of Medicare's PPS.

---
[1]OTA defines medical technology as the drugs, devices, and medical and surgical procedures used in medical care, and the organizational and supportive systems within which they are provided.

Scope of the Report

This report arrays the possible effects of Medicare's PPS on the U.S. health care system and assesses the extent to which these effects can and should be measured. **The effects of PPS most relevant to the performance of the health care system are effects on the *cost* of providing medical care and effects on the *health benefits* received from that care.**

Unfortunately, the direct measurement of health benefits is infeasible; therefore, incomplete, imperfect, and overlapping proxy measures must be used. OTA chose four PPS impact areas to serve as proxy indicators of health benefits: quality of care, access to care, technological change, and clinical research.

These PPS impact areas are discussed separately, but there is a great deal of overlap and interaction among them. The most important concern about the content of care in relation to the health benefits it provides is the quality of that care. Yet quality and access are interrelated, since the same number and mix of services can provide wide variations in access to care if the quality of that care differs widely. Also, the content of medical care (and therefore its costs and benefits) is greatly influenced over time by the direction and rate of technological change and clinical research.

Although the emphasis in this report is on methods for evaluating the ultimate impacts of Medicare's PPS on cost, quality, and the like, changes in the behavior of providers and patients that are brought about by PPS will clearly affect ultimate impacts. This report examines the need for studies of PPS impacts on the organization and utilization of health care services in the context of the ability of such studies to provide useful information on the ultimate benefits and costs of PPS.

Changes in benefits and costs due to PPS are bound to vary among patients, payers, and providers. These redistributions of benefits and costs among the members of society are even more important than PPS impacts on society as a whole, because they have major implications for the equity of PPS. OTA has been mindful of the importance of such distributional impacts in each of the areas discussed.

Certain areas of impact are beyond the scope of this study. PPS has the potential to affect the livelihoods of many people through its influence on patterns of employment in health care and related industries. To the extent that such employment changes affect health costs and benefits, they are captured in this study. But employment shifts require serious public policy attention in their own right. For example, if PPS leads to major layoffs of unskilled hospital personnel, what alternative employment opportunities will be available? Such questions are embedded in larger issues of labor force policy and are beyond the scope of this study.

Also beyond the scope of this study is the effect of PPS on the owners of health care and related businesses. PPS impacts on the health product manufacturing industries, for example, are implicit through their effect, if any, on research and development and, hence, technological change in medicine. Such impacts are not considered for their own sake. Similarly, the effect of PPS on patterns of for-profit versus not-for-profit health care institutions is considered only in the context of PPS impacts on quality and access.

Finally, this report does not directly address the impacts that PPS may have on the quantity and quality of health professions education. These effects could well be both immediate and dramatic. Like all other impacts, however, PPS effects on medical and nursing education are important insofar as they alter the ultimate benefits and costs of health care over the years. Assessment of these ultimate impacts should detect the influence of changes in health professions education. However, the influence of educational changes on health benefits and costs may not be discernible for many years. Thus, although the complexity of the subject precluded detailed discussion of educational effects in this study, the potential delay in detecting their ultimate impacts argues for early attention to the effects of PPS on education, accompanied by an assessment of the implications for health benefits and costs.

Organization of the Report

The rest of this chapter presents a summary of the study findings and strategies and options for evaluating PPS. The body of the report is organized into three parts. Part One (chs. 2 through 4) provides a framework for designing an evaluation strategy, including a statement of what is known about the direction and magnitude of PPS effects from analysis of its financial incentives (ch. 2); a brief review of the sparse evidence available from the first year of operation of PPS (ch. 3); and a discussion of issues that arise in designing an evaluation of PPS (ch. 4).

Part Two (chs. 5 through 9) discusses each of the broad areas in which OTA has assessed needs for evaluative information: expenditures and costs (ch. 5), quality of care (ch. 6), access to care (ch. 7), technological change (ch. 8), and clinical research (ch. 9). Each of the chapters addresses the following topics:

- definitions and measurement issues in the area;
- potential impacts of PPS on the area;
- critical evaluation questions arising from the analysis of potential impacts;
- approaches to addressing the critical evaluation questions; and
- data availability and problems.

Part Three (chs. 10 and 11) examines existing activities of both the Federal Government and private organizations to evaluate and monitor the impacts of PPS (ch. 10) and lays out considerations in the development of strategies regarding the content, organization, and funding of evaluative research activities (ch. 11).

Separate appendixes provide detailed discussions of specific issues, and include descriptions of major population-based databases (app. C), databases that can be used to measure the availability of health services and facilities (app. D), and Medicare Part A data systems (app. E); and data on aggregate measures of technological change (app. F); an analysis of the role of utilization and quality control peer review organizations (PROs) as a component of PPS (app. G); and a description of DRGs and alternative systems for classifying hospital inpatients (app. H).

FINDINGS

Potential PPS Impacts

A central objective of this study has been to identify critical evaluation questions that need to be addressed with respect to PPS impacts on five important dimensions of health system performance:

- expenditures and costs;
- quality of care;
- access to care;
- technological change; and
- clinical research.

Such questions arise from an analysis of the incentives inherent in the structure of PPS relative to cost-based reimbursement. New incentives leading to alterations in the behavior of providers and patients will ultimately affect the performance of the U.S. health care system.

The changes in the health care system brought about by Medicare's PPS will result from a combination of three aspects of PPS:

- that it is a system of expenditure control;
- that it pays hospitals by the case rather than by the day or service; and
- that it uses DRGs as the system of classifying patients for payment purposes.

It is difficult to disentangle the effects of each of these three components of PPS from one another. Many of the changes that occur as a result of PPS might well have come about through any system that successfully controls the aggregate level of Medicare expenditures for hospital care. Other changes, such as reductions in length of hospital stay, can be expected under any per-case payment method. Still other effects on the availability and use of technologies for specific patients can be traced to the peculiar characteristics of the DRG patient classification system.

As a system for classifying hospitalized patients into a limited number of mutually exclusive and exhaustive categories, the DRG system necessarily involves grouping together patients with heterogeneous medical and surgical needs. The DRG patient classification system is based on diagnostic and procedural codes of the International Classification of Diseases, 9th Revision, Clinical Modification (ICD-9-CM). The way in which medical technologies, particularly new ones, are coded under ICD-9-CM and then incorporated into the DRG system determines not only the kinds of patients that are likely to be profitable to hospitals but also the profitability of new technologies. OTA found, for example, that a new technology that reduces per-case cost could actually reduce a hospital's profit if its use places the patient into a lower priced DRG. Conversely, a cost-increasing new technology could increase hospital profits if its use would place a patient into a more highly reimbursed DRG with a sufficiently higher rate of payment. Other patient classification systems—for example, a system based on the physiological condition of the patient at admission—might offer very different specific incentives with regard to the use and adoption of technology.

When the three aspects of PPS just mentioned are taken together, hospitals can be expected to pursue various strategies, among them, for example:

- increasing hospital admissions, particularly those that are profitable under DRGs;
- increasing readmissions and interhospital transfers;
- increasing discharges to nursing homes;
- integrating hospital services with noninstitutional services; such as nursing homes; home health care agencies;
- increasing specialization of services;
- increasing hospital diversification into provision of unregulated health services;
- "upcoding" diagnoses and procedures reported for payment purposes; and
- decreasing cost per admission (through reductions in lengths of stay, ancillary service use, supply prices, or staffing levels).

Table 1-1 summarizes the relationship between the predicted changes in hospital behavior and the five dimensions of health system performance identified earlier. Note that specific PPS incentives, such as the incentive to increase hospital

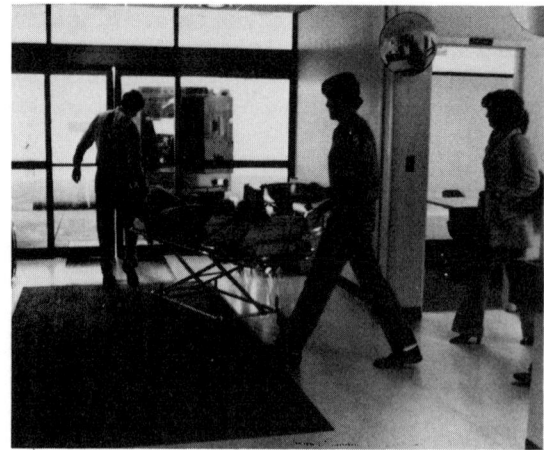

Photo credit: Fairfax Hospital Association

The incentive provided by PPS to increase interhospital transfers may increase quality of care if the receiving hospital is actually a more appropriate source of care for the patient, yet it may decrease quality by overloading stressed hospitals.

admissions, may influence several key dimensions at once. Moreover, the direction of impact is not always completely known or uniform across hospitals or patients. In some cases, the incentives are so complicated or mitigated by other factors that the direction of impact cannot be predicted; in others, negative impacts on some people are matched by positive impacts on others.

The sparse evidence on changes in the health care system after the first year of PPS pertains primarily to changes in the utilization and organization of health services. Furthermore, the evidence from the first year is tentative, because not all hospitals were covered by PPS for the entire year and only 25 percent of hospitals' payments were based on DRG prices. Although none of the observed changes can be solely attributed to PPS, several are strong enough to infer at least partial causation by PPS. The average length of hospital stay for Medicare beneficiaries, for instance, has been declining for over a decade, but it took a further radical drop during 1984 that is probably mainly due to PPS. Changes in hospital management priorities, reductions in staffing, the accelerated move toward automated hospital information systems, and an increase in hospital marketing also appear to have been influenced by

Ch. 1—Introduction and Summary • 7

Table 1-1.—Summary of Potential PPS Impacts on Five Dimensions of Health System Performance

Predicted changes in hospital behavior	Expenditures and costs	Quality of care	Access to health care	Technological change and clinical research
Cost per admission (down)	May either increase or decrease total Medicare program expenditures	May increase or decrease quality	May increase or decrease access	May increase research on and adoption and use of technologies that lower costs by lowering LOS; may decrease development and diffusion of those that raise LOS
Length of stay (LOS) (down)	May either increase or decrease total Medicare program expenditures	May increase psychological benefits to patients and lessen chance of iatrogenic events; but may also result in discharging sicker patients	May decrease access to necessary hospitalization for patients discharged early; but may also increase access for patients who need to get into hospitals with high occupancy rates	May increase development and diffusion of technologies that permit fewer or less frequent ancillary services; may decrease development and diffusion of those that require more
Ancillary services (down)	May either increase or decrease total Medicare program expenditures	May decrease use of unnecessary services and decrease risk of diagnostic tests and invasive procedures; but may also decrease use of necessary technologies	May decrease access to necessary services	
Prices of materials and supplies (down)	Decreases hospital costs	No effect	No effect	May decrease R&D by private industry
Use of less expensive materials and supplies (down)	Decreases hospital costs	May increase use of less effective materials, devices, and supplies	No effect	May increase development and diffusion of supply technologies (such as wound dressings) that lower costs; may decrease development and diffusion of those that raise them
Staffing levels (down)	May either increase or decrease total Medicare program expenditures	May decrease use of specialized personnel when needed	May decrease access to special personnel, such as social workers or speech therapists	May increase research on and adoption and use of technologies that are less labor-intensive; may decrease development and diffusion of those that are more labor-intensive
Admissions (up)	Increases Medicare Part A program and beneficiary expenditures; may increase or decrease Part B expenditures	May build specialty in particular DRGs in hospital; but may also increase iatrogenic events	Increases access to hospital care	May increase clinical research and technology adoption and use in profitable DRGs; may decrease that in unprofitable ones
Readmissions (up)	Increases Medicare Part A program and beneficiary expenditures; may increase or decrease Part B expenditures	May decrease quality if diagnosis or treatment is delayed	May increase or decrease access to appropriate care	No effect
Transfers (up)	Increases Medicare Part A program and beneficiary expenditures; may increase or decrease Part B expenditures	May increase quality through specialization in hospital; but may also decrease quality by overloading stressed hospitals	May increase or decrease access for particular populations, such as poor, very old, alcoholic, or mentally ill patients	No effect
Discharges to:				
Nursing homes (up)	May either increase or decrease total Medicare program and beneficiary expenditures	May decrease use of unnecessary care in hospital; but may also increase severity of illness of patients in nursing homes which could lead to greater demands on nursing staff and lower quality of care	May decrease access to necessary higher levels of care; may also increase access for Medicare beneficiaries to appropriate lower levels of care. Access to lower levels of care for Medicaid beneficiaries may decline	May encourage more clinical research in nursing home settings
Home health care (up)	May either increase or decrease total Medicare program and beneficiary expenditures	May increase psychological benefits for patients and families; but may also result in sicker patients being cared for at home, possibly less effectively	May decrease access for Medicare beneficiaries to necessary higher levels of care; but may also increase access to appropriate lower levels of care	May encourage more clinical research in home settings; may increase development and diffusion of technologies that can be used at home
Vertical integration of services (up)	May either increase or decrease total Medicare program and beneficiary expenditures	May increase use of appropriate level of services; but may also lead to inappropriate placements	May decrease access to necessary higher levels of care; may also increase access to appropriate lower levels of care	May increase diffusion of traditional inpatient technologies into outpatient and home settings
Specialization of services (up)	May decrease per capita health care expenditures	Increases quality through increasing volume of services	May increase access to special services for some patients; but may also decrease access for parts of the population	May encourage research on and adoption of technologies in hospital's area of specialization in order to enhance hospital's reputation
Upcoding (up)	Increases Medicare Part A expenditures	No effect	No effect	May encourage adoption and use of technologies that permit patient to be classified into a higher paying DRG (when resulting additional reimbursement is greater than additional cost

SOURCE: Office of Technology Assessment, 1985.

PPS. On the other hand, the expected increase in hospital admissions did not occur. The failure of this predicted change to occur under PPS implies that certain hospital strategies may take time to develop, that hospital managers' power to influence physicians' behavior may be limited, or that the many other changes taking place simultaneously with the implementation of PPS either enhance or dilute the effects of the new payment system.

The evidence of PPS impacts thus far illustrates the lack of linkages between measured effects (e.g., length of stay, admissions) and the critical impacts (e.g., quality, access). For example, although there is widespread anecdotal evidence that patients are being discharged from the hospital in a sicker condition than before PPS, there is no clear evidence to indicate whether the ultimate impact on the quality of care for those patients is good or bad.

Potential for Evaluation

The ultimate objective of PPS is to reduce Medicare's outlays for inpatient hospital care while maintaining an acceptable level of quality and access to care for Medicare beneficiaries. The intended consequences of the new payment system are the elimination of hospital care that offers too little in the way of patient benefits and the organization of hospital operations to provide the necessary care in the least expensive manner. Thus, PPS rests on the assumption that some part of the health care delivered in hospitals prior to its introduction was unnecessary or was inefficiently produced. A great deal of evidence in the medical literature supports this assumption. If the assumption is true, cost containment might be achieved without sacrificing patients' health or welfare. Indeed, PPS could actually improve quality and access.

How hospitals and other providers actually will respond to the financial incentives inherent in PPS is by no means well understood. Hospitals' responses will depend as much on their own goals and constraints as on the economic incentives of the system. The efficiency with which not-for-profit hospitals—which constitute the vast majority of hospitals—operate, for example, may be more affected by the overall stringency of the Medicare hospital payment system than by the specific design of the prospective payment system. Also, PPS alters hospital incentives in ways that may conflict with each other, thus leading to unintended and possibly undesirable consequences. These interactions are complex and the Nation has little prior experience with payment systems like PPS. **Thus, the magnitude and direction of PPS effects on health care costs and benefits cannot be predicted with confidence.**

The impacts of PPS certainly will not be distributed uniformly across society. Some people

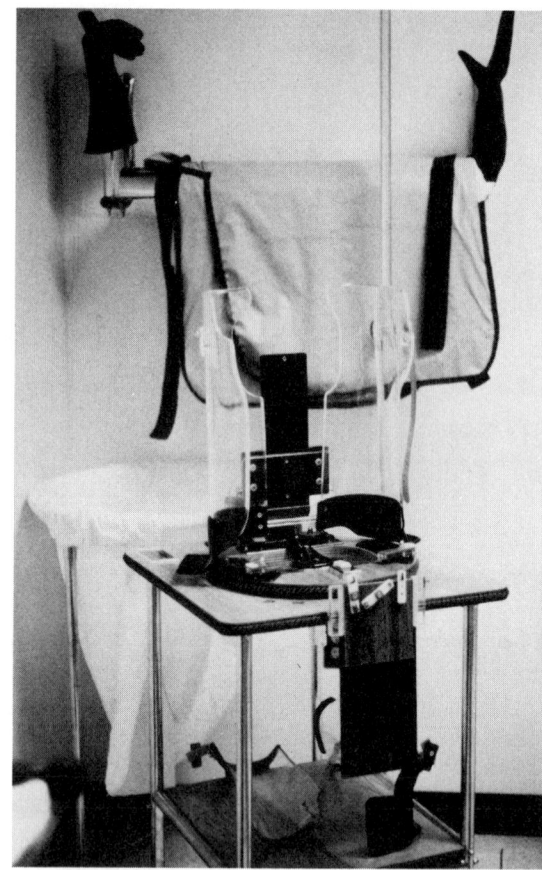

Photo credit: Fairfax Hospital Association

PPS provides an incentive to provide fewer ancillary services, such as radiology, during each inpatient stay.

will be particularly vulnerable to the outcome of PPS incentives. Some vulnerable groups whose access to and quality of care are more likely to be jeopardized under PPS are obvious—very old people, alcoholics and mentally ill people with medical problems, and disabled people. Other groups in particular DRGs or seeking care at particular kinds of hospitals may be equally vulnerable. The distribution of PPS impacts among affected groups is as important as its aggregate impacts. For this reason, **a strategy for evaluating PPS impacts should include specific plans for identifying those groups most likely to be vulnerable to negative consequences of PPS and monitoring its effects on them.**

Since monitoring for negative consequences alone would give a biased picture of PPS, however, **it is equally important in the long run to develop plans for a balanced assessment of the full range of PPS effects, positive as well as negative.**

Any PPS evaluation plan must take into account the fact that the effects of PPS will emerge over time. The adaptation to the new system's financial incentives will require major changes in the way that the health system is organized and in the way physicians and hospital managers behave when providing hospital services. Such alterations in behavior do not occur overnight.

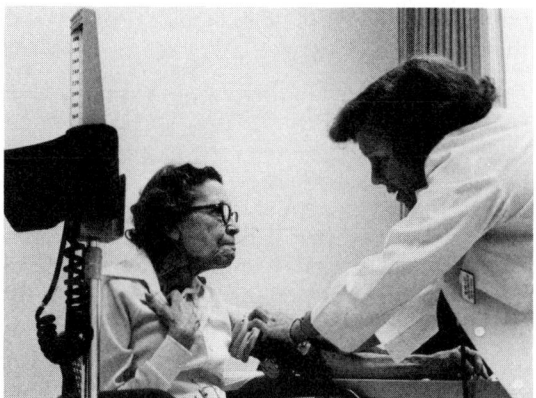

Photo credit: Fairfax Hospital Association

The impacts of PPS will not be distributed uniformly across society. Special attention needs to be paid to those groups most likely to be vulnerable to decreased access to quality care, including very old people, alcoholic and mentally ill people, and disabled people.

Some may take many years to develop. Although certain early changes in the health care system may serve as valid early warning indicators of important long-run effects of PPS, **a mature assessment of PPS can be made only after a substantial period of time has elapsed, perhaps as many as 5 years.** However, now is the time to establish appropriate data collection strategies and monitoring systems so that information is available for such assessments.

The ultimate effects of PPS on health benefits —as represented by quality, access, technological change, and clinical research—and health care costs and expenditures will occur through effects on the utilization and organization of health care services. **Changes in the utilization and organization of health care services are important indicators—but by themselves insufficient measures—of ultimate PPS impacts on health benefits and costs. Without more detailed analyses of how any observed changes in the utilization and organization of services affect the benefits and costs of health care, little can be said about the extent to which PPS has achieved its objective.**

The importance of evaluating PPS notwithstanding, there are many obstacles to achieving an accurate and balanced view of the new system's impacts. Concepts such as quality, access, and technological change are difficult to make operational. The lack of good impact measures necessitates the use of crude measures whose relationship to the concepts of quality or access is often tenuous. Limitations of existing databases require further compromise in the selection of impact measures or, if the limitations are not accepted, expensive studies involving the collection of new data directly from patients or other sources of information.

More importantly, **the feasibility of attributing observed changes in the health care system to PPS is limited by the fact that PPS is not the only change underway in the health care system.** The health care system has been undergoing rapid change in the past 5 years and continues to be dynamic. Simultaneous influences—including changes in the supply of physicians, increasing competition in health care, and concurrent changes in Federal and State health policy—confound researchers' ability to attribute many changes in the health care system directly to PPS. **Consequently, the effects of PPS on the benefits and costs of health care and their distribution throughout society will never be fully understood.** The most that can be expected is that those effects with the strongest hypothesized direct links to PPS can be observed and tentatively related to PPS. Yet verifying the existence of changes in quality, access, etc., is possible and important in its own right. Changes in health benefits and health status frequently require a policy solution, even when the cause of the changes cannot be definitely determined.

Whatever its limitations, evaluation is time-consuming and costly, particularly the kind that attempts to measure changes in quality of care, access to care, and technological change. The design and conduct of such studies require personnel and funding sufficient to support them. Even if federally sponsored evaluation studies are performed by outside grantees or contractors, adequate staffing at sponsoring agencies is required to plan, administer, and oversee the projects. For PPS evaluation to succeed, a commitment is needed to the development and maintenance of databases that can be useful in monitoring the state of the health care system.

At present, the funds and personnel necessary for the conduct of a comprehensive evaluation of PPS do not appear to be available within any Federal agency. The Health Care Financing Administration (HCFA), which has been assigned the responsibility for preparing the congressionally mandated annual impact reports, is using existing databases where possible to address issues of quality and access and has devoted some funds to the development of additional databases and impact measures that can be used for this purpose. However, the amount of funding and number of staff positions currently available for an evaluation of PPS within HCFA are inadequate to meet the information needs identified by OTA. Further budget cuts for HCFA's Office of Research and Demonstrations (ORD) in fiscal year 1986 would exacerbate the problem.

OPTIONS FOR EVALUATING PPS

Several options pertaining to the evaluation of Medicare's PPS are presented below for congressional consideration. OTA has identified two groups of options:

- those pertaining to specific studies that could be undertaken to answer important PPS evaluation questions; and
- those pertaining to the organization of PPS evaluation efforts and the content and organization of databases.

The options for specific PPS studies described below are not specifically numbered as options. Congress could consider any combination of the specific PPS studies described and could mandate or encourage the conduct of the studies it deems sufficiently important. One option would be for Congress to pass legislation mandating and providing funding for the conduct of specific studies by DHHS, the Prospective Payment Assessment Commission (ProPAC), or some other body.

Another option would be for Congress to encourage DHHS (e.g., through oversight, in report language, or through some other mechanism) to undertake certain studies under existing authorities.

In addition to noting options for specific studies, OTA has identified broader congressional options pertaining to the content and organization of databases necessary for PPS evaluation and to the organizational arrangements for the coordination and oversight of PPS evaluation efforts. These options are numbered and are perhaps even more important to consider than the options for specific studies.

Options for Specific Studies

Critical evaluation questions in the areas of PPS impacts on expenditures and costs, quality of care, access to care, technological change, and clinical research are summarized in table 1-2. Because the

Ch. 1—Introduction and Summary • 11

Table 1-2.—Studies and Data Sources Needed To Address Critical PPS Evaluation Questions

Critical evaluation questions	Studies and priority categories[a]	Data sources[b]	Cost
Expenditures and costs:			
To what extent has PPS been successful in controlling Medicare expenditures for inpatient hospital care?	• Analysis of Medicare admission patterns by diagnosis-related group (DRG) [2] • Detailed studies of admissions in DRGs that have undergone substantial changes in volume [2]	• Medicare Part A claims file • Medical records review • Medicare Part A and B claims data	Low High
What effect has PPS had on Medicare expenditures for outpatient and nonhospital services?	• Pre/post comparisons of utilization of nonhospital services by Medicare beneficiaries [2]	• Integrated beneficiary-based Medicare claims files	Medium
What effect has PPS had on Medicare beneficiaries' expenditures for health care?	• Periodic assessment of out-of-pocket expenditures by Medicare beneficiaries [2]	• Direct surveys of Medicare patients who have been hospitalized within a specific time • Patient sample identified through Medicare claims files	High
How well does PPS cover the costs of providing inpatient care to Medicare beneficiaries?	• Studies of revenues and costs of treating Medicare beneficiaries [1]	• Medicare Part A hospital billing file (PATBILL) • Medicare cost reports	Low
To what extent are variations among hospitals in profitability of Medicare patients due to factors beyond the hospitals' control, such as variations in severity of cases, the socioeconomic status of the patients, or input prices?	• Studies of revenues and costs by hospital and area characteristics [1] • Studies of within-DRG differences in case-mix severity among hospital types [1]	• Medicare Provider Analysis and Review file • Medicare cost reports • Medical records review	Low High
Quality of care:			
What, if any, negative effects has PPS had on quality of hospital care for Medicare beneficiaries?	• Pre/post-PPS studies of in-hospital and postdischarge mortality rates [1] • Pre/post-PPS studies of the incidence of drug reactions, decubitus ulcers, postsurgical pneumonia, and falls [1] • Pre/post-PPS studies of reasons for second admissions (e.g., unrelated illness, unsuspected problem, surgical complications, premature discharge) [1]	• Medicare Part A claims files • Hospital Insurance Master file • Medical records review • Medicare claims files to identify readmissions • Medical records review to identify causes	Medium High Low High
What is the net effect of PPS on quality of hospital care for Medicare beneficiaries?	• Pre/post-PPS studies of treatment patterns and outcomes for specific disease conditions and patient complexity (e.g., age, income, severity of illness, health status, and comorbidity) [2]	• Medical records review	High
How has PPS affected the quality of care in nonhospital settings of care?	• Longitudinal studies of cohorts of Medicare beneficiaries to track diagnosis, treatment, and recovery of illness regardless of health care setting [2] • Assessment of patient outcomes such as physical functioning, emotional well-being, capacity for independent living, and effects on family members [2]	• Medicare Part A and B claims • Medical records review • Survey of Medicare patients • Medicare Part A and B claims • Survey of Medicare patients	High High
Access to health care:			
How has PPS affected the availability of inpatient hospital care?	• Pre/post-PPS comparison of number of hospital beds by region, State, and county, urban/rural [2] • Pre/post-PPS comparison of number and geographical distribution of complex facilities (e.g., burn units, intensive care units, and cardiac catheterization labs) [1]	• American Hospital Association (AHA) Annual Survey of Hospitals • State health planning offices (for within-State areas) • AHA Annual Survey • Medicare Provider of Service file	Low Low Low
How have interhospital transfers of Medicare patients changed since the implementation of PPS?	• Pre/post-PPS studies of the number of transfers of Medicare patients [1] • Analysis of the medical, demographic, and socioeconomic characteristics of transferred patients [1] • Studies of the origins and destinations of interhospital transfers by type of hospital [1]	• Medicare Part A claims file • Special survey • Medicare Provider of Service file • Medicare Part A claims file	Low Low to high Low
Has PPS affected the utilization of inpatient care for vulnerable groups (e.g., alcoholic, mentally ill, disabled, or frail elderly patients)?	• Pre/post-PPS comparison of admissions for each vulnerable group [1] • Pre/post-PPS comparison of the utilization of special high cost services for vulnerable groups [1]	• Special surveys to identify vulnerable groups • Medical records review (in the case of alcoholic and mentally ill patients) • Medicare Part A claims file • Population-based surveys	High

Table 1-2.—Studies and Data Sources Needed To Address Critical PPS Evaluation Questions—Continued

Critical evaluation questions	Studies and priority categories[a]	Data sources[b]	Cost
How has PPS affected the availability and utilization of posthospital care for Medicare recipients?	• Pre/post-PPS comparison of the utilization of skilled nursing facility (SNF) days by Medicare beneficiaries [1] • Pre/post-PPS study of the utilization of home health care by Medicare beneficiaries [1] • Studies of the number of SNF beds actually available to Medicare patients within Medicare-certified facilities [1]	• Medicare Part A claims file • Population-based surveys • Medicare Part A claims file • Population-based surveys • Medicare Provider of Service file	Low Low Low
Has the demand for care in Veterans Administration (VA) hospitals increased, and if so, has the increase resulted in longer waiting lists for medical attention?	• Pre/post-PPS comparison of VA Medical Center waiting list reports [2]	• VA central office—hospital inpatient activity reports by each facility, but data not available by age	Low
Technological change: How does PPS affect the extent and direction of research and development that underlies technological change?	• Monitoring of R&D inputs (dollars) in various sectors of the health care field [2]	• National Science Foundation (NSF) survey	Medium
How does PPS affect the development and diffusion of technologies that lower total Medicare costs? That lower health system costs?	• Case studies of specific technologies. Especially amenable to studies of a few individual technologies [2]	Sources to choose technologies for study: • Food and Drug Administration (FDA) and patent databases • Surveys or consensus panels of experts Sources of data on the technologies themselves: • National Hospital Discharge Survey (diagnosis/procedure codes) • Revisions to CPT-4 • Results of cost-effectiveness studies and clinical trials • Surveys of physicians, hospitals, manufacturers, local planning agencies	Medium[c]
How does PPS affect the diffusion of cost-raising but quality-enhancing technologies?	• Case studies of specific technologies [2]		
How does PPS affect the use of technologies that lower quality of health care relative to alternative technologies available?	• Case studies of specific technologies [2]		
Clinical research: How is PPS affecting the level and type of clinical research performed relative to the situation under cost-based reimbursement?	• Analysis of relative costliness of patients on clinical research protocols (compare subject areas) [2] • Analysis of changes in purchasing power of NIH dollars budgeted for clinical trials [2] • Number and proportion of patients over age 65 on clinical trials (compare across research areas) [1]	• Hospital billing data; patient abstract data; Hospital Cost and Utilization Project database; National Institutes of Health (NIH) records of patients participating in research • NIH clinical trial data on dollars spent, number of patients, number of trials, number of participating hospitals and investigating personnel • NIH clinical trial data on patient age	Medium to high[d] Medium[e] Low

[a]Category 1: Studies that can identify major undesirable PPS impacts on the health care system as a whole or on vulnerable groups.
Category 2: Studies that provide a balanced and thorough assessment of PPS impacts on the health care system.
Category 3: Studies whose purpose is to develop methods of measuring important PPS impacts.
[b]Many of these data sources are described in app. E.
[c]Depends on number of technologies studied.
[d]Depending on number and extent of research areas analyzed.
[e]Data exist but are scattered in records of individual institutes and trials.

SOURCE: Office of Technology Assessment, 1985.

range of potential studies to address these questions is a broad one, establishing priorities is necessary.

OTA has identified studies to address these questions and priority categories of studies through an analysis of the strength of the incentives facing providers and their ability or willingness to act on them, the strength of the relationship between these actions and impacts on quality, access, etc., and the feasibility and cost of measuring specific impacts. The result is a three-tiered approach to the identification of studies needed to evaluate PPS:

- *Category 1:* **studies that can identify major undesirable impacts on the health care system as a whole or on vulnerable groups.** These studies are either relatively inexpensive to conduct because they rely on existing databases or are so important that they may justify substantial funding.
- *Category 2:* **studies that provide a balanced and thorough assessment of impacts on the health care system.** These include those intended to examine both positive and negative results. Their cost is generally (but not always) high because of the need for comprehensiveness and balance.
- *Category 3:* **studies to develop methods of measuring important impacts.** These are important for the enhancement of capability to monitor PPS impacts. Cost varies depending on data needs.

Examples of specific studies in the first two categories are summarized in table 1-2. Category 1 (negative impacts) studies should probably be given the highest priority and include both short- and long-run projects. Studies with the potential for surfacing serious negative consequences of PPS could be useful components of a more balanced and comprehensive assessment of PPS impacts. Some Category 1 studies are currently planned or underway as part of HCFA's annual PPS impact reports mandated by Congress. Others, for example, studies of avoidable negative outcomes in hospitals, detailed studies of vulnerable groups, and case studies of new technologies, are neither underway nor currently planned.

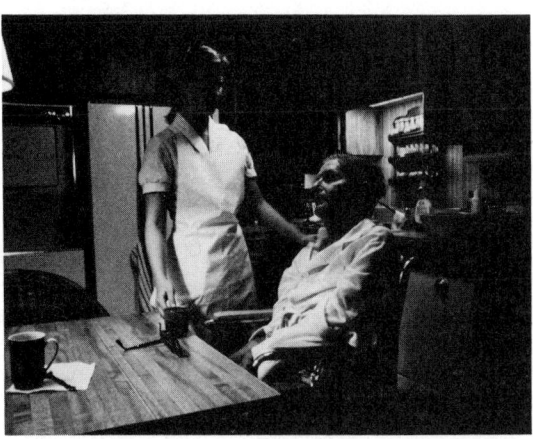

Photo credit: Fairfax Hospital Association

Studies of changes in the use of home health care due to PPS are a necessary part of evaluating the impact of PPS on the entire health care system.

Category 3 (methods development) includes studies in three critical areas:

- *Studies to develop improved methods of classifying patients according to their predicted need for hospital resources.* Although DRGs are at present the patient classification system most practical for use as the basis for a per-case pricing system, their structure has created potential problems in patient selection, fairness to hospitals, and the introduction of new technologies. Moreover, many PPS impact studies require selection of samples of patients with homogeneous resource needs. Improved patient classification systems, even those that may be infeasible for use in payment, could be used in evaluative studies to provide valuable information on the underlying causes of particularly troubling impacts. Comparative studies of the attributes of alternative patient classification systems would enhance this capability.
- *Studies to develop improved techniques for assessing the costs of treating patients.* Current methods of assessing the cost of treating Medicare patients are poor and depend on a cost reporting system that may be inadequate for patient- or DRG-specific estimates. Research into improved methods of

estimating the costs of treating patients in specific DRGs and hospitals would improve the ability of the PPS system to operate fairly.
- *Consensus development on measures and standards of quality of care and access to care.* At present, measures that adequately represent quality and access and that are likely to be sensitive to PPS are insufficiently developed. Also, agreement on the extent to which observed changes in such measures constitute acceptable or unacceptable changes in quality or access is needed. Expert consensus development could assist in identifying appropriate measures and making judgments about their acceptability.

Options for Implementing PPS Evaluation

Databases for PPS Evaluation

Problems in routinely maintained Federal databases complicate the task of evaluating PPS. The Medicare databases are rich sources of evaluative information, but their content and organization make analysis difficult and costly.

The Medicare cost reports that hospitals submit annually to their fiscal intermediaries represent a particular problem. These reports are not available to HCFA in a timely fashion or in automated form. Also, their content is vulnerable to change by HCFA without adequate consideration for their usefulness in addressing critical evaluation questions. There is even some question whether the cost reports will survive at all after 1988, when they will no longer be legally required.

The Medicare claims databases are more timely, but the size of the files and their organization precludes easy access for studies, especially those requiring beneficiary-based histories of utilization or outcomes. The development of integrated beneficiary-based databases would enhance researchers' ability to study systemwide impacts of PPS.

Federal health surveys, particularly those designed to periodically monitor the utilization, expenditures, and health status of the U.S. population, do not live up to their potential usefulness for the evaluation of PPS effects because of funding constraints and inadequate attention to the specific data needs of PPS evaluation.

These problems raise three options for consideration by Congress:

Option 1: Mandate a review of the Medicare cost reporting system.

The basis for Part A Medicare payment under cost-based reimbursement was the Medicare cost report, which was specifically designed to provide the information necessary to calculate Medicare's payment obligation to the hospital. The cost report format changed with revisions and refinements in the cost-reimbursement method over the years; its content has always been dictated by the need for data for purposes of paying hospitals.

Under PPS, the need for cost data is changing. To the extent that PPS becomes a pricing system, with prices tied to the general economy and not to actual costs, the need for hospital-specific cost data to administer the program will be reduced. (Cost reports will be needed only for estimating passthrough items such as capital, direct teaching, and outpatient costs.) Although the Social Security Amendments of 1983 expressly prohibited the total abandonment of the cost reports before 1988, their content can be changed at the discretion of HCFA (with the approval of the Office of Management and Budget).

As a unique source of cost data at the hospital level, the Medicare cost reports are critical to evaluating the financial effects of PPS on different kinds of hospitals, patients, and payers. Although hospitals differ in some reporting details, the cost reports impose a reasonably uniform format on all hospitals and thereby permit comparative analyses. The level of detail of reporting required for PPS evaluation has not been investigated in detail. The 1984 version of the cost report, for example, includes expenses reported at the departmental level. Whether this level of detail is necessary for accurate estimation of costs by DRG, hospital, and payer or whether an even greater level of detail would be useful are important questions.

A review of the content of the Medicare cost reports by experts in hospital finance, accounting, and economics could lead to a streamlined reporting format that is still responsive to the need for information to evaluate the financial impacts of PPS.

Aside from content issues, there is a problem with the timely availability of data from the cost reports at HCFA. An automated cost report information system, referred to as the Hospital Cost Report Information System (HCRIS), has been incompletely implemented. Cost reports are available from the system with a substantial time delay (at least 3 years at present). Currently, only the final audited reports are entered into the system at HCFA, a practice which delays the availability of data by at least 12 months. More timely cost data would be available from the reports submitted by hospitals prior to auditing, and it appears that these preliminary cost reports would be reasonably accurate for purposes of evaluation.

A review of the Medicare cost report information system, including the HCRIS system, by experts both within and outside of the Federal Government could identify further needs for system developments. In addition, such a group could review the submission and auditing time schedules laid out in law and regulations for their reasonableness under PPS and could consider the advantages and disadvantages of alternatives to universal mandatory cost reporting by hospitals.

Option 2: Mandate the development of integrated, beneficiary-based Medicare Part A and Part B databases.

The Medicare databases currently available include data on the use of institutional services (Part A) or physician and other services (Part B), but not both. These unintegrated databases place serious restrictions on attempts to analyze the impacts of PPS on services to beneficiaries systemwide. Only a beneficiary-based database that links Part A and Part B medical claims and enrollment data could follow and compare the entire history of utilization of health services for a sample of beneficiaries. For such a database to be feasible, adequate funding would be necessary.

An integrated Part A-Part B database would be especially important to studies of the impact of PPS on the quality of medical care and on Medicare and expenditures for such care. Studies of PPS impacts on quality of care require a spectrum of data on the full range of services provided to beneficiaries, including hospital admissions, out-of-hospital care, and physician visits. Without this spectrum of data, studies such as analysis of the impact of shorter length of hospital stay on future patient outcome cannot be conducted program-wide. Studies comparing beneficiary and Medicare expenditures across services are likewise hampered by the lack of an integrated database. Studies comparing expenditures systemwide, or linking hospital with nonhospital expenditures, cannot be undertaken without a database that includes the full experiences of Medicare beneficiaries in the health care system.

The only file that combines data from Parts A and B at present is the continuous Medicare History Sample File. This file, which contains the utilization history of a 5-percent sample of Medicare beneficiaries, is limited in several respects. First, the inpatient stay section of each beneficiary's record contains only the principal diagnosis and surgical procedure; accurate DRG assignments are therefore not possible. Second, the ambulatory care record contains no diagnostic or procedural data. Third, as a 5-percent sample, the Medicare History Sample File does not easily lend itself to analyses that require a large sample of beneficiaries with specific combinations of characteristics and medical conditions, as would be required for detailed pre/post-PPS comparisons of quality, access, and expenditures. Finally, there is a substantial time lag in the creation of the file. The latest file available as of June 1985 covered calendar year 1981.

One data system, not yet operational, that promises to link Parts A and B in a flexible way is the Medicare Automated Data Retrieval System (MADRS). This system will retrieve the full array of claims on any beneficiary each year from the various HCFA files, making analysis of systemwide impacts much easier for both intramural and extramural research.

Although MADRS will enable studies on health services, utilization, and expenditures to make comparisons across settings of care, this system has three problems. First, MADRS is a data retrieval and organizing system, not a new database. It links accessible data together and makes them available in one place, but if those data are incompatible or incomparable, it cannot make them less so. Second, MADRS organizes data by year, so examination of the entire history of a Medicare beneficiary still requires tedious organizing of data by beneficiary across all applicable years. Third, even when MADRS becomes operational, its files will include data only from fiscal year 1980 on, thus precluding many comparative studies across time and limiting its usefulness to fairly recent beneficiary history.

Option 3: Encourage DHHS to review procedures for national health surveys.

The national population-based health surveys periodically conducted by the Federal Government for statistical purposes are valuable sources of data, but improvements in their content, sampling designs, and completion schedules could make them more useful for the evaluation of PPS impacts. Appending the appropriate information to the Hospital Discharge Survey records, for example, would allow data from this survey to be arrayed by type of hospital.

Some efforts are already underway to improve national estimates of the use and expenditures for health care services. The sponsoring agencies (the National Center for Health Services Research and Health Care Technology Assessment (NCHSR&HCTA), the National Center for Health Statistics, and HCFA) of the 1987 National Medical Expenditure Survey, the successor to the National Medical Care Utilization and Expenditure Survey, proposed to the Office of Management and Budget to: sample a higher than average proportion of the elderly population; provide more detailed information on community-based long-term care; and release their first published reports after 1 year, in order to allow for a timely assessment of the impact of PPS. This type of review could be generalized across all national surveys.

A review of national health surveys for changes that would accommodate the needs of evaluation could be accomplished by an interagency task force or by an agency responsible for coordinating PPS evaluation, if one were to exist. Of course, changing national health surveys or making them available on a more timely basis would involve additional costs associated with instrument design, sample selection, and pretesting. Changes also might cause further delay in the timeliness of these surveys, which is already a problem. Thus, the organization responsible for reviewing the surveys would need to weigh the value of additional information against these costs.

Organizational Arrangements for PPS Evaluation

Three questions arise with respect to the organization of PPS evaluation:

- What organizations within or outside of the Federal Government should be responsible for conducting PPS studies?
- What funding mechanisms should be used to carry out the needed research?
- How can the total PPS evaluation effort be coordinated?

The first two questions must be answered on a study-by-study basis. At present, HCFA maintains the major responsibility for evaluation of PPS impacts, since it has been assigned the congressionally mandated annual impact reports within DHHS. As the agency with the most detailed knowledge of and access to the critical databases, HCFA is a natural selection for many PPS studies. Yet some PPS studies might better be handled by other agencies whose interests are not so closely aligned with the implementation of PPS. For example, NCHSR&HCTA has the staff skills and grant mechanisms to manage PPS evaluation studies and is already conducting some research in this area. Of course, the budget of this agency would need to be augmented if NCHSR&HCTA were to substantially expand its capacity without jeopardizing other areas of health services research. In addition, the role of ProPAC in evaluating the impacts of PPS is unclear, but ProPAC has been strongly encouraged by at least one congressional committee to take on this task and intends to comply to the extent that its budget allows.

The most important organizational question is the third. The difficulty of ensuring that appropriate studies are undertaken, available data are used efficiently, the knowledge of those most qualified and objective is tapped, and adequate resources are devoted to evaluation suggests that continual coordination and oversight of the evaluation process is desirable.

The importance of PPS evaluation can be underscored by congressional recognition that the impacts of PPS will continue to work themselves out well beyond 1987, the date of the last mandated annual impact report. The observations above lead to options 4 and 5 below.

Option 4: Appoint one Federal agency to coordinate and oversee the organization of PPS evaluation.

The functions of a coordinating organization could include the following:

- assessing the feasibility and cost of alternative studies in relation to their importance;
- developing an annual PPS evaluation agenda;
- recommending an annual PPS evaluation budget;
- identifying the most appropriate organizational sponsors for specific studies;
- recommending the most appropriate funding mechanisms;
- recommending funding levels for individual studies;
- overseeing and coordinating access to needed data;
- overseeing and coordinating changes in data systems to enhance the ability to evaluate PPS;
- reviewing the content of specific studies for their scientific validity; and
- serving as a clearinghouse for both public and private sector studies.

If an executive branch agency were to be appointed, the most logical candidates would be agencies within DHHS. The Office of the Assistant Secretary for Planning and Evaluation has traditionally maintained a coordinating role with respect to evaluation research. Two other possible organizations within DHHS are NCHSR& HCTA and HCFA. NCHSR&HCTA has extensive experience in supporting intramural and extramural research of this kind, has staff with technical skills to carry out the function, and is currently coordinating the PPS-related research of the Public Health Service. However, NCHSR& HCTA is low in the DHHS organizational hierarchy and might therefore have difficulty undertaking an oversight role. HCFA has both program and research expertise. However, if HCFA or any of the other components of DHHS is assigned the task of coordinating the PPS evaluation, it will be important to consider their inherent lack of objectivity, since they are part of the Department implementing PPS.

Congressional agencies, such as the Congressional Budget Office, the Congressional Research Service, the General Accounting Office, or OTA, would be capable of providing the oversight that is necessary, particularly if staff with program evaluation skills were assigned the responsibility, but the missions of these offices are not generally congruent with such a responsibility.

ProPAC has an informal congressional mandate to provide a comprehensive evaluation of PPS (Report 98-911 on H.R. 6028), but ProPAC has a budget that cannot begin to meet these expectations. As a substitute for such a full-scale PPS evaluation, ProPAC's legislated function could be expanded to include coordination and oversight of PPS evaluation activities throughout the Federal Government. As the body with responsibility for recommending relative and absolute DRG prices, however, ProPAC would not be totally disinterested in the outcome of an evaluation of PPS.

Private organizations with experience in health policy research and evaluation are probably not good candidates for the role of coordinator. Such organizations would have low access to information and databases held by Federal agencies and inadequate influence over the evaluation process.

Any organization that is assigned the coordination and oversight functions will need highly skilled staff, adequate resources, and sufficient influence over the evaluative process if it is to perform the functions successfully.

Option 5: Extend the requirements for the PPS annual impact reports by DHHS beyond 1987.

The annual impact reports mandated in the Social Security Amendments of 1983 were intended to provide critical information on PPS impacts. Eliminating them after 1987, as is now mandated, seems to waste an opportunity to complete a PPS evaluation because the impacts may develop over a longer period of time.

Potential problems with extending the impact reports for a longer period of time include the administrative burden and the cost of such reports. If one Federal agency were coordinating and overseeing all PPS evaluation, however, this burden might be somewhat alleviated (see option 4). At this time, the Secretary of DHHS is required by law to submit the annual impact reports to Congress. The responsibility for preparing the reports has been delegated to HCFA, but it does not necessarily have to remain there, especially if a coordinating agency other than HCFA were appointed.

Part One
A Framework for Evaluation

Chapter 2
Predicted Effects of Medicare's Prospective Payment System

Contents

	Page
History and Description of Medicare's PPS System	23
The Goals of PPS	24
Provider Incentives Under PPS	25
Dimensions of PPS Impact	29
The Distribution of PPS Impacts	30
Conclusions	32

TABLE

Table No.	Page
2-1. DRG Weights and Ranks for Selected Coronary Heart Disease, Calendar Year 1981 and Fiscal Year 1985	28

Chapter 2
Predicted Effects of Medicare's Prospective Payment System

HISTORY AND DESCRIPTION OF MEDICARE'S PPS SYSTEM

From its inception in 1965 until late in 1982, Medicare paid hospitals for inpatient services rendered to its beneficiaries on the principle of "reasonable and necessary costs." Hospitals seeking Medicare reimbursement submitted annual cost reports detailing expenses incurred and apportioning them between Medicare and other patients. These cost reports were audited by Medicare's fiscal intermediaries[1] to arrive at the allowable costs for final reimbursement. Allowable costs included operating and capital costs[2] and the net costs of approved educational activities. Prior to 1982, the only limit applied to reimbursement of allowable costs was the cap on reimbursement for inpatient routine operating costs known as "Section 223 limits." First applied in 1974, this cap limited Medicare reimbursement for inpatient routine operating costs to 120 percent of the mean of such costs in a similar group of hospitals. Between 1975 and 1982, the cap was gradually reduced to 108 percent of the mean cost per day in the peer group hospitals. Nonroutine operating costs such as ancillary services and capital costs were exempted from the Section 223 limits.

The death-knell of cost-based reimbursement for hospitals under Medicare was first sounded in 1982, with the passage of the Tax Equity and Fiscal Responsibility Act of 1982 (TEFRA) (Public Law 97-248). In addition to extending the existing Section 223 limits to include the operating costs of ancillary departments and special care units, TEFRA imposed a hospital-specific maximum limit (i.e., a target rate) on the amount of inpatient operating costs per case that would be reimbursed. The hospital's reimbursement for operating costs was capped at the lower of the target rate or 120 percent[3] of the mean cost per case for hospitals of the same type, with adjustments up or down by an index of the hospital's case mix.[4] The hospital could keep a small portion of any savings it could generate. TEFRA put no limit on capital costs, the direct costs of medical education, or outpatient services. These remained "passthrough" items.

A more sweeping revision of Medicare's hospital payment system was signed into law in April 1983. The Social Security Amendments of 1983 (Public Law 98-21) mandated the phasing-in over a 3-year period of a prospective payment system (PPS) for inpatient hospital services. In October 1986, at the close of the 3-year transition period from TEFRA to PPS, Medicare payment for inpatient care will be based on a national set of per-case prices for patients in 468 diagnosis-related groups (DRGs).

DRGs are a patient classification system developed to reflect differences in predicted resource use among different kinds of hospital patients. Under the DRG-based PPS, Medicare payment for inpatient hospital services is made at a predetermined, specific rate for each DRG. During the 3-year transition period from TEFRA to PPS, a declining portion of the total prospective rate is to be based on a hospital's historical costs in a given base year, and a gradually increasing portion is to be based on a blend of federally determined regional and national DRG rates. Beginning in the fourth year, Medicare payment for inpatient care will be based on a set of national DRG rates. The price for a DRG will be adjusted for the hospital's urban or rural location and area

---

[1]A fiscal intermediary is an organization under contract to the Health Care Financing Administration (HCFA) to process claims from hospitals and other institutional health care providers.
[2]Capital costs include depreciation, interest expenses, and return on equity. Return on equity is limited to for-profit institutions.
[3]This limit would be reduced over 3 years to 110 percent.
[4]Case mix refers to the relative frequency of admissions of various types of patients, reflecting different needs for hospital resources. The case-mix index used for TEFRA is calculated on the basis of diagnosis related groups (DRGs).

wage rate. Additional payments will also be made for the indirect costs of medical education.

The DRG payment rates apply to all Medicare inpatient discharges from short-term acute care general hospitals in the United States, except for a small number of discharges (set by statute at 5 to 6 percent of the total Medicare hospital payments) with unusually long lengths of stay or high charges. The rates of payment for these "outlier" cases are increased by a predetermined amount thought to reflect the extra costs of care.

Several types of hospitals (psychiatric, long-term, children's, and rehabilitation hospitals) and hospital units (distinct psychiatric and rehabilitation units) are exempted from Medicare's PPS. For the present, these hospitals and units continue to be reimbursed on the basis of reasonable costs. Capital costs and the costs of direct medical education remain passthrough items under PPS at present, although the law creating the new payment system anticipated the eventual inclusion of payment for capital costs.

The initial set of DRG prices was based on the 1981 average inpatient operating cost per case for each DRG in a 20-percent sample of Medicare claims. The law requires that the DRG prices be updated regularly in two ways. First, an overall annual rate of increase, referred to as the "annual update factor," is applied to all DRG prices. Second, the relative prices of DRGs (i.e., the ratio of the price of one DRG to another) must be assessed and adjusted at least once every 4 years, with the first adjustment scheduled for October 1985. The adjustment must reflect changes in treatment patterns, technology, and other factors that alter the relative use of hospital resources among DRGs. The Prospective Payment Assessment Commission (ProPAC) established by the law is responsible for making recommendations regarding the annual payment increase and relative prices and for evaluating any such adjustments made by the Secretary of the Department of Health and Human Services.

The law requires Medicare to participate in any State-legislated alternative prospective payment program that: 1) covers at least 75 percent of the State's population; 2) makes provisions for competitive health plans; 3) assures the Federal Government that access to hospital care for Medicare and Medicaid beneficiaries will not decline; and 4) assures the Federal Government that hospital costs will not be higher under the State program. Four States—New York, New Jersey, Massachusetts, and Maryland—currently hold waivers from the national Medicare program.[5]

---

[5]New York's waiver expires in December 1985; the State has elected not to seek a renewal of the waiver.

THE GOALS OF PPS

The ultimate objective of PPS is to reduce Medicare's outlays for inpatient hospital care while maintaining an acceptable level of quality and access to care for beneficiaries. This goal is to be sought through a fundamental restructuring of the financial incentives facing hospitals. Consequently, PPS is intended as a long-run cost-containment measure, not as a quick solution for hospital cost inflation. PPS was appended to the provisions of TEFRA, whose controls actually govern the rate of increase in hospitals' Medicare revenues during its 3-year life through a "budget neutrality" provision in the PPS law.

PPS rests on the assumption that some part of the health care delivered in hospitals prior to its introduction was unnecessary or was produced inefficiently. A great deal of evidence has accumulated in the medical literature to support this assumption (57,74,375,387,389). If the assumption is accurate, cost containment might be achieved without sacrificing patients' health or welfare, provided that the incentives inherent in PPS lead to appropriate changes in hospitals' and physicians' behavior.

The intended consequences of PPS are the elimination of hospital care that offers little or nothing in the way of patient benefits and the organization of hospital operations to provide the necessary care in the least expensive manner. By paying a per-case rate, PPS gives hospitals new incentives (relative to cost-based reimbursement) to conserve resources during a person's stay in the hospital and to shift care to less costly settings.

The extent to which hospitals actually respond to these incentives depends on their managers' and physicians' goals and constraints. In the case of not-for-profit hospitals—and these represent the vast majority (87 percent at present (13)) of hospitals—the strength of the incentive to operate more efficiently may depend largely on the overall level of financial pressure the hospitals face. Thus, changes in hospital behavior may depend as much on the restrictiveness of the system as on the structure of DRG prices. Moreover, PPS alters hospital incentives in some ways that may conflict with each other, thus leading to unintended and possibly undesirable consequences. Accurate prediction of the effects of PPS on the health care system requires a detailed assessment of the full range of incentives PPS offers as well as an understanding of how these incentives interact with one another and with providers' objectives and constraints in altering their behavior. Because these interactions are complex and there is little prior experience with payment systems like PPS, the magnitude of all and the direction of some effects remain empirical questions.

PROVIDER INCENTIVES UNDER PPS

As a per-case pricing system, Medicare's PPS creates new financial incentives for hospitals and other providers of health care to behave in ways that are markedly different from those of cost-based payment. Hospital managers and physicians face three basic incentives:

1. to reduce the cost per admission;
2. to increase the number of admissions, particularly those that promise to be profitable; and
3. to develop new sources of profit or surplus by offering services not subject to payment restrictions.

These three basic incentives translate into a number of potential strategies for hospitals and their staffs. Whether a particular strategy is actually followed will probably depend on the size of the potential gains in net revenue, the cost and feasibility of implementing the strategy, the implications for patient care, and the objectives of hospital managements and their physician staffs.

The profitability of any particular admission depends on the price paid for it, which is determined in part by the system used to classify patients. Any patient classification system will assign patients with varying needs for care into a single category. How the assignments are made defines which patients are profitable and which are not. PPS relies on DRGs to classify patients and therefore establishes a particular pattern of profitability among patients. Any other patient classification system (including revised DRGs) would do the same, but the pattern of profitability would be different. Thus, the specific incentives inherent in PPS result both from its general structure as a per-case system and from the selection of DRGs as the patient classification system.

Many observers have speculated or provided anecdotal evidence that in the search for *per-case cost reductions*, hospitals will pursue the following strategies:

- adopting general management efficiencies (298);
- reducing lengths of stay (80,102,176);
- reducing rates of use of ancillary services (95,161,171,210);
- reducing the total ratios of personnel to patients (165,171,246,379);
- providing services formerly provided during the stay before and after the hospital stay (i.e., unbundling);
- reducing rates of increase in employee wages and fringe benefits;
- purchasing hospital supplies more prudently (7,202); and
- reducing discretionary activities (e.g., continuing education; clinical research) (60,271).

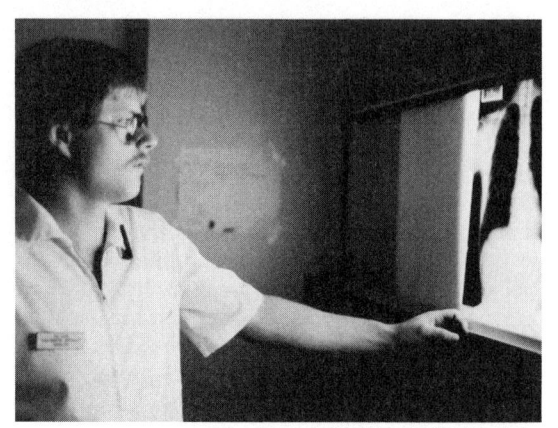

Photo credit: Fairfax Hospital Association

One strategy for reducing the cost per hospital admission is to provide fewer ancillary services, including radiology.

Strategies to *selectively increase admissions* would include attempts by hospitals to do the following:

- treat patients as inpatients who might otherwise be treated on an ambulatory basis (97, 218);
- break hospital stays up into multiple admissions (24);
- identify and attract relatively healthy patients within any given DRG by encouraging services associated with those patients (112,280);
- expand medical staffs in certain specialties and reduce them in others (42,221);
- adopt marketing practices aimed at relatively healthy patients (262); and
- encourage physicians to refer patients posing an expected financial burden to other hospitals, particularly, to Veterans Administration (VA) and other public hospitals (110).

Finally, PPS encourages hospitals to expand services to areas that are less financially constrained or more profitable. The hospital is at a particular advantage in marketing pre- and posthospital services to its patients in the hospital. The existence of a largely captive market for posthospital home health services, for example, has led many hospitals to set up their own home care agencies (53,190).

Another area that may see substantial expansion as a result of PPS is hospital-based outpatient surgery. Medicare pays hospitals for outpatient surgery on a cost basis. In addition, the 1980 Budget Act (Public Law 96-499) gave physicians financial incentives to perform certain surgical procedures (e.g., cataract surgery, biopsies, endoscopies, dilation and curettage) in outpatient surgical facilities. Hospital managers should be eager to attract surgical procedures from physicians' offices to outpatient units as a way of spreading overhead expenses and may also have a financial incentive to substitute outpatient for inpatient care if the inpatient surgery is unprofitable under PPS. At the same time, physicians have financial incentives to perform certain procedures in outpatient facilities that might otherwise have been performed either in their office or on an inpatient basis. An additional impetus toward outpatient surgery will be given by the utilization and quality control peer review organizations (PROs), which have contracts with the Health Care Financing Administration (HCFA) to review inpatient surgical admissions for their appropriateness. Taken together, these factors imply that outpatient surgery is likely to grow in the future.

Hospitals are likely to approach decisions regarding the introduction of new medical technology under PPS in ways that differ from those used under cost-based payment. Before PPS, the additional costs of new technologies were fully covered; hospitals therefore had no financial incentives to refrain from adopting costly new technologies and had few financial incentives to adopt cost-reducing technologies. Under PPS, new technology that raises the cost of treating a case will have to compete with alternative uses of funds, such as employee wage and benefit increases, additional nursing staff, etc. Costly new technology often has the disadvantage of offering uncertain benefits in the early stages of diffusion (249). The implications are obvious: With limited resources, hospitals will need to assess new technologies more closely and ration resources more carefully.

Nevertheless, the introduction of promising new technologies, particularly those that are cost-reducing, but even some that are cost-raising to the hospital, will be attractive to hospitals as they

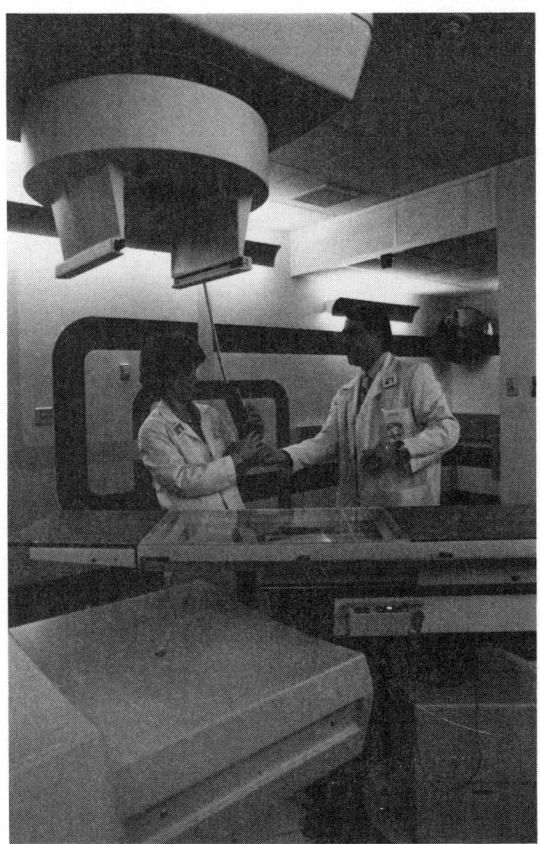

With limited resources, hospitals will need to assess new technologies, particularly those that are costly, more carefully than prior to the implementation of PPS.

compete for physician loyalties and, ultimately, the admissions they represent (23). Thus, for example, despite its high capital and operating cost, magnetic resonance imaging, a new medical technology still largely a research tool, may be highly desirable to hospitals that seek to protect their admissions base from encroachment from other hospitals (279). The importance of this incentive as a constraining force to the previous incentive is unknown. Thus, though PPS does not imply that technological change will approach a standstill, the directions of such change are likely to be altered, and the adoption of technologies that are cost-raising to hospitals is likely to decline by an unknown quantity.

Of course, physicians make the major decisions regarding placement of patients and ordering of services once patients are hospitalized. Although physicians may be disposed to cooperate with hospital managements in their effort to avoid deficits or increase surpluses (276), there may be important limits to this cooperation. First, defensive medicine[6] operates to an unknown extent to discourage physicians from reducing the intensity of services provided (290). Second, hospitalization is an important source of income for physicians. In 1981, 64 percent of physicians' Medicare services were provided in the inpatient setting, although only 24 percent of Medicare beneficiaries were hospitalized in that year (50). One physician visit for each day of hospitalization is the custom for nonsurgical cases, which comprise about two-thirds of the total admissions for the Medicare program (194). With so much income riding on hospitalized patients, physicians may be reluctant to cooperate with all strategies to reduce costs.

Hospitals also have an incentive to assign patients to DRGs that will provide the greatest possible revenue (280). DRG assignments are made by a computer program called GROUPER that uses the diagnostic and procedural codes and patient age reported on the hospital bill. In the past, accurate diagnostic and procedural coding was not crucial to the payment process, and many errors in coding, particularly omission of surgeries, appear to have occurred (392). Hospitals now have an incentive not only to improve the accuracy of coding, but also to report codes that will maximize payment levels.

Hospitals under PPS may encourage physicians to consciously consider the payment implications of their medical recordkeeping and the assignment of principal diagnosis upon discharge (232). Although there are bound to be limitations on the extent to which "upcoding" takes place and upcoding is likely to occur early in the implementation of PPS, it remains in the interest of the hos-

---

[6]Defensive medicine refers to the physician practice of providing services and ordering tests primarily for the purpose of avoiding possible claims of malpractice.

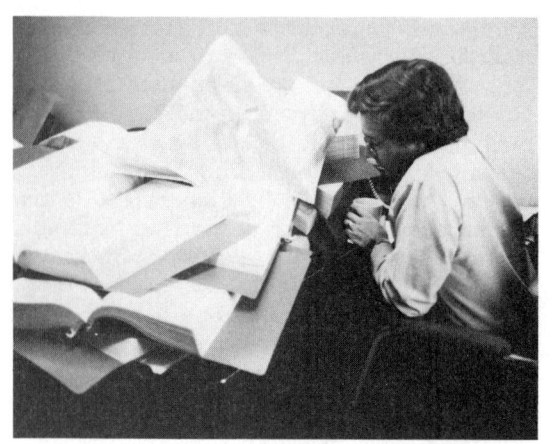

Under PPS, hospital managers have an incentive to improve the quality of their medical and financial information systems.

pital always to obtain the most favorable DRG assignment.[7]

An example involving coronary heart disease illustrates the complexity of the coding issue. For patients with chest pain indicative of heart disease, coding the principal diagnosis as atherosclerosis rather than angina pectoris not only increases the DRG weight (from 0.75 to 0.85) but also "makes perfect medical sense" (152) (see table 2-1). Indeed, there is virtually no financial incentive ever to assign a patient to DRG #140 (angina) or DRG #143 (chest pain) (152). Although it raises the per-case cost to some extent, cardiac catheterization of such patients further increases the DRG weight to 1.62, virtually doubling payment for the admission.

Table 2-1 shows the reported percent of Medicare hospital discharges in these DRGs in calender year 1981 and fiscal year 1985.[8] Cardiac catheterization (DRGs #124 and #125) jumped from 0.2 percent of discharges in 1981 to 1.3 percent in 1985, reflecting in part higher rates of catheterization and in part more accurate reporting of the procedure. Undoubtedly, a large (but unknown) proportion of patients assigned in 1981 to DRGs #132, #133 (atherosclerosis), and #140 (angina) were catheterized and were therefore wrongly assigned. The data in table 2-1 also show a dramatic increase in the proportion of discharges in DRG #140 (angina), despite the fact that the financial incentives of PPS argue strongly for reclassification of such cases to DRG #132 (atherosclerosis). The reasons for the disparity between the incentives and actual behavior are not well understood.

---

[7]Evidence of upcoding has already appeared, and the implications for Medicare expenditures are serious. A review of 1984 Medicare hospital claims revealed reported DRG assignments that would produce 5.85 percent greater revenue for hospitals than those expected using 1981 case-mix information. Payment amounts had originally been reduced by 3.38 percent in anticipation of coding improvements. The Department of Health and Human Services (DHHS) attempted to neutralize the expenditure impacts of this by reducing all DRG weights for fiscal year 1985 2.4 percent. Because reported codes could have changed due to actual case-mix changes, DHHS yielded to industry pressure and compromised with 1.05 percent.

[8]This period includes October 1, 1984 to July 26, 1985.

Table 2-1.—DRG Weights and Ranks for Selected Coronary Heart Disease, Calendar Year 1981 and Fiscal Year 1985

DRG No.	Name	Weight[a]	Calender year 1981 Percent of discharges	Rank	Fiscal year 1985[b] Percent of bills	Rank
124	Cardiac catheterization, complex diagnosis	2.1969	0.02	338	0.5	50
125	Cardiac catheterization without complex diagnosis	1.6284	0.2	127	0.8	28
132	Atherosclerosis (age >69 and/or c.c.[c])	0.9087	3.6	3	0.6	41
133	Atherosclerosis (age <70 w/o c.c.)	0.8510	0.8	27	0.1	242
140	Angina pectoris	0.7470	1.9	11	3.3	3
143	Chest pain	0.6743	0.7	31	0.8	31

[a]Weight assigned in first year of PPS operation.
[b]Bills received by Medicare between Oct. 1, 1984 and July 26, 1985.
[c]c.c. = comorbidities and complications.

SOURCE: U.S. Department of Health and Human Services, Bureau of Data Management and Systems, Health Care Financing Administration, unpublished data, 1985.

DIMENSIONS OF PPS IMPACT

The incentives under PPS set in motion provider strategies that have consequences for the costs and quality of health care and their distribution throughout society. Some behavior changes may improve the performance of the health care system; some may reduce it. Other changes may have little ultimate impact. Some of the consequences should occur early on, others only after a substantial period of time has elapsed. Some may be one-time adjustments; others may continue. Some may be highly visible and easily measured; others may be discernible only indirectly by observing changes in behavior of patients or providers to which they are closely linked.

The impacts of PPS will not be distributed uniformly across society. Some groups or individuals will gain more or lose less than others. The distribution of PPS impacts among affected groups is as important as the aggregate impacts. Thus, in discussing the consequences of PPS, it is necessary to identify specific groups for whom such impacts should be separately tracked.

The most important effects of PPS are on the *cost* of providing health care and on the *health benefits* such care bestows.[9]

- *Health care costs*: The impacts of PPS on the costs of both the Medicare program and health care in general is obviously of great importance. In discussing these impacts, a distinction can be made between costs and expenditures. The "cost" of a health service is the value of the productive resources (e.g., personnel, materials) used in the production of the service. The "expenditure" is the amount actually paid in exchange for the service. At the national level, health care costs and expenditures can be equated. However, the cost of serving a set of patients may be different from the expenditures made by them or on their behalf if cross-subsidization is occurring or if providers are making high profits.[10] Thus, it is important to measure both the expenditures borne by specific kinds of consumers (or the third-party payers who insure them) and the costs of actually treating them.
- *Health benefits*: Patients receive two basic kinds of benefits from health care—improvements in health status and prognostic information. When health status is defined broadly to encompass the quality as well as the length of people's lives, then palliative care can be as important as curative or restorative services. Also, even if health care were completely unable to interrupt or reverse the natural history of any disease, accurate diagnosis would still be valuable for its ability to inform or reassure patients and their families. The benefits deriving from health care involve many dimensions, including rates of mortality, morbidity, disability, and satisfaction. Tracking changes in these benefits is difficult and inevitably requires the selection of incomplete and imperfect proxy measures.

Health program evaluations, rather than focusing directly on health benefits, usually measure a program's effects on subsidiary concepts such as access to care, quality of care, utilization of services, and organization of care (44,127). These proxy measures provide partial and overlapping views of the benefits and costs of health care and are discussed in the chapters that follow.

"Access" refers to the "potential and actual entry of a given population group to the health care delivery system" (4). It raises the question of how much health care each person is able to receive

---

[9]PPS also has the potential to affect the livelihoods of a large number of people through its influence on patterns of employment in health care and related industries. To the extent that such employment changes affect health costs and benefits, they are captured in the benefit/cost framework here. But employment shifts raise issues of public policy in their own right. For example, if PPS leads to major layoffs of unskilled hospital personnel, what alternative employment opportunities will be available? Or, what are the implications of PPS for Federal subsidy of medical and allied health sciences education? These questions are embedded in larger questions of labor force management and, while important, are beyond the scope of this study.

[10]In a perfectly competitive health care system, profits would be reduced through competition to the minimum required to keep providers in the market. Any profits above this minimum return are referred to as "economic rents," and represent a net transfer of wealth from the consumer to the provider as a result of the provider's market power.

and the terms on which he or she receives it. Thus, access is closely related to, but not identical with, utilization, which refers to the quantity and mix of services actually provided and to patient's out-of-pocket expenditures. Access is also affected by the content of the care actually received, for even if they use the same number and mix of services, people can have very different levels of access if the quality of those services differs widely.

"Quality of care" is a term that is widely used but rarely defined. One often cited definition of quality care is the kind of care which is expected to maximize an inclusive measure of patient welfare, after one has taken account of the balance of expected gains and losses that attend the process of care in all its parts (86). Deviations from this ideal represent degradations in quality. Such deviations can occur if the patterns of utilization of services or their content are suboptimal. Quality is also affected by changes in access to care. Indeed, some discussions of quality of care treat access as a constituent element of quality (223).

Cost, access, and quality of care are all affected by the organization of services—the configuration of setting, location, and management by which care is provided—through its influence on the utilization and content of care. For example, many hospitals with low occupancy rates may convert acute care beds into long-term care beds. The increased supply of long-term care beds could markedly improve Medicare patients' access to long-term care at the same time that it encourages hospitals to become more selective in their acute care admission strategies.

In the long run, PPS may affect health benefits and costs through its influence on the process of technological change—the periodic introduction of new medical technologies and abandonment of some existing ones. If PPS alters the rate and direction of introduction of new medical technologies and the rate and depth of their adoption by providers and consumers, then the stream of health benefits and costs over time will inevitably be altered. Whether the ultimate effects on health benefits and costs resulting from any alteration in the patterns of technological change are negative or positive and what the magnitude of such effects is remain questions for empirical investigation.

Technological change itself rests partly on an underpinning of research and development (R&D) conducted largely by academic health researchers and the health products industry, which is also likely to be affected by PPS (151). An important component of R&D that some have claimed will be particularly sensitive to PPS is clinical research—investigations conducted on patients. If clinical research is altered, knowledge about the relative effectiveness of alternative medical technologies will be affected.

THE DISTRIBUTION OF PPS IMPACTS

As mentioned earlier, Medicare's PPS will not affect everyone uniformly. Changes in benefits and costs will vary among classes of patients, payers, regions of the country, and providers of care.

Medicare patients with particularly complicated health problems, for example, may receive lower quality care than will those with relatively simple medical problems. Medicare patients who might have received nutritional support during the hospital stay under cost-based reimbursement may now be required to obtain these services outside the hospital as a Part B benefit which requires 20-percent patient copayment. Medicare patients may also find their access to some services reduced relative to non-Medicare patients. For example, admission to hospitals' special care units could conceivably become more selective for patients under PPS than for patients covered by cost- or charge-based reimbursement. On the other hand, Medicare patients could reduce the access of Medicaid patients to nursing home beds, because Medicare is more generous with nursing home reimbursement than are most Medicaid plans.

Shifts in the burden of health expenditures among Federal programs, third-party payers, and consumers are also likely. Even within the Medicare program, PPS may lead to expenditure shifts from Part A (Hospital Insurance) to Part B (Supplementary Medical Insurance). It is difficult to predict how PPS will affect either Part A or Part B expenditures in the aggregate. The objective of the new payment system, of course, is to reduce the rate of increase in Medicare's expenditures for inpatient hospital services. Since the law sets a cap on the annual increase in per-case prices, Medicare's aggregate PPS expenditures can increase more or less quickly than that rate only if the number or reported mix of hospital cases change.[11] Thus, interpretation of PPS impacts on Medicare's hospital expenditures will require a detailed examination of inpatient utilization rates and case-mix changes.

For other Part A services—for example, services in skilled nursing facilities and home health services—some predictions of directions of effect are possible. Medicare expenditures for home health services and skilled nursing care, for example, are likely to increase as a result of the incentives inherent in PPS. Yet the magnitude of such effects is highly uncertain, because it is simply unknown how providers and patients will react to PPS.

The same uncertainty exists regarding the impact of PPS on Part B expenditures. PPS may move some services, such as cataract surgery, to outpatient settings, with consequent increases in Part B expenditures. Conversely, the incentive to increase hospital admissions under PPS may move certain procedures from an outpatient to an inpatient setting. Shorter lengths of hospital stay may reduce the number of physician visits to hospitalized patients, resulting in lower payments to physicians.

How PPS will affect expenditures for other Federal health care programs, such as VA and Medicaid, is also uncertain. Reductions in Medicare Part A payments may increase the demand for VA medical care (110), but how Congress responds in providing appropriations to the VA system to meet that demand will determine the actual expenditure effects. The Medicaid program, too, has limited eligibility; only if PPS increases the demand for Medicaid services by joint Medicaid/Medicare beneficiaries will these expenditures increase. This would happen, if, for instance, PPS forces poor patients out of the hospital into nursing homes where Medicaid benefits are required.

Expenditures for patients who are privately insured could either increase or decrease as a result of PPS. To the extent that PPS forces hospitals and their physicians to become generally more efficient in their use of hospital resources, privately insured patients will have reduced total outlays (premiums plus copayments). For example, reductions in average length of hospital stay in 1983 were observed in all age groups, not just in the Medicare population. On the other hand, PPS can lead to cost-shifting, in which hospitals increase their prices to cost- or charge-paying consumers to make up for shortfalls from serving Medicare patients. Whether hospitals have the market power to raise prices at will is debatable (126) and probably varies from place to place depending on the degree of competition for patients. About 33 million people in the United States were uninsured in 1983 (282), and many privately insured people have incomplete coverage for hospitalization, so some sensitivity to prices probably exists, especially in the areas with substantial excess hospital capacity.

The introduction of PPS promises to redistribute surpluses[12] among hospitals, with some suffering losses and others gaining. To the extent that this redistribution is related to the hospitals' relative efficiency in patient care, it is desirable and may be temporary in many hospitals. To the extent that inefficient hospitals cannot adjust to PPS, such hospitals may decline or even close. Hospital closure due to inefficiency would be a desirable consequence of PPS.

However, hospitals with certain attributes may find themselves at a financial disadvantage under PPS—for example, if they are classified as ru-

---

[11]In its first annual report, the Prospective Payment Assessment Commission recommended that the average DRG price be adjusted downward to account for any changes in reported case mix due to upcoding (as opposed to real case-mix changes), but the Commission neither estimated the size of this adjustment nor suggested a method by which DHHS should arrive at such an estimate (237).

[12]Surplus (or profit) refers here to the difference between a hospital's revenue and the cost of operation. Although the concept of surplus is clear, its measurement depends on the methods used to account for costs.

ral hospitals when they must pay wages and other costs that are essentially urban (232); if they systematically receive the most seriously ill patients within DRGs; if they systematically treat patients whose home environments or economic circumstances make early discharge infeasible; or if they substantially engage in clinical research. Such hospitals would be likely to have costs that exceed DRG payments. Hospitals without these attributes would be likely to have below-average costs.

The redistribution of financial resources among hospitals due to these factors would be undesirable for two reasons. First, it would affect the distribution of health care resources, and hence, of health benefits among patients; and second, it would simply be unfair to the owners, managers, and employees of the hospitals who lose under the system. Assessments of the extent of such systematic redistribution of profits and surpluses among hospitals is therefore of critical importance.

CONCLUSIONS

The response by health care providers to the new incentives under Medicare's PPS will inevitably affect the costs and benefits of health care. While it is reasonably straightforward to catalog many of the incentives inherent in PPS relative to Medicare's previous cost-based hospital reimbursement system and to array possible provider behaviors emanating from the new incentives, it is difficult to predict which strategies will be followed, the degree to which they will be followed, and the effects they will have on the benefits and costs of health care.

Two conclusions can be drawn. First, the effects of PPS are likely to occur over time, with some appearing quite early and others taking much longer to work themselves out. A mature assessment of the impacts of PPS will require continued observation over the years. Effects due to changes in patterns of medical practice, organization of care, or the rate of technological change may take years to develop.

Second, the effects of PPS are likely to fall unevenly across patients, providers, and payers. Patients with certain conditions, life situations, or residing in certain areas may find the access to and quality of their care lower than others. Some hospitals may be financially penalized because they systematically treat a higher than average number of these patients. And some patients or their third-party payers may find themselves paying a greater proportion of the cost of their care than others as a result of PPS. Identification of such inequities in the impacts of PPS is absolutely critical to evaluation.

Since PPS represents a dramatic reversal of incentives away from the encouragement of more care in the hospital at higher cost toward less care at lower cost per hospitalization, it would appear prudent to focus evaluation on changes in the amount and distribution of care given and the settings in which it is rendered. Yet information on the effects of PPS on the quantity and location of care is inadequate if it is not related to health benefits and costs. To know that the organization of health care delivery and patterns of utilization of services and technologies have changed is simply not enough. These changes must be related to their impacts on benefits and costs. The assessment of impacts of PPS on expenditures and costs, quality of care, access to care, technological change, and clinical research, is an admittedly imperfect, but necessary, substitute for the direct measurement of health benefits and costs. Part Two of this report discusses the evaluation of each of these critical impact areas.

Chapter 3
Preliminary Evidence of the Impacts of PPS

Contents

	Page
Introduction	35
Evidence From the First Year Under PPS	35
The Nature of the Evidence	35
Distribution of Financial Effects Among Hospitals	36
Utilization of Hospital Services	37
Hospital Staffing, Supplies, and Equipment	40
Hospital Management and Organization	42
Evidence of the Effects of Other Prospective Payment Programs	44
State Ratesetting Programs	44
New Jersey's DRG-Based Hospital Payment System	45
Medicare's End-Stage Renal Disease Program	46
Conclusions	47

LIST OF TABLES

Table No.		Page
3-1.	Predicted Distribution of Financial Effects of PPS on Hospitals	37
3-2.	Distribution of PPS Bills by Discharge Status, October 1983 to September 1984	39
3-3.	DRGs Representing the Most Frequent Causes of Hospital Admission in Fiscal Year 1985, Fiscal Year 1984, and Calendar Year 1981	42
3-4.	Medicare-Certified Home Health Agencies by Type of Agency	43

LIST OF FIGURES

Figure No.		Page
3-1.	Average Length of Hospital Stay for Medicare Patients, 1967-84	38
3-2.	Average Length of Hospital Stay: U.S. Short Stay Hospitals, 1974-83	39
3-3.	Medicare Hospital Admissions, 1967-84	41

Chapter 3
Preliminary Evidence of the Impacts of PPS

INTRODUCTION

A useful early step in the development of a strategy for evaluating a program is to identify what is and is not known about it. Medicare's prospective payment system (PPS) established by the Social Security Amendments of 1983 (Public Law 98-21) completed on October 1, 1985, the second year of its 3-year phase-in period. Some evidence of its impacts during the first year of its implementation is available but is tenuous at best.

As discussed in this chapter, some changes have occurred in the U.S. health care system that appear to be related to the adoption of PPS. In certain cases, strong evidence of changes that are coincident with the adoption of PPS suggest that at least part of the changes are due to the new payment system. Although in the absence of sophisticated analyses observed changes in behavior cannot be confidently ascribed to PPS, preliminary evidence of changes in the health care system can suggest whether the effects predicted by analyses of the financial incentives of PPS are occurring.

Because the evidence available from the first year of Medicare's PPS is so sparse, it is also useful to examine evidence from other prospective payment systems. The second part of this chapter reviews the evidence on the effects of three kinds of hospital prospective payment systems to assess the extent to which providers actually do change behavior in ways consistent with new financial incentives:

- State ratesetting programs that do not use per-case prices based on diagnosis-related groups (DRGs);
- New Jersey's DRG-based prospective payment system; and
- Medicare's End-Stage Renal Disease program, which has essentially set prices for hemodialysis services since 1974.

The findings from studies of these programs might be better thought of as indicators than as evidence. The payment systems the studies analyze, even those that are nominally similar to PPS, differ enough from Medicare's PPS that few findings can be directly applied to the latter. What the findings from these studies can do is indicate, first, that certain impacts *may* apply to PPS; and second, the conditions under which the behavior of providers is likely to be sensitive to the financial incentives of PPS.[1]

[1] For a recent and more thorough summary of evidence from the Maryland and New Jersey payment systems, see F.J. Hellinger, "Recent Evidence on Case-Based Systems for Setting Hospital Rates," 1985 (131).

EVIDENCE FROM THE FIRST YEAR UNDER PPS

The Nature of the Evidence

The first year of Medicare's PPS, October 1983 to September 1984, had two features that are important in understanding the system's measured effects. First, since PPS took effect at the beginning of each hospital's fiscal year, hospitals entered the system gradually throughout the year. Although some hospitals entered the system on October 1, 1983, others did not do so until mid-1984. Second, the implementation of PPS was only partial. Only 25 percent of each hospital's per-case payment amount during the first year was based on regional average costs of treating Medicare patients; the remainder was based on the hospital's own historical costs. The gradual implementation of PPS means that hospitals may not yet need to adjust fully to the new system's incentives. On the other hand, many hospitals may be changing behavior now in anticipation of the system's full implementation. PPS-related trends may even be exaggerated in some cases because hospital managers and staff are reacting to their expectations of the new payment system rather than to the system itself.

Evidence from the first year under PPS does not give direct information regarding the new system's impacts on expenditures and costs, quality of care, access to care, technological change, or clinical research. The evidence that is available can be broadly separated into four categories:

- evidence on the distribution of financial effects among hospitals;
- evidence on utilization of hospital services;
- evidence on hospital staffing, supplies, and equipment; and
- evidence on hospital management and organization.

Observed changes in overall Medicare hospital expenditures in the first year of PPS cannot be attributed to the new payment system. The reason is that these expenditures were capped in the first year of PPS's implementation by the budget neutrality provisions of the Social Security Amendments of 1983.[2]

The nature and quality of the available evidence on the new system's impacts varies widely. Some "evidence" on the distribution of financial effects among hospitals, for instance, is derived from studies that use pre-PPS Medicare data to simulate a PPS situation and compare it with cost-based reimbursement. Although these simulation studies do not reflect actual experiences under PPS, they do identify the patterns of redistribution of resources that would occur in the absence of any compensating responses by hospitals. Other evidence, particularly that on staffing and utilization, is based on actual experiences of hospitals under PPS, and levels and trends can be compared with those of the pre-PPS period. These data reflect real post-PPS experience and can provide relatively objective measures of hospital behavior, though changes in these measures cannot be confidently attributed to PPS.

Finally, there is a great deal of subjective information on hospital behavior under PPS. Some information derives from surveys of or interviews with State health officials, hospital administrators, physicians, and other knowledgeable affected people. Market research surveys fall into this category, as do surveys and many studies by government and professional organizations (see ch. 10 for a compendium of surveys and studies of PPS). The validity of evidence relying on the perceptions of individual respondents is questionable. Nevertheless, anecdotal evidence is important in identifying individual changes or behaviors that may be due to PPS.

Distribution of Financial Effects Among Hospitals

Baseline Data From Simulation Studies

Simulation studies that compare Medicare revenues of hospitals under cost-based reimbursement with a hypothetical outcome if those hospitals had been under PPS (fully implemented) at the time provide baseline data on the distributional effects of PPS on hospitals' surpluses or profits. Table 3-1 summarizes the results of three such studies, all based on either 1980 or 1981 Medicare cost and billing data.

As shown in the table, all three studies predicted that small hospitals would fare well under PPS while large hospitals would fare relatively poorly. Teaching hospitals that qualified for large Medicare teaching allowances were generally expected to fare better than nonteaching hospitals. Government-owned hospitals were also predicted to do relatively well, possibly because many government-owned hospitals are also teaching hospitals. Urban hospitals and hospitals in the Northeast and South were predicted to fare better than rural hospitals and hospitals located in the North Central and West regions.[3]

These simulation studies are important because they predict PPS effects and suggest hypotheses that can be tested, but they do not themselves reflect real changes in hospital behavior or finan-

---

[2]The PPS law (Public Law 98-21) specifies that payments for Medicare inpatient hospital services through fiscal year 1985 must be "budget neutral," i.e., no more (or less) than would have been paid under the Tax Equity and Fiscal Responsibility Act of 1982 (Public Law 97-248). The 1982 act placed payment limits and a rate of increase ceiling on Medicare cost-based reimbursement.

[3]The latter regions tend to have markedly lower average lengths of hospital stay than the former, but the implications of this for hospital performance are not entirely clear (265).

Table 3-1.—Predicted Distribution of Financial Effects of PPS on Hospitals

Hospital type	Vaida, 1984[a]	Vaida, 1984[b]	CBO, 1984	Wennberg, 1984
Size:				
0-49 beds	+		+	+
50-99 beds	+		+	0[c]
100-299 beds	–		–	
300+ beds	–	–[d]	0	–[e]
Teaching status:				
Teaching:	–			
Minor[f]			–	
Major[g]			+	+
Nonteaching	+			–
Ownership:				
Church			–	–
Other nonprofit	+			–
For-profit	–	–		
Government	+			+
Location:				
Urban	+			+
Rural	+		–	–
Northeast	+			+
North Central	–		–	–
South	+			+
West	0		–	–

KEY: "+" indicates that hospitals in that category are predicted to do well under PPS relative to cost-based reimbursement.
"–" indicates that hospitals are predicted to do relatively poorly under PPS.
"0" indicates that hospitals are predicted to do about the same under either payment system.
[a] Projection of hospital bonuses and shortfalls.
[b] Regression analysis.
[c] Medium-size hospitals, 50 to 250 beds.
[d] A greater number of beds was correlated with poorer performance.
[e] Large hospitals (more than 250 beds).
[f] Teaching hospitals with small intern- and resident-to-bed ratios, and thus relatively small Medicare teaching allowances.
[g] Teaching hospitals with large intern- and resident-to-bed ratios, and thus relatively large Medicare teaching allowances.
SOURCES: M. Vaida, "The Financial Impact of Prospective Payment on Hospitals," Washington, DC, *Health Affairs* 3(1):112-119, Spring 1984; U.S. Congress, Congressional Budget Office, "Impact of Medicare's Prospective Payment System," memorandum, Nov. 30, 1984; and J.E. Wennberg, "Small Area Variations in Hospitalized Case-Mix," final report, Department of Community and Family Medicine, Dartmouth Medical School, Hanover, NH, Oct. 31, 1984.

cial outcomes. In fact, changes in either hospital behavior (e.g., staff layoffs), hospital characteristics (e.g., case mix), or the structural aspects of PPS (e.g., the Medicare allowances to teaching hospitals) could invalidate their results. Also, these studies are one-dimensional. For example, small hospitals are predicted to do well, but rural hospitals are expected to fare poorly. Even if most rural hospitals are small, it is possible for these results to hold as long as a few large rural hospitals suffer very heavy losses or as long as enough small urban hospitals do very well.

Baseline predictions of differences in financial status among hospitals are available from other sources besides these studies. For example, one study of hospitals in five large metropolitan areas, based largely on 1981 Medicare billing and cost report data, found that inner-city hospitals had higher average costs per patient than did suburban hospitals, implying that the former may be "losers" relative to the latter under PPS (82).

Evidence Since the Introduction of PPS

The only strong evidence of actual hospital financial status since PPS is from the American Hospital Association's (AHA) "National Hospital Panel Survey Report," which found that hospitals as a group saw a larger financial gain in 1984 (an $8.3 billion surplus) than in any year since 1963, when the survey began (21). Geographically, hospitals in the West South Central and Mountain regions of the United States experienced a financial decline (146). Small hospitals' operating margins[4] also dropped, and the smallest hospitals (those with fewer than 25 beds) suffered absolute losses (21). This evidence suggests that large hospitals were able to cut costs rapidly, while small hospitals were not. Nonetheless, hospitals as a group did well under the first year of PPS and have continued to do so into 1985 (177). The caution to this conclusion is that further cost reductions may prove to be much harder, even as PPS becomes fully implemented.

Several observers have predicted that PPS may pose financial hazards to rural hospitals (284, 384), and the American Medical Association's DRG Monitoring Project suggests that this may actually be so (18). There is no published, objective evidence on how rural hospitals have fared, although given that many of them are small they probably have not prospered.

Utilization of Hospital Services

Average Length of Hospital Stay

The most pronounced change in hospital utilization among Medicare patients in the early 1980s is a decrease in the average length of hospital stay

---
[4] A hospital's margin is the percent of its revenue retained after expenses (i.e., revenue minus expenses, divided by revenue) (21)).

(ALOS). PPS seems to have contributed to this trend. The ALOS of the Medicare population in short-stay hospitals[5] decreased before the implementation of Medicare's PPS from 13.4 days in 1968 to 10.2 days in 1982, an annual rate of decrease of 1.9 percent. By the end of 1984, it had dropped to 8.8 days (see fig. 3-1), for an average annual rate of decrease of 7.1 percent between 1982 and 1984. The difference between PPS and non-PPS Medicare stays is even more striking. Between October 1983 and September 1984, the first year of PPS phase-in, Medicare ALOS in all short-stay hospitals (including those under PPS) was 8.9 days, but the ALOS of Medicare patients in hospitals under PPS alone was 7.5 days (332).

[5]"A short-stay hospital is one in which the average length of stay is less than 30 days. General and special hospitals are included in this category" (326).

PPS is not the only factor that has contributed to shorter lengths of stay in acute-care hospitals. Hospital ALOS has been decreasing in both the Medicare and non-Medicare populations for some time. Between 1974 and 1983, the ALOS in the under-65 population dropped from 6.6 to 5.8 days; the ALOS in the over-65 population dropped from 11.9 to 9.8 days (see fig. 3-2).[6] However, this trend was almost certainly accelerated by the

[6]The over-65 population differs slightly from the Medicare population, since Medicare covers many disabled individuals under 65 and does not cover all persons over 65. Since the Health Care Financing Administration does not collect national utilization data on the non-Medicare population, however, age-based data are the only easily available means of providing a rough comparison between Medicare and non-Medicare admissions and lengths of stay. Age-based utilization data are available from several sources, including the American Hospital Association and the Commission on Professional and Hospital Activities (see app. C). The data used here were compiled by the National Center for Health Statistics.

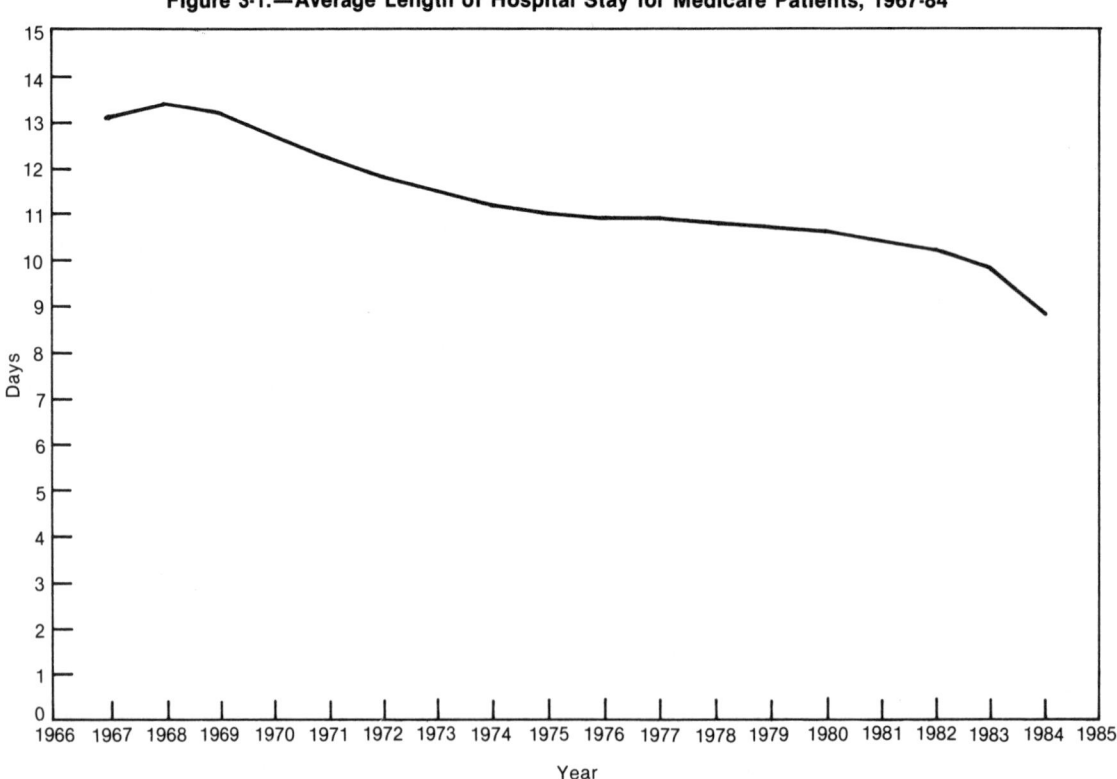

Figure 3-1.—Average Length of Hospital Stay for Medicare Patients, 1967-84

NOTE: Data for 1967-77 based on hospital discharges; 1978-79 on admissions; 1980-84 on APM.
SOURCE: G. Lintzeris, Bureau of Data Management and Strategy, Health Care Financing Administration, U.S. Department of Health and Human Services, Baltimore, MD, personal communications, Dec. 4, 1984 and Jan. 11, 1985.

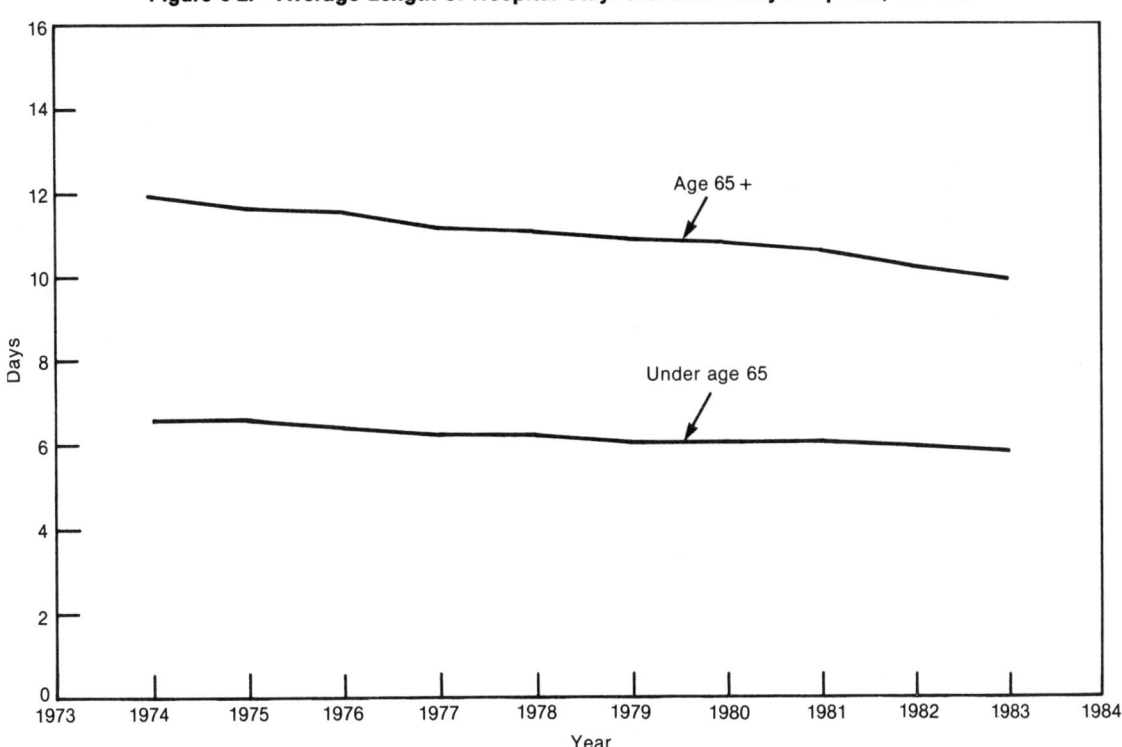

Figure 3-2.—Average Length of Hospital Stay: U.S. Short Stay Hospitals, 1974-83

SOURCE: E. McCarthy, National Center for Health Statistics, Public Health Service, U.S. Department of Health and Human Services, Hyattsville, MD, personal communication, Mar. 28, 1985.

introduction of PPS. ALOS seems to be stabilizing somewhat in 1985 (148).

Interpretation of the impact of PPS on ALOS is complicated by factors other than the underlying trend. Reported ALOS is influenced by two separate PPS incentives, each with different policy implications. First, if hospitals are able to attract patients with less serious conditions, ALOS will decline. (Conversely, ALOS could rise in some DRGs if all but the most severely ill are treated as outpatients.) Second, reported ALOS will decline if patients are discharged earlier to other settings. During the first year of PPS, 13.7 percent of Medicare patients discharged from hospitals were discharged to some form of continuing care besides self-care (see table 3-2).[7] No com-

[7]There is reason to believe that some data on hospital discharge status may be unreliable. The General Accounting Office is currently investigating inconsistencies between hospital and utilization and quality peer review organization (PRO) data on discharges to home health services (34).

Table 3-2.—Distribution of PPS Bills by Discharge Status, October 1983 to September 1984

Discharge destination	Percent
Home (self-care)	80.8%
Short-term hospital	1.7
Skilled nursing facility	5.4
Intermediate care facility	2.7
Other facility	0.9
Home health service	3.0
Discharged against medical advice	0.2
Died	5.3
Total	100.0%

SOURCE: U.S. Department of Health and Human Services, Health Care Financing Administration, "Background Paper," Baltimore, MD, December 1984.

parable data are readily available from a pre-PPS period, though it is probably possible to derive baseline data from the Commission on Professional and Hospital Activities' files (see app. C).

Results from a General Accounting Office study (297) and a congressional survey (303) support the hypothesis that Medicare patients are being discharged from the hospital in a poorer state of health than before PPS and that the demand for posthospital skilled nursing care has increased as a result. Interpretation of these results must proceed cautiously, since they were based on small surveys of professional opinions; they may reflect the anticipation as well as the actual realization of earlier patient discharges. However, they are supported by indications that outpatient and home occupational therapy seem to have increased under PPS (122). They are also supported by widespread anecdotal evidence of early hospital discharges (134,150) and reports of inappropriate discharges identified by utilization and quality control peer review organizations (PROs) (288).

What these apparent discharge patterns mean for the ultimate outcomes of health care is not clear. If patients can receive adequate care outside a hospital, then earlier discharge (even if patients are in a sicker condition) may be acceptable or even beneficial. If these patterns of hospital behavior are accompanied by poorer outcomes of care, on the other hand, they have serious implications for Medicare policy.

Hospital Admissions

Contrary to expectations, Medicare hospital admissions during the first year of PPS actually declined. In the States participating in Medicare's PPS,[8] Medicare admissions to short-stay hospitals were more than 4 percent lower in fiscal year 1984 (the first year of PPS) than in fiscal year 1983. By contrast, admissions had risen over 2 percent in the previous year (338). Figure 3-3 shows the hospital admission trends in the United States for Medicare patients from 1967 to 1984.

Aggregate admissions are not the only area of change; admissions in specific DRGs also suggest that hospitals may be changing their behavior in response to PPS. Table 3-3 lists the DRGs describing the 25 most frequent causes of hospital admission in fiscal year 1985 and indicates their relative ranking in fiscal year 1984 and calendar year 1981 for the purpose of comparison. Changes in DRG rankings, which are based on the relative number of admissions in each DRG, do not always show the anticipated effects. As noted in chapter 2, for instance, the DRG for angina pectoris ranked higher as a proportion of total admissions in 1985 than in 1981 and the DRG for atherosclerosis ranked lower, yet a cursory analysis of the financial incentives predicts the opposite situation (152) (see table 2-1 in ch. 2). The extent to which these changes in frequency of admission are due to changes in technology and medical practice, hospital admission practices, coding practices,[9] or simply changes in disease patterns is unknown.

The fact that admissions declined in the first year of PPS, rather than rising as predicted, suggests three hypotheses: 1) that there may be strong counteractive forces; 2) that strategies aimed at increasing admissions take time to be developed; or 3) that admissions are difficult for hospital managers to influence directly. It may be easier, at least initially, for hospitals to increase outpatient visits (reimbursed on a cost basis) than to increase inpatient admissions in profitable DRGs. Strategies to admit patients twice (e.g., once for diagnosis and once for treatment) may also take time to develop. No data on hospital readmissions under PPS have yet been analyzed, but the decline in overall admissions implies that the readmission rate has probably not increased significantly. Data on readmissions before PPS indicate that under cost-based reimbursement, approximately 22 percent of Medicare patients discharged from the hospital were readmitted within 60 days (24).

Hospital Staffing, Supplies, and Equipment

A decrease in hospital occupancy frequently corresponds with a decrease in staffing, and there is clear evidence that hospitals have been reduc-

---

[8]Nonparticipating, or "waivered," States are Maryland, Massachusetts, New Jersey, and New York.

[9]Changes in the way hospitals code diseases and procedures can result in the appearance of patients being admitted with more serious illnesses than before PPS, even if there is no real change in case mix. This has apparently taken place (55). It is unknown how much of the coding change is due to hospitals' efforts to maximize reimbursement, since more accurate coding would increase the admissions in higher paying DRGs in any case. Analysis of Medicare data from two States revealed that, while incomplete or inaccurate surgical coding frequently led to classification into a lower paying medical DRG, the reverse virtually never occurred (392).

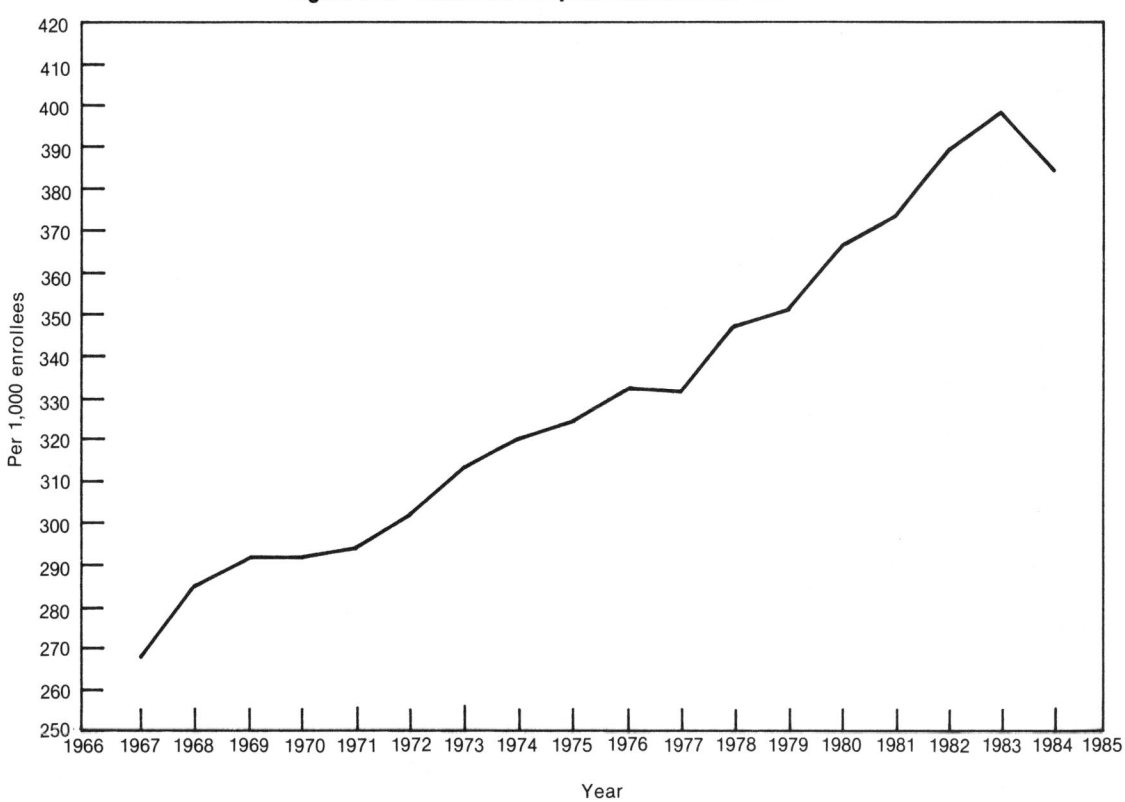

Ch. 3—Preliminary Evidence of the Impacts of PPS • 41

Figure 3-3.—Medicare Hospital Admissions, 1967-84

NOTES: 1967-81 are calendar years; 1982-84 are fiscal years. 1967-77 are discharges, not admissions. (1967-81: aged only. 1982-84: includes disabled.)
SOURCE: G. Lintzeris, Bureau of Data Management and Strategy, Health Care Financing Administration, U.S. Department of Health and Human Services, Baltimore, MD, personal communications, Dec. 4, 1984 and Jan. 11, 1985.

ing their staffs during the past 2 years. AHA survey data indicate that the level of full-time equivalent (FTE) employees in U.S. community hospitals declined by 2.2 percent between May 1983 and May 1984, primarily because of a decrease in full-time employees (379). The number of part-time workers decreased by only 0.2 percent during the same period. The American Nursing Association reports that there has also been a shift away from licensed practical nurses towards the more highly trained registered nurses (20).

Data from specific States and regions reinforce this picture of hospital cost containment through staff reductions. In Wisconsin, for example, total hospital employment dropped 4.9 percent between 1982 and 1984 (398). Major staff layoffs have also been reported in Pennsylvania, California, Florida, Ohio, Michigan, and Washington D.C. (25,109,246,251,379). It is important to note that since strategies for staff reduction include hiring freezes and attrition, the extent of staff reduction activities is probably much higher than the layoff figures alone indicate. On the other hand, the trend toward staff reductions began before many hospitals came under PPS. Thus, although PPS has probably encouraged the trend, it is by no means the only cause.

A reduction in staffing does not necessarily mean less staff time per hospitalized patient. Because of the recent trends towards fewer admis-

Table 3-3.—DRGs Representing the Most Frequent Causes of Hospital Admission in Fiscal Year 1985,[a] Fiscal Year 1984, and Calendar Year 1981

DRG No.	Description	Fiscal year 1985 rank[a]	Fiscal year 1984 rank	Calendar year 1981 rank
127	Heart failure and shock	1	1	1
089	Simple pneumonia and pleurisy	2	6	7
140	Angina pectoris	3	5	11
182	Esophagitis, gastroenteritis, miscellaneous digestive disorders	4	2	2
014	Specific cerebrovascular disorders	5	4	6
096	Bronchitis and asthma	6	12	16
138	Cardiac arrhythmia and conduction disorders	7	8	13
296	Nutritional and miscellaneous metabolic disorders	8	10	21
039	Lens procedures	9	3	4
088	Chronic obstructive pulmonary disease	10	9	5
243	Medical back problems	11	7	12
015	Transient ischemic attacks	12	11	15
209	Major joint procedures	13	14	26
336	Transurethral prostatectomy	14	13	25
174	Gastrointestinal hemorrhage	15	15	23
122	Circulatory disorders with acute myocardial infarction	16	16	9
320	Kidney and urinary tract infections	17	17	19
210	Hip and femur procedures	18	20	32
121	Circulatory disorders with acute myocardial infarction and cardiovascular complications	19	22	NA[b]
087	Pulmonary edema and respiratory failure	20	24	45
294	Diabetes	21	18	10
468	Unrelated operating room procedure	22	19	8
148	Major small and large bowel procedures	23	23	38
082	Respiratory neoplasms	24	21	18
141	Syncope and collapse	25	30	47

[a]Bills received through July 1985.
[b]Calendar year 1981 rank not available because previously combined with DRG #122.
SOURCE: D. Wood, Bureau of Data Management and Strategy, Health Care Financing Administration, U.S. Department of Health and Human Services, Baltimore, MD, personal communication, August 1985.

sions and shorter lengths of stay, the number of FTE employees per 100 patients actually increased between May 1983 and May 1984 (379).

There is no objectively measured evidence of PPS impacts on nonstaffing inputs, i.e., supplies and equipment. The general environment is one of cost competition; hospital suppliers are engaging in price wars and diversifying into other markets, while hospitals are forming group purchasing organizations to increase their buying power (14). The extent to which PPS is influencing this competitive environment, however, is unknown.

Cost competition also appears to be affecting the medical equipment market. Anecdotal evidence suggests that manufacturers are pursuing strategies such as developing equipment that is less labor-intensive (260). An analysis of the diagnostic imaging market suggested that government efforts to contain cost, including PPS, are slowing sales (48). Manufacturers are responding to a constriction of the market by increasing research and development efforts that will make current equipment obsolete through small incremental improvements; focusing efforts on the few areas of the market that promise to expand; and attempting to reduce the costs of producing those systems that are technologically stable (48).

Hospital Management and Organization

Medicare's PPS appears to be having an unambiguous impact on hospital information systems and their use in management. The use of DRGs as the basis for payment has led to a proliferation of computer packages aimed at helping hospitals estimate their actual costs per case and predict the reimbursement levels per patient (51,106).

The medical records departments of hospitals have also assumed great importance under PPS, since accurate records processing is necessary for prompt maximum reimbursement (154). One result of this incentive has been an increase in automated medical records processing; one market research survey showed that use of automated processing among sampled hospitals jumped from 28.3 percent in 1981 to 48.1 percent in 1984 (222). Once again, this recent rapid trend toward automation is probably not entirely due to PPS, because increases in computerized information applications have taken place in many industries. Nevertheless, the information requirements and incentives of PPS have certainly been a contributing factor.

Lower hospital occupancy and incentives to increase admissions may be contributing to trends in the hospital industry toward increasing competition for patients, through strategies such as increases in hospital advertising (8,112,290). In the American Medical Association's DRG Monitoring Project, a compilation of physicians' comments on PPS, 73 percent of respondents stated that hospital admission and discharge policies had changed since the introduction of PPS (18).

Along with new discharge policies and the incentive to shorten ALOS comes an incentive under PPS for hospitals to benefit from extending their services to other settings. The evidence suggests that hospitals are doing this, though again the trend began before the inception of PPS. The number of hospitals offering posthospital services (home health care, skilled nursing care, or other long-term care) increased between 1982 and 1983 and has increased even more since; 17 percent more hospitals were offering home health care services in 1984 than in 1983 (382). The number of Medicare-certified hospital-based home health agencies increased by more than 50 percent during 1984 (see table 3-4). Furthermore, three-quarters of hospital administrators responding to one recent survey said they planned to add or expand their home health services, outpatient surgery services, or both (204).[10]

---

[10]PPS may be affecting the organization of health care through more than incentives for hospitals to expand to new services. Some have postulated that the present health care environment, of which PPS is a part, encourages for-profit hospital chains that can cut costs through mechanisms such as bulk discounts (94). There is certainly abundant evidence of the activities of such enterprises, and in specific cases there seem to be links to PPS (285). However, there have been no general surveys or studies of PPS-specific effects in this area.

Table 3-4.—Medicare-Certified Home Health Agencies by Type of Agency

Type of agency	December 1979	September 1981	December 1982	December 1983	December 1984
Visiting nurses association	511	513	517	520	525
Combination (government/voluntary)	50	55	59	58	59
Government	1,274	1,234	1,211	1,230	1,226
Rehabilitation center based	NA[a]	11	16	19	22
Hospital based	349	432	507	579	894
Skilled nursing home based	NA	10	32	136	175
Proprietary	165	287	628	997	1,569
Private nonprofit	443	547	632	674	756
Other	66	38	37	45	21
Total	2,858	3,127	3,639	4,258	5,247

[a]NA = Not available; home agencies in these categories were classified as "other" in 1979.
SOURCE: D. Milstead, Health Care Financing Administration, U.S. Department of Health and Human Services, Baltimore, MD, March 1985.

EVIDENCE OF THE EFFECTS OF OTHER PROSPECTIVE PAYMENT PROGRAMS

State Ratesetting Programs

Over the past decade, a number of States have instituted some form of prospective payment as a means of controlling hospital costs. All of these State programs are characterized by payment rates that are set before services are actually rendered and that need not be a mere reflection of the costs actually incurred in serving patients (88). In other respects, the programs differ greatly. The most important differences are whether hospital participation is mandatory or voluntary; whether compliance is mandatory or voluntary; whether all payers are covered or only a few; how rates are set; and the basis of payment. Payment rates may be set, for instance, through the application of a formula or through review of a hospital's budget, which, once approved, is translated into rates sufficient to generate enough revenue to cover it (89). The unit of payment may be per stay, per day, per specific service, or based on the allocation of the approved hospital budget among third-party payers according to their anticipated share (89).

The State programs whose experience is most relevant to PPS are those in which hospital participation and compliance are mandated by law. These include programs in the four States currently holding Medicare waivers from PPS (New Jersey, Massachusetts, New York,[11] and Maryland) and in a few States without waivers (notably Washington, Connecticut, and western Pennsylvania). Two of these States—New Jersey and Maryland—have had some experience with both per-case payment and a case-mix classification method similar to Medicare's DRG system. However, only New Jersey has required that all hospitals use the same classification system; Maryland has allowed hospitals to choose from a number of systems.

The one finding common to nearly all studies of State prospective payment programs is that programs with mandatory participation and compliance have controlled rates of increase in hospital costs. States with such mandatory programs have succeeded in keeping their increases in hospital costs and expenditures below increases of other States. The findings with regard to whether State programs with voluntary participation have controlled costs are inconclusive (35,60,268,269).

The finding that mandatory State ratesetting programs have helped control increases in hospital costs must be interpreted carefully. First, with the exception of Washington, the States with strict prospective payment programs had much higher costs than the national average; only the *increases* in cost were lower than States without such programs (385). Rather than being the cause of all observed differences, State ratesetting programs may have been implemented because of preexisting differences between State health care systems. Second, in most cases, these effects on cost became apparent only after the programs had been in place for a few years (35,269). Third, the comparability between State ratesetting programs and Medicare's PPS is debatable. Experience with the State program that is perhaps the most comparable to PPS, New Jersey's DRG-based program, is discussed further below.

Cost containment may come at the expense of efficiently run hospitals as well as inefficient ones. One study found that hospitals with particularly high expenditures before ratesetting were likely to remain high (22). It was not clear whether this occurred because hospitals with high expenditures convinced regulators that in fact they were efficient, because the State did not find it cost-effective to pursue them, or because the hospitals could not reduce the inefficiencies despite financial pressure.

Worthington and Piro, analyzing the effects of State ratesetting programs from 1969 to 1978 on hospital utilization, found that occupancy levels were generally higher (and increased faster) in ratesetting States than in other States (401). States that regulated per diem rates had the most predictable outcomes; as hypothesized, length of stay was significantly increased in all three such States.

---
[11]New York's waiver expires at the end of 1985.

A more surprising finding was that in three States in which rate regulation decreased the cost per admission it nevertheless increased the ALOS. One explanation for this finding is that in the early years of rate regulation, hospitals tended to control costs by reducing service intensity rather than by reducing ALOS even where they were not paid per diem (401). For example, much of the cost savings per admission in the New Jersey program has been achieved through inpatient ancillary service savings, with possible coincidental cost-shifting to nonregulated outpatients (250).

Prospective payment programs do seem to affect health care employment. States under prospective payment tend to reduce the number of FTE employees per inpatient day (166). In New York, Maryland, and Massachusetts, prospective payment lowered the demand for licensed practical nurses and, to a lesser degree, for registered nurses as well (113). Average net physician incomes have also grown more slowly in States with strict hospital regulatory programs than in those without (406).

There is evidence of State prospective payment effects on the diffusion of medical technologies, but the evidence is often inconsistent. The observed changes may be due to specific characteristics of the individual States rather than to the existence of ratesetting programs. One analysis found that State ratesetting programs generally discouraged computed tomography scanning in hospitals, leading in a shift in the location of scanners from hospitals to physicians' offices (157). But other analyses have found very State-specific effects on technology adoption and use. One study found that New York's program appeared to depress the availability of all types of services; New Jersey's tended to reduce the availability of most complex services; and other States' programs showed no consistent impact on service adoption at all (70). Another study of the impact of prospective payment on capital equipment adoption in five States found that New York hospitals tended to adopt more cost-saving and less cost-raising equipment, but programs in Maryland and Indiana showed no such consistent effects on hospitals' adoption behavior (249). A third study found that ratesetting had no effect on the diffusion of most surgical technologies but did slow the adoption of the expensive coronary bypass procedure (270). However, about half of the rate-setting hospitals analyzed for this study were in New York, and the conclusion may be simply that New York has characteristics that sometimes slow technological diffusion.

New Jersey's DRG-Based Hospital Payment System

New Jersey is the only State to have implemented a prospective hospital payment system, uniform across all hospitals and all payers, in which the unit of payment is per-case and patients are classified according to DRG. New Jersey's program was first implemented in a small number of hospitals in 1978 and then was expanded to the entire State in 1980. The design of the program differs in several important details from Medicare's PPS. Nevertheless, New Jersey's hospital payment system is closer to Medicare's PPS than any other State system, and because of that, it has received quite a bit of attention.

An evaluation of New Jersey's DRG-based hospital payment system was completed by the Health Research and Education Trust of New Jersey in 1982. The study's findings regarding the organizational impact of the DRG-based system were as follows (130):

- Hospitals under New Jersey's DRG-based payment system expanded the type and quantity of management information gathered. Clinical data improved in accuracy but also took more time to produce.
- Decisionmaking was more decentralized in hospitals under the DRG-based payment system than in non-DRG hospitals.
- The importance of medical records departments increased dramatically in hospitals using DRGs.
- The medical staffs in hospitals using DRGs became much more involved in managerial decisions than they had been before the DRG-based payment system was implemented.
- Hospitals under DRG-based payment tended to be more output-oriented than non-DRG hospitals.

The Health Research and Educational Trust also found a number of financial and economic impacts of DRGs that have implications for PPS:

- The direct costs of implementing DRG-based payment was high because of the need to improve hospital data collection and billing (131).
- In the initial year of DRG implementation, hospitals under DRG-based payment actually received more revenue than they would have under the previous ratesetting scheme. Most hospitals benefited financially from the case-mix classification system (131).
- The evaluators estimated that it would be several years, if ever, before the overall cost containment objective could be attained (192).

Finally, the 1982 evaluation of New Jersey's system noted that the ALOS seemed to be affected very little by the use of DRGs; it dropped only 0.03 percent between 1979 and 1980 (131).

Some of the effects of New Jersey's hospital payment system are likely to be artifacts of its specific design. Each DRG price is computed as a blend of the hospital's own costs and the average cost of treating patients in specific hospitals (123). Hospitals are cushioned by this system from incurring severe losses in any DRG. Also, New Jersey's program apportions payment for uncompensated care among the payers. This approach reduces financial problems for hospitals at high risk for bad debts.

Thus, the lessons from New Jersey for Medicare's PPS are limited. They do suggest, however, that hospitals will respond to per-case payment in ways that are predicted by theory.

Medicare's End-Stage Renal Disease Program

Since 1973, Medicare has covered approximately 93 percent of the people in the United States suffering from end-stage renal disease (46). From July 1973 until August 1983, Medicare reimbursed for hemodialysis[12] services and supplies to these patients at a rate of 80 percent of the average cost to a hospital-based dialysis facility (up to a specified limit); 80 percent of reasonable charges for a freestanding facility (also up to a limit); and 80 percent of allowed costs for supplies and equipment for home dialysis (100 percent after 1978) (248). By 1982, nearly all freestanding facilities were being paid at the limit of $138 per treatment.[13] Most hospital-based facilities, on the other hand, had been granted exceptions to the specified payment limit, and the average payment to hospitals by 1980 was about $159 per treatment. Since 1974, then providers of dialysis services have faced prospectively set rate limits. Hospital-based providers had few incentives to keep costs below the payment rates because they could not retain surpluses. Freestanding facilities, in contrast, were able to keep any profits. Under these conditions, providers of dialysis services and supplies proliferated, and costs multiplied, though most of the increase in costs was due to an increase in the eligible population (96,115,245).

The End Stage Renal Disease Amendments of 1978 (Public Law 95-292) established a new prospective payment method for dialysis facilities. Under this new program, effective August 1, 1983, hospital facilities are paid an average of $131 per dialysis session, and freestanding facilities are paid an average of $127, regardless of whether dialysis occurs in the center or at home (48 FR 21254). Hospitals may keep payment surpluses but must absorb losses when costs exceed price.

The prospective payment method does seem to have stimulated some cost competition in the supply market. Since its implementation, there has been little increase in the price of dialysis supplies. Prices for at least one key product, dialyzers, have actually fallen (248). Reuse of dialyzers, one way of lowering costs,[14] has increased rapidly in re-

---

[12]Hemodialysis is a process that substitutes for normal kidney function. Blood is pumped from the patient's body into a dialyzer, cleansed of waste products, and returned to the body.

[13]Payment for dialysis from 1974 until mid-1983 was limited to a maximum of $133 per treatment. "If routine laboratory services were included in the facility's costs, the screen [limit] was raised by $5; if the supervisory services of a physician were included in the facility's costs, the screen was increased by $12 more to $150" (248).

[14]The extent to which this apparent cost savings comes at the expense of safety has not been resolved, although reuse seems to be safe most of the time if the dialyzer is properly reprocessed and not overused (248).

cent years, suggesting that this trend is encouraged (though not necessarily caused) by prospective payment. It is expected that the prospective payment program will also continue the trend to home dialysis and encourage the proliferation of dialyzing devices used in that setting (248).

CONCLUSIONS

An overview of the evidence on the impacts of Medicare's PPS during its first year of implementation indicates the breadth and depth of evaluation necessary, helps identify evaluation resource needs, and supports the formulation of critical questions.

The evidence presented here is sparse and demonstrates how little we know at present about the ultimate effects of PPS on the health care system. Its weakness is due in part to the fact that hospitals moved to PPS at the beginning of their own fiscal years, so the first year in which all Medicare participating hospitals are under PPS began October 1, 1984. Also, in the first year of the program, the portion of payments based on regional and national average DRG costs was small (25 percent) compared to the historical hospital-based portion (75 percent). The evidence is further weakened by the fact that there are few causal links that can be demonstrated between observed changes in the health care system and PPS. *The greatest deficiency in the evidence, however, is that most of it is not conceptually linked to the ultimate outcomes of health care.* It is simply not possible to assess, for example, whether the observed changes in length of stay have had any impact—for good or bad—on the quality of care given to Medicare beneficiaries. To answer that question, more refined analyses, using better indicators of quality, will be required.

What little evidence is available from the first year under PPS tends to confirm some predictions based on analysis of financial incentives and contradict others. For instance, contrary to expectations, admission rates in PPS hospitals decreased slightly since the payment system was instituted. There is evidence in line with predictions, however, that PPS is influencing the already decreasing ALOS for Medicare patients. Staffing trends also have followed expectations; the number of FTE personnel has declined. Because admissions have decreased, the number of FTE employees per 100 patients has increased, but those employees may be treating sicker patients than they were treating before PPS.

The only compelling evidence of significant behavioral changes in the first year of PPS is the drop in ALOS, which is probably only partly due to PPS; and extensive hospital investment in information systems, which is probably due primarily to PPS.

Many of the predictions about the impacts of Medicare's PPS are based on evidence from other prospective payment programs. Analyses of these programs yield three general conclusions relevant to PPS. First, many of the impacts of prospective payment systems take time to develop. Second, the impacts may vary considerably according to the specific characteristics of each program. And, third, while many effects can be predicted by theory, some important impacts may be unexpected and some expected impacts may never materialize. A successful evaluation strategy for PPS must reflect these lessons.

Chapter 4
Issues in Designing an Evaluation of PPS

Contents

	Page
Introduction	51
Fundamental Issues Underlying the Development of a PPS Evaluation Plan	51
Specifying the Perspective of Evaluation	51
Specifying the Standard of Comparison	51
Defining the Objectives of Evaluation	52
Determining the Evaluation Time Schedule	53
Alternative Evaluation Research Designs	53
Aspects of PPS Affecting Research Design	55
PPS as a Moving Target	55
Simultaneous Influences in the Health Care System	55
Data Availability	57
Conclusions	57

FIGURE

Figure No.	Page
4-1. Comparison of the Feasibility, Affordability, and Validity of Alternative Designs for Evaluating the Impact of PPS on the Health Care System	54

Chapter 4
Issues in Designing an Evaluation of PPS

INTRODUCTION

This chapter examines issues that arise in developing a strategy for evaluating the impact of Medicare's prospective payment system (PPS). These issues are of two kinds:

- fundamental choices that must be made with respect to the kinds of questions that are asked about PPS; and
- tradeoffs that are necessary in the selection of specific research designs for answering the questions.

In this report, the term "evaluation" as applied to PPS refers to any effort to associate changes in characteristics of the health care system with the implementation of PPS or its components. The usefulness of an evaluation in guiding policy and program changes varies directly with the quality of evidence on which such associations are based and the confidence with which causal inferences can be made.

FUNDAMENTAL ISSUES UNDERLYING THE DEVELOPMENT OF A PPS EVALUATION PLAN

Important choices are necessary before critical PPS evaluation questions can be developed. These choices involve specifying the kinds of information that are important in guiding policy and program changes. OTA made such choices in developing the critical evaluation questions summarized in chapter 1. Considerations underlying these decisions are discussed below.

Specifying the Perspective of Evaluation

One of the first questions to be addressed in developing a PPS evaluation plan is whose perspective is important in the evaluation. The impacts of PPS on Medicare expenditures was, of course, critical to the passage of the law establishing PPS, and these effects need to be assessed. But such a narrow program perspective is inadequate in evaluating a program with the wide range of effects of PPS.

PPS will have varying effects on Medicare beneficiaries, other cohorts of the population, providers of health care, suppliers of medical products, employees, educators, and researchers. An evaluation could proceed from the perspective of one or a combination of these groups. A comprehensive evaluation would be one that would balance the effects on these different groups and take the interests of society as a whole into account. This report recognizes the tradeoffs among affected groups and lays out evaluation questions regarding the distribution of such effects across members of society.

Specifying the Standard of Comparison

A second question involves the standard against which PPS effects will be judged. PPS contains three central elements: 1) a system of expenditure control carried forward from the Tax Equity and Fiscal Responsibility Act (TEFRA) (Public Law 97-248); 2) a restructuring of financial incentives from cost-based reimbursement to per-case payment; and 3) the use of diagnosis-related groups (DRGs) to classify patients for the purposes of payment.

Some of the effects of PPS might occur in any system that controlled revenues going to hospitals. If one wanted to compare the results of Medicare's PPS with the results of alternative systems of expenditure control, one could analyze evidence in the four States—Maryland, Massachusetts, New Jersey, and New York—currently holding waivers from Medicare's PPS.[1] As noted in chapter 3, the ratesetting systems in these States are different from PPS in major and minor aspects of program design. The State systems are generally all-payer systems, the unit of payment in some is not the admission, and the method of arriving at the payment rates differs in each State. The State systems are required by their waiver contracts, however, to hold expenditures to levels that are no higher than those that would have occurred under PPS. Consequently, comparative analyses of experience under PPS and under the State waivers can be highly revealing of the specific gains and losses from a system like PPS compared to other kinds of expenditure control.

For immediate policy, understanding the impacts of particular elements of PPS, such as the special treatment of teaching hospitals or the use of DRGs as the patient classification system, may be even more important than understanding the overall effects of PPS relative to cost-based hospital reimbursement. Yet it is nearly impossible to identify the specific aspects of PPS that are responsible for any observed changes in the health care system. Indeed, as the remainder of this report shows, attributing any changes in the health care system to PPS as a whole will be difficult enough. Thus, it is probably infeasible to evaluate the impact of specific components of PPS on the behavior and outcomes of the health care system. In general, then, this report deals with approaches to evaluating the effects of PPS as a whole relative to Medicare's former cost-based hospital reimbursement system.

One component of PPS that is particularly critical to the incentives in the system is the use of DRGs as the system of classifying patients for payment purposes. Other approaches to patient classification have been or are under development, and DRGs themselves are likely to be refined as time goes by. (The DRG and alternative patient classification systems are described in app. H.)

Under Medicare's DRG-based PPS, the financial desirability of any given patient is established in part by his or her assignment to a particular DRG. Patient classification systems other than the DRG system would group patients in different ways, changing the amounts paid for, and therefore the relative profitability of, some patients. The patient classification system can also influence the financial incentives involving the use of existing medical technologies and the introduction of new ones. Patient classification systems such as DRGs, which assign patients at least partly on the basis of whether a specific technology is used, can encourage or discourage the introduction of new technologies whose use would change the patient's category (see ch. 8 for examples). Classification systems that assign patients to categories on the basis of clinical condition alone, not resource use, create very different incentives for new technologies. The focus of this study is on the incentives inherent in Medicare's DRG-based PPS relative to cost-based reimbursement, but comparative studies of the effect of alternative approaches to patient classification on hospital behavior regarding admissions strategies and technology use and adoption would be useful as well.

Defining the Objectives of Evaluation

A third major issue is the relative importance of various desirable features of an evaluation of PPS. One has to address the tradeoffs among the following, partially competing, objectives:

- to act as an early-warning system for serious, unintended consequences of PPS;
- to obtain a balanced view of PPS effects, including both positive and negative impacts;
- to quantify any observed effect with precision;
- to attribute any observed effect to PPS with confidence;
- to afford the research effort; and
- to choose feasible evaluation approaches.

The affordability and feasibility of using particular impact measures and research methods are determined largely by the kinds and quality of data sources available, the cost of obtaining the data, and the administrative or ethical barriers to their use. Feasibility is also limited by the lack of comprehensive and balanced measures of quality of care (see ch. 6) and access to care (see ch. 7). In the meantime, the measures that do exist,

---
[1]Together, these four States account for 533, or 9 percent, of the non-Federal community hospitals in the United States (13).

if chosen carefully, may give an acceptably accurate picture of how the health care system is changing in this regard.

The feasibility of attributing observed effects to PPS is limited by several factors. One problem is that because PPS has been implemented universally among non-Federal community hospitals (except in the four States with waivers), the opportunities for comparison are limited. Another problem is that PPS is not the only change underway in the U.S. health care system; simultaneous influences, which can often be accounted for only by the passage of time, confound attempts to directly attribute many changes in the health care system to PPS.

Despite such difficulties, it is still possible to conduct pre/post-PPS analyses that offer strong suggestive evidence about the impacts of PPS or its components. Success hinges on careful a priori analysis of the likely magnitude and direction of influence of other factors so that the effects of PPS may be reasonably well inferred.

Determining the Evaluation Time Schedule

An evaluation plan must take into account the fact that the effects of PPS will unfold only over time, as the health care system gradually adapts to the new payment environment. Some changes may occur early and continue throughout the lifetime of PPS; some may occur early but disappear as PPS goes on; others may not surface until much later. Reductions in personnel staffing levels, for example, appear to take place almost immediately as hospitals have sought quick responses to the incentives of PPS (379), but these changes may not be long-lived. Or, the incentive to move patients out of the hospital early to reduce length of stay may not be acted on in the short-run if facilities to care for these patients are in short supply. As time goes by, however, if the health care system responds with an increase in the supply of long-term care facilities, shifts in the settings of care may be more dramatic.

One of the most fundamental changes encouraged by PPS is also likely to take a number of years to occur. Physicians' attitudes may gradually become more positive toward the appropriateness of taking cost into consideration in clinical decisionmaking (275). Increasing interest in issues of cost-effectiveness of medical practices will lead to more research into these questions and ultimately more information available to physicians. Yet, these developments are likely to be quite gradual, showing their influence on patterns of medical care utilization only after years.

A strategy for monitoring and evaluating PPS should take account of the timing of effects as well as the ultimate impacts. Certain observable changes in the health care system may be able to serve as valid early warning indicators of important long-run effects of PPS; the challenge is to choose them correctly when little evidence of such validity is available.

ALTERNATIVE EVALUATION RESEARCH DESIGNS

A question that transcends all areas of impact is how to design an evaluation that will provide sufficiently valid answers about the impacts of PPS at reasonable cost and in a timely manner. A range of evaluation designs can be considered, each with its own strengths and weaknesses.

In selecting an evaluation design, one must consider the potential validity of the findings against the cost (or, alternatively, the affordability) and the feasibility of the approach. The validity of a study is defined here as the extent to which explanations other than the program under study can be ruled out as responsible for the observed effect (internal validity); and the extent to which the findings can be generalized beyond the study sample (external validity) (54). Often, the level of validity obtainable with a particular research design varies directly with cost and inversely with feasibility.

Figure 4-1 summarizes the performance of alternative evaluation designs on the dimensions of feasibility, affordability, and validity. *Controlled*

Figure 4-1.—Comparison of the Feasibility, Affordability, and Validity of Alternative Designs for Evaluating the Impact of PPS on the Health Care System

Feasibility/ affordability	Validity		
	Low	Medium	High
Low		Studies using comparison groups	Controlled random experiments
Medium		Pre/post-program comparisons	
High	Opinion surveys, anecdotes	Case studies	

SOURCE: Office of Technology Assessment, 1985.

experiments typically have high validity (particularly internal validity) because they are carried out prospectively and generally involve the random assignment of subjects to an experimental program or to a control group (or program). Since both groups are exposed to whatever simultaneous influences occur, differences in study outcomes can reasonably be ascribed to the experimental program. Unfortunately, program evaluations can rarely take place in such an environment. In the case of PPS, the program has been implemented universally, with waivered States generally unrepresentative of the rest of the country.

Quasi-experimental research designs move back from the strict requirements of controlled experiments to the use of *comparison groups* whose representativeness has not been established or to *pre/post-program comparisons.* Only if the analyst has a high level of confidence that the comparison groups are likely to be representative or that observed effects are unlikely to be due to simultaneous influences can these designs offer much validity.

More informal approaches, such as detailed *case studies,* are systematic efforts to identify behavior or outcomes that can be linked in very specific circumstances to the program under study. Case studies of decisionmaking in hospitals, for example, can uncover behavior that is in direct response to PPS. Case studies of the development and diffusion of medical technologies provide an excellent means of identifying aspects of the payment system that affect technological change (see ch. 8 for more detail). These approaches to evaluation can be enlightening, but they pose threats to validity that need careful attention. Most important, bias in the selection of subjects for case studies, a phenomenon that is difficult to guard against, can call attention to some effects of PPS and ignore others that are equally important.

As chapter 3 of this report illustrates, much of the information currently available on the impacts of PPS consists of *anecdotes and opinions* (sometimes systematically collected through surveys). Often, observed changes in a measure of effect may be ascribed to PPS on the basis of opinion. For example, changes in employment patterns in hospitals since PPS have been documented. Whether or to what extent such changes are due to the implementation of PPS is unknown, however. A survey might ask hospital administrators for their opinions regarding the importance of PPS relative to other factors in bringing about these changes.

Evidence consisting of anecdotes and opinions has the lowest validity for obvious reasons—the opinions may be biased and the anecdotes rare outliers—but it is not necessarily wrong. In fact, such informal sources of data can be most useful as early warning systems that raise hypotheses about the impacts of PPS. Reliance on these sources without further analysis, however, exposes policymaking to high risks.

ASPECTS OF PPS AFFECTING RESEARCH DESIGN

The most appropriate research design depends on the particular characteristics of PPS that affect the feasibility, cost, and validity of the alternatives laid out above. Three such characteristics are as follows:

- PPS is a moving target;
- PPS is being implemented in an environment of multiple and major simultaneous influences; and
- the availability of data for some kinds of designs is limited.

Each of these aspects is discussed below.

PPS as a Moving Target

A problem common to all evaluations of major programs is that the character of the program itself changes over its lifetime. Evaluations of the effects of a program in its early years may be irrelevant by the time the evaluations are finished. In the case of PPS, major changes are inevitable. The 3-year phase-in period institutionalizes a policy of change. Not only are hospitals finding their revenues increasingly subject to PPS, but the DRG prices themselves are moving from a regional to national basis. Moreover, important components of hospital costs, namely capital and direct medical education expenses, have been excluded from PPS, but there is reason to believe that these exclusions will not persist in the next 5 years. Finally, the overall generosity of PPS, which is largely determined by the annual rate of increase in the average DRG price, may have more to do with impacts on the health care system than any other aspect of the program and is subject to variation over time as cost-containment pressures grow or recede.

These realities argue for a continuous system of monitoring PPS effects that focuses on sensitive and readily available indicators of system performance such as changes in patterns of expenditures, utilization, and organization of care. But information on these indicators needs to be buttressed by research linking them to the important, ultimate impacts on health care benefits and costs.

Simultaneous Influences in the Health Care System

Were PPS the only change underway in the health care system, it would be possible to compare outcomes before and after its imposition in order to infer its impacts. But the health care system has been undergoing rapid change in the past 5 years and continues to be dynamic. Among the most important simultaneous influences are the following:

- *The ratio of physicians to population has been increasing.* The supply of physicians has been rising dramatically in the past decade as a consequence both of Federal policy on medical education and the immigration of foreign-trained physicians. In 1975, there were 179 physicians per 100,000 people in the United States. By 1981, this number had grown to 207 (346). The trend toward higher physician-to-population ratios is expected to continue, with an expected ratio of 264 per 100,000 people by the year 2000 (346).
- *Competition in the health care system has been increasing.* Numerous factors have contributed to an increase in the amount of competition for patients. First, the supply of physicians and innovative health care facilities has increased in the past 5 years and continues to increase. New alternative sites of health care delivery, such as freestanding ambulatory surgical and emergency centers, have been formed throughout the country. For example, between 1979 and 1982, the number of freestanding emergency centers grew from 44 to almost 500 nationwide (292). Hospitals have attempted to compete with freestanding facilities by upgrading hospital-based emergency rooms and providing their own freestanding facilities (292).

Second, increasing pressure on employers to contain the costs of their health benefits has led to changes in health insurance plans, which encourage competition among providers on the basis of price. Increased beneficiary cost-sharing requirements, for example, make patients more price sensitive in selecting their settings of care. The development of preferred provider organizations, which contract with insurers to provide services at a reduced rate, is the latest manifestation of increasing competition (307).

Third, the size of the uninsured population tends to fluctuate with the business cycle but has been on the rise in recent years (283). With more patients lacking insurance, they are likely to become more sensitive to hospitals' prices and hospitalizations are delayed.

- *Various aspects of Federal health policies have undergone changes concurrent with PPS.* Other aspects of Federal health policy have been altered during the time immediately prior to or during the implementation of PPS. For example, the Medicaid program, which is administered by States under general guidelines and financial subsidies from the Federal Government, has given increasing flexibility to the States to define eligibility, scope of covered services, and levels of payments to providers. In fiscal year 1982, after the passage of the Omnibus Budget Reconciliation Act of 1981 (Public Law 97-35), the number of Medicaid recipients per capita and Medicaid payments per recipient declined (111). These declines occurred despite a severe economic recession that would be expected to raise welfare rolls and Medicaid expenses.

The Veterans Administration (VA) is also currently undergoing changes in the way funds for patient care will be allocated among facilities. The VA has begun to implement a new budget allocation system that will tie budgets more closely to standardized work units. For inpatient admissions, the DRG definitions are being used. Facility budgets will come to be more dependent on case mix than in the past, when high occupancy was rewarded regardless of turnover. The new budget systems provide incentives to VA facility managers for cost containment and more selective admission and treatment criteria (110). Consequently, it may be difficult to separate the effects of PPS on the utilization of VA services from the effects of the VA's own administrative changes.

The Medicare program itself has undergone substantial changes in policy concurrent with PPS. For example, the Deficit Reduction Act of 1984 (Public Law 98-369) mandated a fee schedule for ambulatory laboratory procedures, including those performed by hospital laboratories, that may reduce the incentives for hospitals to provide laboratory services to hospital outpatients and physician office practices. The imposition of a freeze on physician fees and changes in Medicare assignment policies also alter the environment in which PPS operates, although the directions and extent of their effect are unknown.

- *State policies have changed concurrently with PPS.* As mentioned above, individual States have acted to contain the costs of their Medicaid programs in a variety of ways (307). State certificate-of-need programs, intended to constrain the supply of hospital and nursing home beds and expensive capital equipment, have waxed and waned with State politics (308). In a few instances, States have enacted laws to make the environment more favorable to competition for health care. California, for example, passed a law in 1982 which permitted the formation of preferred provider organizations, which enhances price competition in the health care market (79). In 1984, an estimated 15 to 20 percent of the State's 25 million people were served by preferred provider organizations (370).

Taken together, these simultaneous influences substantially reduce the validity of pre/post comparisons of measures of effect. They also suggest that differences among States and regions of the country in the health care environment will jeopardize the validity of State-by-State comparisons of health system variables. Only those effects with the strongest hypothesized direct link to PPS can be analyzed in such a way, and even then imperfectly.

For example, all experts agree that PPS should shorten the average length of stay (ALOS) in short-term hospitals. ALOS has been falling gradually for both Medicare and non-Medicare patients over the past 5 years (see ch. 3). One can extrapolate from this previous trend to predict changes in ALOS that would have occurred in the absence of PPS and then compare these predictions with actual ALOS since the beginning of PPS. ALOS may also be compared among hospitals with varying shares of Medicare patients. But neither of these approaches is entirely valid. We cannot know with certainty whether the predicted trend in ALOS is an accurate representation of what would have occurred in the absence of PPS or whether the ALOS might have shifted one way or another on its own. Yet the demonstration of a significant shift in ALOS from previous trends concurrent with or shortly after the implementation of PPS remains strongly suggestive that PPS is having the expected kinds of effects on a critical measure of hospital utilization. Thus, imperfect as the evidence of PPS on ALOS is, it provides an approximate estimate of PPS effects that needs to be linked to the more important questions of PPS impacts on cost, quality, and access.

Data Availability

The choice of research design is inextricably related to the kinds of data that are available and the costs of making necessary data available. The use of data routinely collected by the Health Care Financing Administration to administer the Medicare and Medicaid programs or of data available from organizations with ongoing surveys clearly offers cost advantages over special surveys or other primary data collection methods. Because these systems have not been developed or maintained with an eye to their usefulness as tools for program evaluation, however, they omit important data elements, and some items are so unreliable that analysis cannot proceed.

Moreover, the content and reliability of the data change over time, complicating pre/post-PPS comparisons. For example, prior to 1982, the assignment of diagnostic and procedural codes to Medicare hospital claims data was sloppy, because payment was not based on these items and the data entry procedures were inadequate (213). This information is expected to improve markedly for post-PPS years, but other data items that are not important for payment may deteriorate in quality.[2] Comparisons of billing claims in the post-PPS era with those in the pre-PPS period may be complicated by this problem.

Conversely, pre/post-PPS comparisons of the content of medical care delivered in hospitals would require detailed review and abstracting of medical records, an approach to data collection that is reasonably reliable but very costly (see ch. 6). And observed changes in impact measures could still not be ascribed to PPS with complete confidence.

---

[2] For example, PPS puts a new premium on rapid submission of claims following a patient's discharge. Hospitals may not have an incentive to code discharge status accurately.

CONCLUSIONS

Medicare's PPS is a complex program instituted in an even more complex health care environment. As a radical new approach to hospital payment, it needs to be evaluated for its impacts on health care costs, quality of care, access to care, technological change in medicine, and clinical research. Yet it is important to be realistic about what can be expected from such evaluations.

A variety of research designs are potentially applicable to the evaluation, each with its own strengths and weaknesses. The tradeoff of validity with cost and feasibility is critical to optimal selection of research designs from among the alternatives.

Because the availability of data figures so directly in the choice of impact measures and research designs, the temptation is great to study only those questions that are easy to study because of data availability. The danger of this situation is that it may result in an unbalanced view of the impacts of PPS. Consequently, it is important to identify at the outset the critical evaluation questions that need to be addressed. Serious consideration needs to be given to ways of addressing each of these critical questions, using methods and data that reflect the tradeoff between validity, feasibility, and affordability. Part Two of this report examines each of the five PPS impact areas identified in chapter 1—health care, expenditures and costs, quality of care, access to care, technological change, and clinical research —and identifies the critical evaluation questions in each. It also examines the data available to support analyses of these questions and suggests specific studies that appear to be worth their costs.

Part Two
Critical PPS Impact Areas

Chapter 5
Expenditures and Costs

Contents

	Page
Introduction	63
Potential Impacts of PPS on Expenditures and Costs	63
Expenditure and Cost Shifts	63
Distribution of Financial Effects Among Hospitals	65
Approaches to Evaluating the Impacts of PPS on Expenditures and Costs	66
Critical Evaluation Questions	66
Data Sources	71
Conclusions	72

Chapter 5
Expenditures and Costs

INTRODUCTION

This chapter examines the issues for evaluation raised by Medicare's prospective payment system (PPS) regarding health care expenditures and costs. First, it is necessary to distinguish among the various meanings of the terms "cost" and "expenditure." Though often used as synonyms, these terms actually represent distinct concepts. The *"cost"* of a health service (or class of services) is defined here as the value of the productive resources (e.g., personnel, materials, capital plant and equipment) that are used in the production of the health service. The *"expenditure"* for a health service is the amount actually paid in exchange for the service. To those who pay for health care, expenditures are synonymous with costs. However, the costs of serving a set of patients may be different from the expenditures made by them or on their behalf if one class of patients subsidizes another or if providers of health care make excessive profits (or losses).[1]

The difference between the expenditure for a health service made to a provider (*revenue* to the provider) and the cost of providing the service is referred to here as "surplus" (or profit, if the provider is a for-profit entity). It is worth noting that, in the aggregate, providers' revenues are not necessarily equal to their total *charges*, since some third-party payers, particularly Blue Cross/Blue Shield plans, Medicare, and Medicaid, pay at rates below full charges.

---
[1] In economic theory, profits are expected to be just high enough to induce suppliers of a product to stay in the market to meet the demand. In a perfectly competitive industry, where entry and exit are entirely free and no artificial pricing policies are followed, profits would tend to stay at the minimum level. Excess profits higher than that level can occur when the producers of a service have some measure of monopolistic power.

POTENTIAL IMPACTS OF PPS ON EXPENDITURES AND COSTS

Through a combination of fixed prices for each type of care and limits on the annual rate of increase in the fixed per-case prices, Medicare's PPS forces hospitals to reduce the costs of treating hospitalized patients. As currently structured, however, PPS provides imperfect control over aggregate Medicare hospital expenditures, in part because the number of admissions and the reported or actual disgnosis-related group (DRG) case mix can change.[2] Also, certain kinds of hospitals and hospital units (e.g., psychiatric, rehabilitative, major cancer centers) are currently exempted from PPS. Some admissions could shift into these institutions.

---
[2] Recognizing these potential avenues for increases in aggregate expenditures, the designers of Medicare's PPS charged the peer review organizations (PROs) with the responsibility for monitoring admissions and DRG assignments. Whether these organizations can actually control admissions or DRG assignments remains to be seen. Wennberg and colleagues have demonstrated the existence of substantial geographical variation in admission rates by DRG, suggesting a diversity of clinical standards and potential for admission rate increases that can be easily defended by the medical community (390).

Expenditure and Cost Shifts

In order for PPS to reduce Medicare inpatient hospital expenditures from what they would have been had cost-based reimbursement continued, one or more of three things must occur:

- the cost of treating patients is shifted from hospitals to other settings of care;
- hospitals reduce the cost of treating inpatients; or
- a portion of the cost of treating Medicare patients is borne by third-party payers other than Medicare.

Each of these scenarios has implications for the efficiency and fairness of PPS. Absolute reductions in the cost of treating hospital inpatients without shifting costs to other settings are, of course, most desirable provided that they do not come at the expense of the quality of hospital care. If cost reductions are accomplished by serving patients in settings outside the hospital, which must also be paid for, then the actual control of Medicare's hospital expenditures will be somewhat offset by additional expenditures in other parts of the program (or by patients themselves). If hospitals finance the treatment of Medicare patients by raising charges to other patients, serious questions of equity arise. Of course, it is also possible that hospitals may be able to reduce per-case costs by so much that Medicare inpatients become profitable relative to others, generating a surplus that could be used to subsidize care to other kinds of patients. An evaluation of the impacts of PPS would be incomplete without some understanding of the extent to which each scenario has occurred.

Although PPS offers clear financial incentives to substitute care provided outside of hospitals for care that would otherwise have been provided within, the extent of such substitution and the net impacts on Medicare nonhospital expenditures are difficult to predict. The services apart from inpatient services reimbursed by Medicare include those provided by physicians, outpatient departments, skilled nursing facilities (SNFs), home health agencies, and nonphysician suppliers such as laboratories and durable medical equipment suppliers. In 1982, physicians received 23 percent of Medicare reimbursements; outpatient departments received 5 percent, nonphysician Part B suppliers 4 percent, home health agencies 2 percent, and SNFs 1 percent (341).

The aggregate impact of PPS on Medicare's expenditures for physician services may be small, with a slight decline in the early years.[3] In 1981, 64 percent of physician services paid for by Medicare were provided in an inpatient setting, although only 24 percent of Medicare beneficiaries were hospitalized in that year (50). One physician visit for each day of hospitalization is the custom for nonsurgical cases. If lengths of stay in the hospital are reduced, one would expect a direct effect on the number of physician visits. Shorter stays would also reduce the potential for consultative visits for both medical and surgical discharges. Conversely, if the number of hospital ad-

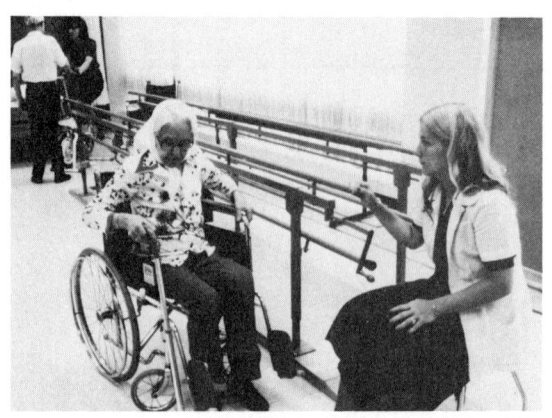

Photo credit: Fairfax Hospital Association

PPS offers incentives to substitute outpatient care for traditional inpatient care for a number of services, including physical therapy. The net impact on system costs of such substitutions is difficult to predict.

missions increases so that total Medicare hospital days of care increase, then physician visits may increase to some extent.

Skilled nursing homes and home health services are often seen as substitutes for hospital services rendered in the postoperative or predischarge phases of the hospital stay. To the extent that they can shorten lengths of stay by discharging inpatients to a lower level of care facility or to their home, hospitals can take full advantage of the incentives of PPS. Hospitals may increase their efforts with respect to discharge planning, potentially increasing the demand for skilled nursing and home care. Yet Medicare coverage of skilled nursing care is quite limited (20 days of care with total coverage, and an additional 80 days with a 50-percent copayment), and there has been a chronic excess demand for nursing home beds. This excess demand is likely to continue, largely because most SNF expenditures for Medicare patients are made by the State Medicaid programs, which have had low reimbursement rates (101). The net expenditure impact of increases in the use of nursing homes by Medicare beneficiaries may be greatest for the beneficiary, who must pay for 50 percent of the cost after 20 days.

Home health services can be expected to increase as a result of PPS. Medicare reimbursement for home health care is largely cost-based, and home health benefits were expanded in 1980 and

---

[3]A recent analysis of the impact of State hospital ratesetting systems on physicians' income revealed that physician incomes grew more slowly between 1980 and 1982 in these States than in unregulated States (407).

1981 to encourage the use of home health care (306).[4] Consequently, these services represent a ready source of diversification for hospitals (53,190,195).

Medicare beneficiaries themselves share in the cost of medical care, but at different rates depending on the type of service. The amount of cost-sharing required of the beneficiary depends on the statutorily defined deductible, the coinsurance rate, and limitations on coverage. Each type of service (hospital inpatient, physician visits, skilled nursing home, etc.) has different rules. Therefore, a change in the mix of services consumed has implications not only for Medicare's expenditures but also for the share of expenditures borne by the beneficiary.

For the approximately 12 percent of Medicare beneficiaries who are also eligible for Medicaid, the increase in the burden on the beneficiary may be largely borne by Medicaid (324). Frequently, Medicare patients become eligible for Medicaid sometime after they are placed in nursing homes for long-term care. To the extent that these patients are moved to nursing homes earlier under PPS than they would have been under cost-based reimbursement, Medicaid obligations will increase. The amount of increase is likely to be small, however.

The ultimate impact of PPS on private third-party payers' expenditures for hospital care is difficult to predict and will probably vary among different kinds of payers. The incentives offered by PPS for hospitals to become more efficient in providing care to inpatients could spill over to other types of patients, thereby reducing the costs of providing services to these patients and possibly the amounts that such patients or their third parties must pay. Also, the first year's DRG prices were based largely on the historical costs of providing hospital inpatient services to Medicare patients. If hospitals can rapidly realize economies in serving those patients—and recent evidence from the first year of PPS suggests that they have

(see ch. 3)—surpluses will increase. These surpluses could be used for a variety of purposes, including reduction in the share of costs paid for by other payers. Some evidence suggests that PPS may actually lead to lower charges for private third-party payers, because under cost-based reimbursement, hospitals raised their charges in response to the rule that Medicare would pay the lesser of costs or charges (75). Yet the apprehension of many private third-party payers is that the effects of PPS will be to lower Medicare reimbursements without reducing hospitals' costs of producing services, thus leading to increases in charges to other payers.

Some third-party payers have greater market power than others and can avoid subsidizing other classes of payer. Blue Cross plans, for example, often pay on the basis of costs or receive a discount from charges (16), and State Medicaid programs have increasingly imposed their own payment limits on hospitals. Patients who must pay for their own care or who have commercial insurance are often in the position of paying the hospital's full charges. To the extent that these charges reflect the costs that go unpaid by Medicare, charge-paying patients will be subsidizing Medicare patients.[5]

Distribution of Financial Effects Among Hospitals

Because Medicare's PPS generally pays each hospital a fixed price per discharge while the use of resources for patients in a specific DRG may vary widely, PPS establishes a pattern of financial winners and losers across Medicare patients and the hospitals that serve them. An uneven distribution of profits and losses across patients has three problems associated with it. First, it creates an incentive for hospitals to position themselves to treat winner cases and to avoid losers (219). To the extent that such cases can be identified before admission, serious implications for access arise (see ch. 7). Second, random and unpredictable variation in costs creates a financial risk that

---

[4]The General Accounting Office is currently addressing the information requirements for assessing the impact of PPS on the long-term care system. A preliminary report under that study described changes observed in six cities that support the contention of rapid growth in the use of home health care resulting from PPS (297).

[5]It is often asserted that charge-paying payers also bear the greatest share of the burden of subsidizing hospitals' delivery of uncompensated care (i.e., care to people with inadequate insurance or third-party coverage) (126,203).

is borne by the hospital. Because this risk varies inversely with the volume of cases, small hospitals or those with low-volume DRGs suffer a disproportionate burden of financial risk associated with cost variation. Third, some hospitals, by virtue of their mission or location, may find themselves serving a disproportionate share of high cost patients. Referral centers and public hospitals for example, may be subject to this kind of bias (384). To make such hospitals bear the financial burden of higher cost patients not only would be inequitable, but also might ultimately lower the quality of care being provided to those served in such institutions.

Revenues vary across hospitals independently of differences in patient characteristics. The reason is that hospitals are paid different rates per DRG depending on their area wage index, their urban or rural location, and (temporarily) the region of the country in which they are located. In addition, teaching hospitals receive an extra payment to account for the extra patient care costs associated with teaching. Presumably, the differences in DRG payment rates mirror differences in the costs of providing care that are outside the hospital's control. However, whether the DRG pricing structure is refined enough to accurately reflect uncontrollable differences in input costs is subject to question. Many hospitals in rural counties on the fringe of major metropolitan areas, for example, have claimed that the urban/rural rate differential financially discriminates against them (232). The Social Security Amendments of 1983 (Public Law 98-21) mandated the elimination of regional differences in DRG payment rates at the end of 3 years on the assumption that any regional differences in costs are due to systematic and un-

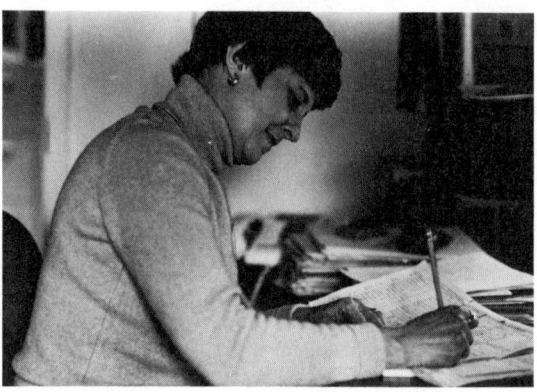

Photo credit: Fairfax Hospital Association

Data on hospital costs remain an important source of information as to whether DRG-specific profits and losses vary across types of hospitals.

justifiable differences in medical practice patterns in different parts of the country. That such differences exist has been thoroughly documented (57), but it is unclear whether hospital managers can adjust to uniform rates by changing their own and their physicians' behavior so quickly, or whether such uniformity in practice style is even a desirable outcome of PPS.

If the DRG pricing structure does not adequately reflect uncontrollable differences in input costs, certain hospitals will systematically have higher or lower surpluses than average. Even simple changes in the method of computing relative DRG prices can produce redistributions of revenue that are unrelated to hospitals' behavior (169). Not only are such arbitrary redistributions of revenue unfair to the hospitals that lose, but the patients who tend to be treated in such hospitals may have their access and quality of care jeopardized.

APPROACHES TO EVALUATING THE IMPACTS OF PPS ON EXPENDITURES AND COSTS

Critical Evaluation Questions

The previous discussion raises five critical questions regarding the impact of PPS on health care expenditures and costs:

- To what extent has PPS been successful in controlling Medicare expenditures for inpatient hospital care?
- What effect has PPS had on Medicare expenditures for outpatient and nonhospital services?
- What effect has PPS had on Medicare beneficiaries' expenditures for health care?
- How well does PPS cover the costs of providing inpatient care to Medicare beneficiaries?

- To what extent are variations among hospitals in profitability of Medicare patients due to factors beyond the hospitals' control, such as variations in severity of cases, the socioeconomic status of the patients, or input prices?

Potential approaches to addressing each of these questions and problems that might arise are discussed below.

Evaluating the Effects of PPS on Medicare Expenditures for Inpatient Hospital Care

Since Medicare pays a single per-case price for each DRG, once the average price is set, total Medicare expenditures for hospital care will vary with three factors that can be deliberately manipulated by hospital administrators and physicians:

- the total number of admissions to hospitals subject to PPS;
- the reported distribution of PPS admissions across DRGs; and
- the total number of admissions to hospitals and units exempted from PPS.

Estimating the contribution of each of these three factors to the observed rate of change in Medicare hospital expenditures is a straightforward task, but interpreting such changes is difficult. The three factors can be expected to vary from year to year with changes in characteristics of the Medicare population, the introduction of new medical technologies that alter the demand for hospital care, and random variations in the incidence of illness. The challenge is to estimate the extent to which changes in the pattern of admissions and case mix result from deliberate actions by hospitals to maximize the surplus obtainable from Medicare.[6] If PPS is unable to adequately control Medicare hospital expenditures, it is unlikely to survive in the long run.

Hospitals' ability to manipulate patterns of admissions and reported case mixes is limited not only by the oversight of PROs, but by ethical, legal, and practical constraints: perfectly healthy people will not be hospitalized; an admission for cataract surgery will not purposely be coded as cardiac surgery; patients will not be admitted to psychiatric hospitals for treatment of asthma. Moreover, what changes in admission patterns and case-mix reporting do occur are likely to be concentrated in the early years of PPS as hospitals adjust policies and procedures to the new financial incentives.

To address the question of whether changes in admissions and coding practices occur, annual data are needed on Medicare admissions by DRG and type of hospital and on characteristics of the Medicare population (e.g., age distribution) for a period before and after the introduction of PPS. Pre-PPS data can be used to establish preexisting trends and variations for comparison with post-PPS experience. Admissions data based on hospital bills are readily available at the Health Care Financing Administration (HCFA) for a period extending from the mid-1970s to the present, but the accuracy of DRG assignments made on pre-PPS bills is questionable. Prior to fiscal year 1983, diagnostic and procedural coding was not necessary for payment, so hospitals had no incentive to provide complete information. Surgical procedures were probably underreported; the distribution of admissions, therefore, was skewed toward medical DRGs (194). This kind of bias in diagnostic and procedural coding complicates analysis of admission patterns. It suggests that observed changes in patterns of admissions by DRG may be difficult to interpret from Medicare billing data alone and that more detailed studies are warranted of selected DRGs that appear to have undergone substantial changes in admission rates.

Evaluating the Effects of PPS on Medicare Expenditures for Nonhospital Services

As discussed above, Medicare expenditures for services other than inpatient care will be affected by PPS, but the extent and, in some cases, the direction of such effects cannot be predicted well. To know whether PPS is meeting its cost-containment objectives, however, these effects must be known.

Aggregate statistics on Medicare program expenditures are readily available by program cat-

---

[6]A recent analysis of the 8.4-percent increase in hospitals' reported DRG case mix between 1981 and 1984 estimated that changes in coding practices accounted for about 75 percent of the increase and actual changes in medical practices for only 25 percent (55).

egory (home health agency, physician services, SNF, etc.). Comparing post-PPS rates of growth in these expenditure categories with pre-PPS rates offers little insight into the contribution of PPS, however, because each category has undergone substantial changes in Medicare policy concurrent with the phase-in of PPS. For example, in 1983, Medicare tightened the rules governing the allowed frequency of skilled nursing visits by home health care agencies (136). It is virtually impossible to separate the effects of this change in policy from PPS effects by analyzing time trends in aggregate expenditures for home health services.

Patient-based studies of changes in the patterns of utilization of hospital and nonhospital services will be needed to identify PPS effects with greater accuracy. Because the most immediate effects of PPS are likely to involve changes in hospitalization rates, it would be useful to compare pre- and post-PPS patterns of nonhospital care for Medicare patients who have been hospitalized. Such detailed patient-specific analyses of hospitalized patients would provide an opportunity to isolate the effects of PPS more fully, though not perfectly.

To analyze the complete pattern of utilization of services and health care expenditures for a sample of beneficiaries who were hospitalized, Medicare billing records for both Part A and Part B providers would have to be integrated by beneficiary. Since each beneficiary has a unique identifier number, the development of integrated files for analysis is technically feasible. A later section of this chapter discusses the current ability of Medicare data systems to produce data of this kind.

We should, nevertheless, not expect too much precision from detailed statistical analyses of the full Medicare utilization and expenditure impacts of PPS. At best, such analyses are likely to provide upper or lower limits on estimates of expenditure effects, and a great deal of judgment will be required to interpret statistical findings. These difficulties argue in favor of involving multiple independent investigators in the analysis of out-of-hospital utilization and expenditure effects of PPS.

Evaluating the Effects of PPS on Out-of-Pocket Expenditures by Medicare Beneficiaries

Because PPS is likely to lead to shifts in settings of care, some Medicare beneficiaries may be particularly at risk for large increases in out-of-pocket expenditures. Since Medicare coverage for nursing homes is limited[7] and nursing home care is expensive—the average per-day cost of Medicare-certified homes in 1980 was approximately $72 (324)—patients discharged to nursing homes earlier than they would be under PPS would bear a heavy additional financial burden.

Unfortunately, estimating the total out-of-pocket expenditures of Medicare beneficiaries themselves is not possible using Medicare claims records. Medicare claims data can identify beneficiaries who are at risk for high expenditure burdens, such as those who have been discharged from hospitals to nursing homes, but the complete utilization or expenditure history is not available through claims data. Once Medicare benefits run out, the Medicare program may not receive bills from either patients or providers.

A comprehensive estimate of out-of-pocket expenditures by Medicare patients for all services would require a population-based survey of a sample of Medicare beneficiaries sufficiently large to identify pre- and post-PPS differences in expenditure patterns. But such a survey is unlikely to be either economically or technically feasible. Out-of-pocket expenditure burdens would be concentrated among a small population of Medicare beneficiaries who are high users of medical care. Detection of rare events requires large sample sizes. Also, surveys of health care utilization and expenditure are often subject to systematic underreporting (187) unless meticulous procedures to verify responses are followed.

A special survey of a sample of patients discharged to nursing homes could be used to collect information on the duration of nursing home stays both before and after PPS. In addition, data

---

[7]Medicare covers 100 percent of the cost of care in skilled nursing facilities (SNFs) for a period of 20 days, and 50 percent of care between the 21st day and the 100th day. Medicare coverage ends after the 100th day.

from the National Nursing Home Survey conducted in 1977 and 1984 (and scheduled for 1990) may provide data on patterns of utilization of nursing homes by Medicare beneficiaries (see app. C for a description of the survey).

Evaluating How Well DRG Payment Rates Cover the Cost of Serving Medicare Patients

Because there is concern that PPS may lead to unintended subsidies across payers, it is important to know how closely the inpatient revenues hospitals receive from Medicare match the costs of serving those patients. Although the first DRG prices were based on the estimated costs of serving Medicare patients, it is possible and, indeed, likely that costs and prices will diverge over time.

To some extent, such divergence is desirable, because it allows hospitals to reap the benefits of any economies they are able to make. However, too great a divergence either way is risky. If costs are substantially higher than revenues, some hospitals may be financially stressed, and other payers may subsidize Medicare. If costs are much lower than revenues, Medicare will be paying for care delivered to other patients, investments in expanded capacity or technology, or high profits to the owners of for-profit institutions. Consequently, the relationship between Medicare hospital expenditures and costs should be assessed periodically.

In theory, it is straightforward to compare Medicare payments made for hospital care with the costs of treating Medicare patients. In practice, limitations of cost-finding methods and data availability create impediments to precise estimation of the true costs of treating different kinds of patients. Rough estimates are probably the best obtainable.

The hospital can be thought of as a multiproduct firm that uses certain resources to produce a variety of different products. The resources are personnel, materials, equipment, and buildings; the products are treatments delivered to inpatients. (Each hospital stay is, in essence, a unique blend of hospital products.) Allocating the costs of the resources used among the specific products necessarily involves cost allocation techniques which can vary substantially. For example, the cost of nursing services can be allocated among patients according to the length of stay, the total patient charge, or a measure of relative need for nursing services (289). Allocations using the first two measures are relatively easy to execute; the third measure may require an assessment of the severity of illness of each patient. Moreover, the resulting cost allocations are likely to look quite different from one another (289). Properly executed, an estimate of need for nursing services may most fully account for cost differences among patients, but the administrative costs of employing this allocation procedure are high. Approximate measures often must suffice.

The most readily accessible source of hospital cost data is the Medicare cost report prepared and submitted annually by hospitals to Medicare intermediaries (see app. E for a description of the Medicare cost reporting system). The cost reports allow a substantial amount of flexibility to hospitals in cost allocation methods. Under cost-based reimbursement, hospitals had an incentive to manipulate cost allocations to maximize revenue from Medicare (75).[8] Moreover, the fully allocated costs of each department were apportioned between Medicare and other patients on the basis of the ratio of Medicare charges to those of other patients, which may not reflect the true cost differentials between Medicare and other patients.

More direct cost-finding techniques are available, but these are expensive and typically hospital-specific. Several hospitals have developed sophisticated cost-finding systems to estimate the true costs of serving certain kinds of patients (196, 397). Results of hospital-specific costing exercises could be useful in studying the problems inherent in using the Medicare cost report as a basis for estimating the costs of treating Medicare inpatients.

---

[8]In some States, hospitals must submit cost reports to a State rate-setting or regulatory authority. The reporting requirements may differ somewhat from the Medicare cost reports, but the principles of cost allocation are fundamentally similar. In a recently published study of cross-payer subsidies in hospitals in New York State, a sophisticated cost-allocation technique was applied to data from the State's cost reporting system (191). The study found that under cost-based reimbursement, Medicare paid 100 percent of the estimated costs of treating its patients.

Even with accurate allocation of costs across different kinds of patients, the question arises as to what costs Medicare should pay for. If Medicare is a prudent buyer, then it should pay only for the costs of providing efficient care. Average per-stay costs may be artificially high if hospitals are systematically inefficient in caring for patients. If DRG prices are based on average costs calculated on the basis of substantial inefficiency in the system as a whole, including that based on excess capacity, then PPS will essentially be financing this inefficiency and may not adequately encourage more efficient operation of the hospital industry. (Were the industry not largely composed of voluntary hospitals, concern over continued inefficiency would be replaced with concern over excess profits or excess capacity in the system. As largely not-for-profit entities, however, hospitals may use their revenues in other ways, including the financing of inefficient operations.)

Should Medicare pay its fair share of the cost of inefficiency (including excess capacity) in the system, or should it let third-party payers and self-pay patients with less market power bear the full cost of inefficiency in the hospital industry? This is a basic question of equity which cannot be answered here, but which has ramifications for the kind of cost estimation methods that should be used to compare the costs of treating Medicare patients with those of non-Medicare patients. Either way, the data exist on the Medicare cost reports to estimate, albeit imperfectly, the cost of treating Medicare patients compared to the revenues actually received by hospitals.

Evaluating Variations in Hospital Profits Under PPS

A prospective payment system that rewards efficiency and penalizes inefficiency in hospitals also redistributes profits among hospitals. The important question in evaluating the fairness of such a payment system is whether the patterns of profit redistribution are related to causes outside the hospital's control. The contention by some observers that DRGs do not adequately measure severity of illness bears on this question (see, for example, ref. 140). However, even if DRGs were able to measure severity of illness perfectly, unjustified systematic losses and gains could still occur in some patient categories because of unmeasured differences in the costs of inputs (e.g., regional differences in the cost of nonlabor inputs) (174).

Of course, interhospital differences in profits due to systematic variations in patient resource needs or input costs must be distinguished from those due to differences in the relative efficiency of hospitals. The best way to distinguish between systematic and efficiency-based cost differentials is to examine the distribution of costs of serving Medicare patients in specific DRGs across various classes of hospitals. Classes of hospitals could be defined by combinations of the following characteristics:

- volume of low-income Medicare patients;
- teaching status;
- inner city/suburban/rural location;
- Standard Metropolitan Statistical Area size;
- proprietary/public/voluntary ownership; and
- region of the country (nine census regions).

If the costs of serving patients in specific DRGs are found to be relatively high for hospitals in a particular class, especially when other characteristics such as the size of the hospitals or the complexity of their facilities are accounted for,[9] there is suggestive evidence that patients vary systematically across hospitals in their resource needs. However, differences in costs might also result from historical patterns of availability of funding for different kinds of hospitals, with some hospitals having had to "make do" with fewer resources.

At present, hospital revenues under PPS vary with teaching status, urban or rural location, area, and regional location of the hospital. Thus, the first step in determining whether hospitals (and the Medicare patients they serve) are being treated

---

[9]Large hospitals have certain inherent advantages in coping with PPS. They can take advantage of whatever economies of scale exist in the production of hospital services; they may have more sophisticated management; and they can spread financial risks over a larger number of patients. However, recent analysis also suggests that the complexity of a hospital's services may increase average costs because of the substantial excess capacity that exists with expensive, unused technology (143). An analysis of cost differences by size and related variables creates a context for understanding the impacts of other factors.

fairly under PPS is to compare hospital-specific costs with their relevant DRG payment rates.

Several organizations have examined the potential redistribution of surplus that would be brought about by PPS if the distribution among hospitals of patient characteristics and the costs of treating those patients were to stay the same as they were prior to PPS (295,369,388). These profit simulations have compared average revenues under PPS with the costs of treating Medicare patients (as estimated from Medicare cost reports and claims data) by hospital size, urban or rural location, teaching status, ownership, and region of the country.

The results of these simulations (shown in table 3-1 in ch. 3) are limited as predictors of ultimate redistributions of surplus and losses due to PPS. First, they assume that PPS brings about no change in patient characteristics or in hospital operations, when in fact PPS is specifically intended to induce such changes. If certain kinds of hospitals systematically have greater flexibility in patient selection or were operating less efficiently than others at the start of PPS, the actual surplus redistribution could look quite different from the predicted one.

Second, and more important, the comparison of surpluses across types of hospitals fails to differentiate between differences due to patient characteristics or input costs and those due to the relative efficiency of different kinds of hospitals. This is, of course, the central dilemma in interpreting such differences.

To truly differentiate efficiency problems from those due to uncontrollable factors, much finer analyses of patient characteristics are required. If, for example, public hospitals come to be financial losers under PPS, detailed comparisons of patient severity in these institutions compared to others might be warranted. A number of patient classification systems other than DRGs exist that can provide information on within-DRG differences in patient characteristics (see app. H for a description of existing patient classification systems). Although all such systems may not be practical for direct use in prospective payment they can provide valuable information on systematic differences in patient distributions across types of hospitals. Such studies would be expensive, as reclassification of patients according to a new system generally requires primary data collection from the medical record, but the expense may well be justified if this is the only way to settle this important question.

Data Sources

Medicare's Part A and Part B data systems provide a rich base for monitoring Medicare expenditures for all kinds of health services and for estimating hospital costs (Part A data systems are described in app. E). Because these data systems were developed and designed for use in the administration of the Medicare program, however, their content, quality, and timeliness is governed by the administrative requirements of the past. These data systems are largely limited to providing information on the Medicare program and Medicare beneficiaries. However, they also contain data on health care providers who serve Medicare patients, and these data can be used to a limited degree to assess the general issue of cost-shifting among payers.

Patient bills are the basis for data on utilization and expenditures for hospital and other covered services for Medicare beneficiaries. Medicare hospital expenditures per enrollee and per DRG can be obtained from the patient billing files. Medicare expenditures for other kinds of services (e.g., physicians, SNFs) are also easily monitored by these data systems, but an integrated beneficiary-based claims data file, which would link Part A and Part B claims for purposes of analysis, does not exist at present.

Medicare claims data cannot pick up out-of-plan expenditures made by or on behalf of Medicare beneficiaries. Thus, for example, out-of-pocket or Medicaid expenditures for nursing home care rendered to Medicare beneficiaries cannot be tracked through the Medicare databases.[10] Direct surveys of Medicare patients who have been hospitalized may be the only practical way to obtain this information.

---

[10]Unfortunately, the Medicaid data available at the national level do not provide for easy tracking of these expenditures either.

Data on hospital costs are available in the Medicare cost reports submitted annually by hospitals to Medicare intermediaries. Because virtually all non-Federal short-term hospitals participate in Medicare, data on hospital costs are available for the universe of such hospitals. (Cost data on other kinds of providers, such as SNFs or home health agencies, are not nearly so universal.)

It is possible to apportion hospital costs between the Medicare and non-Medicare populations using the Medicare cost report data, but finer breakdowns of cost among different kinds of non-Medicare payers (e.g., Blue Cross vs. commercial insurance firms) are not possible. The cost reports also contain data on costs and charges by department for Medicare and non-Medicare patients.

When combined with hospital billing data, the Medicare cost reports provide a reasonable but imperfect source of data on hospital specific costs by DRG. Indeed, the Medicare cost reports, along with Medicare billing data, were used to generate the first set of DRG prices. The cost of each department was apportioned between Medicare and non-Medicare patients according to the charges each patient incurred in the department. The weight of each DRG was computed as the average cost of cases in the DRG divided by the average cost across all hospitals. As DRG prices increase according to administrative or legislated formulas, they can be compared to DRG costs recalculated in this way, thus providing generally valid information on the distribution of profits and losses by DRG and across hospitals.

The Medicare cost reports present two problems. One problem is that these reports are available in automated form only after a substantial delay. A second problem is that the content of data required in the reports has changed over time as the details of Medicare payment have changed. New report formats can be (and are routinely) developed by HCFA. One concern is that HCFA could reduce data reporting requirements without adequate consideration for their usefulness in estimating the costs of serving Medicare and other kinds of patients.

The importance of knowing whether and how DRG-specific profits and losses vary across types of hospitals argues for the continued availability of Medicare cost report data at least at the level of detail that was available for the construction of original DRG weights. At present, HCFA's data processing systems do not allow for timely access to the cost-report data to support the monitoring function. The long delay in the availability of Medicare cost report data in automated form at HCFA limits the ability to monitor this important issue.

CONCLUSIONS

The five critical questions on the expenditure and cost impacts of PPS present conceptual, methodological, and data problems. In each area, the methods available for analysis are imperfect and data sources are limited. Judgment will be needed both in the selection of methods for analysis and in the interpretation of findings.

Interpreting changes in Medicare hospital expenditures, on its surface the most straightforward task, will require judgment in separating out the causes of changes in patterns of admissions and coding if the effects of PPS are to be distinguished from effects that are beyond the control of the hospital.

The full effect of PPS on Medicare's nonhospital expenditures and on Medicare beneficiaries' out-of-pocket expenditures cannot be known with accuracy. There is simply too much going on throughout the health care system to be able to attribute changes in some categories of expenditures (especially physician services) to PPS. Yet the use of some settings—notably home health care and SNFs—is bound to be altered dramatically as a result of the strength of the PPS incentives. Attention should be paid to these components of Medicare and out-of-pocket expenditures. Estimating the magnitude of these changes will require data that will allow tracing the complete history of medical use by beneficiaries. Medicare claims data from different kinds of providers need to be integrated by beneficiary for use in such analyses.

Measuring hospital surplus under Medicare, both to monitor the degree to which Medicare pays the full costs of treating its beneficiaries and to identify financial winners and losers among hospitals, will be difficult. A primary reason is that cost-finding techniques are limited by the data available on the Medicare cost reports. Also, conceptual issues such as whether to include the costs of excess capacity in such calculations will complicate the interpretation of the findings. Nevertheless, the overwhelming importance of these two questions argues for careful attention to their study and to further development and maintenance of data files that can offer insight into them.

Thorough analysis of the reasons for differences among hospitals in the costs of treating Medicare patients will require detailed comparisons of patient characteristics in different kinds of hospitals.

Patient classification systems other than DRGs, that account for a higher proportion of observed variation in the resources used, can be used for such detailed analyses of cost differences. Although such studies are costly, they represent the best way to address this important distributional issue.

The availability of data on hospital costs and Medicare claims is critical to adequate assessment of all of the questions raised in this chapter. The main data sources are Medicare's routinely maintained Part A and Part B databases. The Medicare cost reports play a central role in tracking the expenditure and cost impacts of PPS on hospitals and payers. And, provided they are organized into beneficiary-based files, claims data are promising sources of information on shifts of utilization from inpatient hospital to nonhospital settings. Problems in the content, quality, and timeliness of these databases that exist at present will seriously restrict analytic capability.

Chapter 6
Quality of Care

Contents

	Page
Introduction	77
Defining and Measuring Quality of Care	78
Definitions of Quality of Care	78
Measures of Quality of Care	78
Potential Impacts of PPS on Quality of Care	80
PPS Incentives That May Affect Quality of Care	81
Distribution of PPS Effects on Quality of Care	81
The Influence of PROs on Quality of Care	83
Approaches to Evaluating the Impacts of PPS on Quality of Care	84
Critical Evaluation Questions	84
Data Sources	87
Conclusions	91

LIST OF TABLES

Table No.	Page
6-1. Potential Effects of Provider Financial Incentives Under PPS on Quality of Care	82
6-2. Data Elements in Patient-Based National Databases	88

Chapter 6
Quality of Care

INTRODUCTION

Medicare's prospective payment system (PPS) has intensified concern with the complex relationship between cost and quality of medical care. Although in ideal terms the best care is that which is most effective, in practical terms some tradeoff between cost and quality is unavoidable. The possibility of such a tradeoff has been anticipated in many quarters, prompting attention to the quality-of-care issue from the General Accounting Office (GAO), OTA, Prospective Payment Assessment Commission, and the Health Care Financing Administration (HCFA). One manifestation of this concern was the establishment by Congress of utilization and quality control peer review organizations (PROs) as the successors to professional standards review organizations (PSROs).

Assessing PPS impacts on quality of care is critical for several reasons. First, if PPS succeeds in containing expenditure growth for the Medicare program, its effect on the quality of care will be a deciding factor in the program's continued survival. (Another will be its effect on access to care, as discussed in ch. 7.) Second, PPS incentives for the amount and mix of inpatient services provided to the elderly differ markedly from the incentives of cost-based payment, yet the Nation has little experience with the effects on quality of such prospective payment systems.[1] Third, widespread concern among professional groups, including physicians', nurses', and hospitals' associations, and among representatives of the elderly that PPS might pose a substantial threat to quality of care has made quality a highly visible issue (280,302, 310,381).

Complicating the task of evaluating PPS impacts on the quality of care is the fact that PPS impacts vary along at least four dimensions: their seriousness, their timing, their measurability, and their distribution among the elderly. These dimensions vary in ways that make evaluating PPS, and particularly its effects on quality, very difficult to plan and carry out.

Highly visible or easily measured effects on quality of care are likely to be the most serious, especially if they involve deaths, inappropriate readmissions, and the like. They are also likely to be concentrated in a few groups of patients. More subtle effects, such as effects on the quality of life for Medicare beneficiaries, are likely to be both more difficult to measure and less serious.

How effects on quality of care will emerge over time is difficult to predict, but the more serious effects may not appear for a number of years. Indeed, PPS may not have much discernible effect at all on quality of care for 2 to 3 years. Initially, PPS impacts on quality may be small because many hospital management efficiencies may have no appreciable impact on clinical practice; such efficiencies may even enhance outcomes for Medicare beneficiaries. As slack in the system is taken up, however, PPS could force economies that are inconsistent with maintaining quality of care as now known. Some problems may arrive sooner for hospitals with low financial reserves, for those in areas of high labor or nonlabor costs, or for those facing other problems external to PPS. In short, although some PPS effects on quality of care may surface relatively early, others that ultimately are equally or more important may take some years to be detected or documented.

Most important to understand is that PPS is likely to change the quality of care in both positive and negative ways. More skillful hospital management may lead to desirable administrative or clinical efficiencies, such as improved choices of diagnostic or therapeutic interventions (87). Nevertheless, PPS incentives for hospitals to reduce inpatient services are strong enough to raise fears that the lives or health of at least some Medicare beneficiaries could be endangered.

---

[1]Several States had prospective hospital ratesetting programs before PPS, but they differ in structure from each other and from the current national program; in any event, a report on the impact of these State programs on quality of care (and other topics) has not yet been released (59).

The remainder of this chapter is organized into four sections. The next section examines the concept of quality of care, highlighting the difficulties of both definition and measurement. The third section describes how PPS may affect the quality of care, and the fourth section sets out the critical evaluation questions in this area, with attention to what data sources are or might be available to support evaluation activities. The final section reviews strategies for evaluating PPS effects on quality of care.

DEFINING AND MEASURING QUALITY OF CARE

Definitions of Quality of Care

Medicare is expected to purchase quality health care for its beneficiaries, but what constitutes "quality" remains poorly defined. One definition is "...the kind of care that maximizes an inclusive measure of patient welfare after one has taken account of the balance of expected gains and losses that attend the process of care in all its parts" (86). The term "benefit" could easily replace "welfare" in this definition without markedly changing the essential meaning. Hence this definition has intuitive appeal, for it is consistent with the benefit and cost framework for PPS evaluation laid out in chapter 2.

Two terms frequently used in the literature on health care quality—"quality assessment" and "quality assurance"—need to be distinguished from one another. "Quality assessment" refers to the measurement and evaluation of quality of care for individuals, groups, or populations. "Quality assurance" refers to integrated programs that attempt to protect or raise quality of care by conducting assessments, taking action to correct problems found, and following up corrective actions.

Quality assurance programs historically focused on changing the behavior of individual providers through educational interventions or payment sanctions. The major quality assurance efforts for Medicare have been the PSRO program and its successor, the PRO program.

Because quality assurance programs rest on assessments of the care delivered to individual patients, the terms quality assurance and quality assessment are sometimes used synonymously. In this report, however, the two terms are used quite differently. A major focus of this report is on the assessment of changes in the quality of care due to a health care financing program, namely, Medicare's PPS. This report is only indirectly concerned with the ability of PROs to assess and assure quality. Quality assessment data developed for quality assurance programs, particularly the PROs, are of interest in this report primarily for their potential usefulness in evaluating the impacts of PPS (including the PRO program) on the quality of care.

Measures of Quality of Care

Measures of quality of care fall into three categories: structure, process, and outcome (85). "Structure" refers to the relatively fixed and stable parts of the medical care delivery system, such as numbers, types, and qualifications of professional personnel, physical facilities, and medical technologies. Criteria for such structural factors, which may be set by professional associations, regulatory bodies, or legislation, are often used for accreditation, licensing, and Medicare certification purposes.

"Process" measures reflect what is done to and for the patient: the application of medical procedures, drugs, nursing care, counseling, and the like. Typically, the process of care is evaluated against implicit or explicit criteria that reflect professional norms of practice; often such criteria are stated in terms of particular diagnostic or therapeutic practices at specific points in an episode of illness. Ultimately, however, assessing quality in terms of process gives an incomplete picture of patient benefits. The reason is that links between much of the process of medical care and eventual patient outcomes have not been clinically demonstrated (46).

"Outcomes," the results of patient care, are more direct reflections of patient benefits. They are measures of changes in the patient's actual health status. Health status itself has many dimensions: the level of functioning in daily or usual activities, capacity for physical activity, emotional health, physiologic functioning of body organs, perceptions of and expectations of one's own general health, and even satisfaction with care. Most broadly, health status has been defined to include the physical, mental, and social well-being of individuals, not just the absence of disease (400).

Ideally, the benefits of medical care should be viewed in terms of effects on patients' outcomes—i.e., health status. At a fairly crude level, health status can be evaluated in terms of death or presence of serious illness or disability. Health status can also be assessed with respect to short-term physiologic factors, such as the presence or absence of fever or infection, or the level of functioning of a specific organ (e.g., kidney). These are relatively unambiguous measures, but they tend to be insensitive to small or incremental changes in medical practice.

A wide array of health status scales and indexes has been developed over the past 15 years (31,47, 378). Health status indexes typically focus on the physical and mental aspects of health and are constructed from separate items or measured by direct examination, interview, or self-administered questionnaires. Many have been shown to be highly reliable and valid, meaning that they will give reproducible results when administered more than once and that they provide information about the aspect(s) of health status they are purported to measure, not something else. Nonetheless, no one set of health status indexes currently available will comprehensively measure health outcomes for persons in the Medicare population.

Despite the fact that patient outcomes are the most desirable benchmark against which to assess quality of care, outcome measures have several drawbacks. One is that outcomes need to be evaluated over time: the patient's health status at the time of discharge from hospital may or may not indicate his or her health status in a week, a month, or a year. Another is that the collection of data on outcomes may be very expensive and intrusive, if, for instance, patients must be interviewed or examined directly.

Although process measures are more tentative indicators of quality, some do correlate directly with outcomes. Handwashing reduces infection, so use of surgical scrubs will improve surgical outcomes. Immunizations reduce the threat of communicable diseases such as influenza. Pap smears improve the likelihood of detecting and adequately treating cervical cancer. Followup of abnormal laboratory tests such as serum glucose levels may have dramatic implications for eventual patient outcomes. Administering an appropriate antibiotic based on a bacterial urine culture usually cures a urinary tract infection. Nursing care can prevent or reduce bedsores and skin ulcers. In these and other cases, explicit criteria for judging the quality of the process of care can be (or have been) developed through either the consensus of experts (usually physicians), the accumulation of evidence from clinical practice, or clinical trials and research.

For every example of a probable process-outcome link, however, there is one for which the evidence is equivocal. Hospital length of stay is a case in point. A recent OTA study concluded that variations in length of hospital stay for five diseases had not been shown to be related to differences in health outcomes (57). Patients with acute myocardial infarction or elective surgery who were discharged "early," for instance, fared no worse than those with traditionally longer lengths of stay. For psychiatric disorders, the evidence favoring shorter lengths of stay was strong. The medical literature, however, does not provide clear clinical criteria for *appropriate* lengths of stay (57). In this situation, judging quality by the process measure (i.e., length of stay) provides no indication of likely outcomes.

Previous evaluations of quality impacts of health care have used specific measures in all three categories (structure, process, and outcome). In-hospital mortality rates by specific patient condition or severity of illness are frequently used outcome measures in studies of the quality of hospital care (107,108,403). Population-based mortality rates by age, sex, and race have been used in broader analyses of the effects of health care programs (47,125). Other outcome variables have

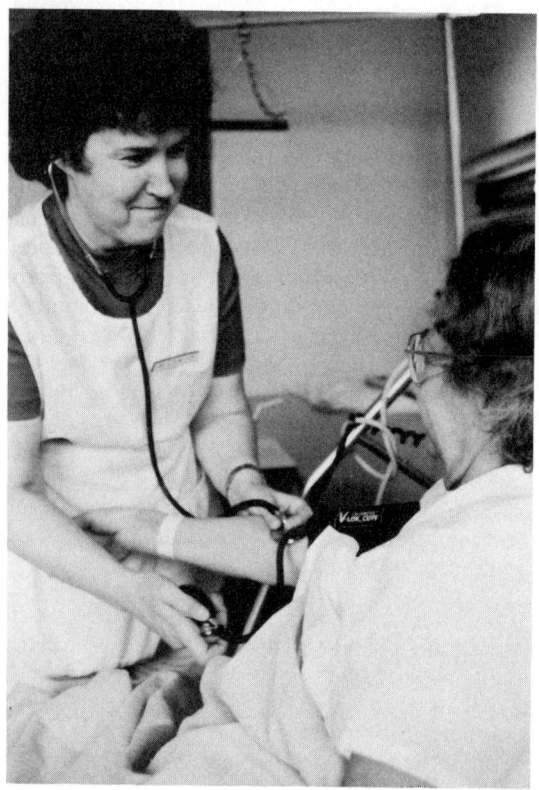

Determining the impact of changes in nursing care on patient health outcomes is an important component of evaluating the impact of PPS on quality of care, yet this impact is difficult to measure.

included health status indexes (44,47), patient satisfaction (44,47), and hospital readmission rates (403). Typically, these analyses are conducted for specific "tracer" conditions, identified as medical conditions whose outcomes are likely to be sensitive to the administrative or clinical decisions of health care providers (44,313,403).

Structural variables and process criteria have been used in some evaluations of health care programs but with a great deal of caution. Structural quality measures, such as accreditation status, staffing levels, or availability of specific services, have been used occasionally (403). Process criteria have been used more often (225,313,403). The method of selecting process criteria and validation of process criteria against outcomes takes on great importance in studies using these quality indicators. For example, in a study of the quality impacts of State-level hospital ratesetting programs, the intensity of ancillary service[2] utilization and length of stay were selected as process measures of quality (403). Yet, documentation of either increases or decreases in these variables says little about the ultimate quality of care. Indeed, if there were substantial evidence of a strong relationship between general measures of intensity of care and patient outcome, the ratesetting programs under evaluation, whose primary purpose is to reduce service intensity, would probably not have been initiated in the first place.

To summarize, a balanced assessment of quality of care requires attention to both process and outcomes; this may be especially true for any evaluation of Medicare's PPS. PPS will change medical and hospital care in as yet unknown ways and to unknown degrees. Focusing exclusively on process means learning very little about the impacts of PPS on Medicare patients. Conversely, measuring only outcomes means learning very little about which changes wrought by PPS had good, bad, or neutral impacts—information that will be critical in planning or implementing further changes in the Medicare program.

---

[2]Ancillary services are technologies used in the hospital that are typically billed separately from routine services. They include diagnostic radiology, radiation therapy, clinical laboratory, and other special services.

POTENTIAL IMPACTS OF PPS ON QUALITY OF CARE

This section explores the potential effects of PPS on the quality of care for Medicare beneficiaries through an analysis of the financial incentives inherent in PPS. As the section will demonstrate, some effects are likely to be positive, others deleterious to quality. And some people may benefit from PPS in the quality of care they receive, while others suffer.

This section also examines the ways in which the PRO program can be expected to enhance or moderate the basic effects of PPS. Because PROs are an integral part of PPS, charged both with containing Medicare outlays through the review of hospital admissions and with assuring the quality of hospital care for Medicare beneficiaries, they are likely to have strong direct and indirect impacts on quality. Appendix G contains a detailed discussion of the current role and potential effects of PROs in this regard.

PPS Incentives That May Affect Quality of Care

Table 6-1 presents the major financial incentives of PPS that may affect the quality of care received by Medicare patients. The eventual net impact of these incentives depends heavily on physician practice patterns, preexisting levels of inefficiency in hospital care, current levels of quality in hospitals and other medical care delivery sites, and physicians' and hospital managers' willingness to respond to financial incentives given their competing goals and constraints.

Specific PPS financial incentives (e.g., to lower length of stay, increase admissions, specialize in particular services, or induce unprofitable patients to seek care at other sites) will have both positive and negative effects on quality of care. The main goal of PPS is to encourage hospitals to adopt more efficient ways of delivering patient care. Chief among these ways is to reduce the number and kinds of services provided to patients. As shown in table 6-1, quality might well be improved through such cutbacks. With earlier discharge from the hospital, for instance, patients may face a lower risk of iatrogenic events[3]; they may also enjoy a more comfortable and psychologically beneficial recuperation at home or in a short-term nursing facility.

However, quality of care could be affected negatively by PPS. Premature discharges may neces-

[3]Iatrogenic events are misadventures occurring because patients are hospitalized. They include broken bones from falls (either out of bed or because elderly ambulatory patients are unattended), decubitus ulcers from insufficient nursing attention (turning, bathing, and the like), infections from bacteria indigenous to hospitals, and problems related to drugs or medications (interactions of incompatible drugs; improper dosages, etc.).

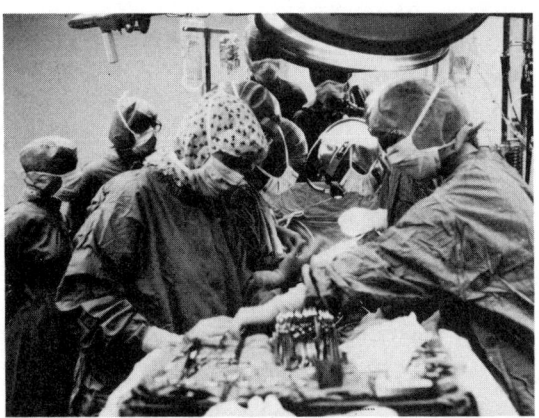

Photo credit: Fairfax Hospital Association

The fact that PPS may spur specialization in particular types of services may increase quality of care, especially for surgical procedures (e.g., coronary surgery) where high volume is correlated with high quality.

sitate readmissions (or cycles of discharges and readmissions); illnesses treatable at an early stage could progress undetected to a much more serious degree; patients could be forced to acquire followup care in inappropriate settings, with ramifications for both their physical and mental well-being. If total PPS expenditures are constrained to a point where adequate care simply cannot be rendered, outcomes could be seriously compromised.

Distribution of PPS Effects on Quality of Care

Some regions or institutions will undoubtedly find it harder than others to cope under Medicare's PPS; in these regions or institutions, quality of care is likely to be more severely affected. Under PPS, Medicare payments to hospitals for patients in specific diagnosis-related groups (DRGs) are based on average resource use, and the dispersion around that average can be very wide. Within any DRG, elderly patients may require resources close to the average, well above the average, or well below it. Hospitals that admit mostly patients whose needs are at or below the average, even inefficient hospitals, may make money. Those that admit patients whose needs are mainly at or above the average may lose money.

Table 6-1.—Potential Effects of Provider Financial Incentives Under PPS on Quality of Care

Financial incentive	Behavior depends on	Possible positive effects	Possible negative effects
To reduce length of hospital stay	• Physician practice patterns • Hospital management practices	• May increase psychological benefits for patients • May lessen chance of iatrogenic events	• May lead to discharge of sicker patients (may lead to pattern of admission/discharge/admission)
To increase admissions	• Physician practice patterns • Ratio of DRG price to cost	• May build specialty in particular DRGs in a hospital	• May increase psychological costs for patients • May increase possibility of iatrogenic events
To avoid admitting "unprofitable" patients	• "Unprofitable" DRGs • Ability to identify severely ill patients at admission	• May increase specialization by eliminating some services	• May decrease access for some patients
To decrease use of services or change mix of services	• Physician practice patterns • Hospital management practices • Hospital purchasing decisions	• May decrease use of unnecessary services • May decrease risk from diagnostic tests and invasive procedures	• May decrease use of necessary technologies • May increase use of cheaper and less effective materials, devices, and supplies • May decrease use of specialized personnel where needed
To shift patients to nonhospital sites of care	• Physician practice and patient acceptance	• May lessen chance of iatrogenic events • May increase access to other appropriate types of care	• May decrease access to appropriate hospitalization
To increase hospital specialization	• Physician specialties within the hospital • Ratios of DRG price to cost	• May increase volume in specific services (high volume often correlates with high-quality outcomes)	• May decrease access for certain patients (locations may not be accessible) or for particular diseases (no hospital will want to specialize in a DRG that loses money overall)

SOURCE: Office of Technology Assessment, 1985.

Hospitals feeling little or no financial threat from PPS may thus be in a good position to maintain or even improve the quality of care rendered, especially if by doing so they can attract more cases into DRGs that are "profitable" for them. Improvements in quality of care may well spill over to all patients admitted into these institutions. In contrast, hospitals with patient populations that put them in serious financial straits under PPS may have to cut back on services to a degree that compromises quality of care, not just for those patients with higher-than-average needs but for all their patients. In the absence of some form of balancing, this phenomenon can become a self-perpetuating downward cycle for some hospitals and for the patients served by those institutions.

Some DRGs are very heterogeneous, with numerous diagnostic and treatment options that may differ widely in cost. For instance, the two DRGs concerned with gastrointestinal bleeding (DRGs #174 and #175) include patients who are bleeding from anywhere in the gastrointestinal tract, and appropriate diagnostic and therapeutic options range very widely (152). Care that is correct for the average patient with gastrointestinal bleeding, if adopted as the standard for patients admitted in these DRGs, may produce poor outcomes for those patients with both more and less serious problems.

Even efficient hospitals can lose money when DRGs consistently do not cover the costs of needed services. This may happen if a DRG has been priced incorrectly or when the average level of severity of illness within one DRG increases without a corresponding drop in severity of illness within a similarly priced DRG. It may also occur if the natural evolution of medical practice leads to more outpatient management of patients who formerly would have been admitted, leaving only the more severely ill to be hospitalized without corresponding changes in DRG prices. Recalibration of DRG prices that occurs only infrequently may not forestall the negative impacts on quality imposed by these problems.

The Influence of PROs on Quality of Care[4]

The PRO program was established by the Tax Equity and Fiscal Responsibility Act of 1982 (Public Law 97-248) as a direct successor to the PSRO program; it was modified the following year by the Social Security Amendments that inaugurated PPS (Public Law 98-21). PROs, which are administered by HCFA, have substantial responsibilities for monitoring and controlling changes in hospital admissions, readmissions, and transfers that are predicted to increase in response to PPS incentives; PROs are also expected to carry out quality-of-care review. They are not required to review the quality of care delivered by nonhospital providers.

Most of the responsibilities delegated to PROs by HCFA pertain to the review of hospital admissions and use of invasive procedures, largely for cost-containment purposes. However, PROs are also required to identify and meet specific objectives in five general areas relating to quality of care.[5]

Several admissions review activities required of PROs have stringent numerical objectives, as do all five quality-of-care areas. The general quality objectives for the first 2-year contract period, which are common to all PRO contracts, were defined by HCFA. Within them, however, PROs were given flexibility to identify local problems and devise local approaches to solve them. The actual quantitative objectives were arrived at during contract negotiations with HCFA.

---

[4]This section is based on app. G, which is taken from K.N. Lohr, "Peer Review Organizations (PROs): Quality Assurance in Medicare," prepared for the Office of Technology Assessment, U.S. Congress, Washington, DC, July 1985.

[5]The five quality-of-care areas are: 1) reducing unnecessary hospital readmissions due to previously substandard care; 2) reducing the risk of mortality associated with selected procedures and/or conditions requiring hospitalization (211) (recently changed by HCFA from "decreasing avoidable deaths"); 3) lowering unnecessary surgery; 4) curtailing avoidable postoperative or other complications; and 5) assuring provision of medical services which, if not given, would have significant potential for causing serious patient complications.

The direction in which the PRO program influences the quality of care depends not only on the extent to which PROs make appropriate choices in the selection of specific quality assurance issues, but also on how they carry out admissions review functions. Some critics have argued that PROs may treat both the quality and admissions objectives as quotas for limiting Medicare hospitalizations irrespective of whether or not they are appropriate. In that case, PROs could actually reduce rather than enhance the quality of care rendered to some Medicare beneficiaries. Thus, despite the explicit recognition of a quality assurance role for the PROs, the simultaneous existence of other cost-containment objectives and HCFA's reliance on numerical objectives for the evaluation of PRO contracts leaves the net impact of PROs on quality of care largely unpredictable.

The limitations of PROs as a quality assurance mechanism are heightened by funding issues. PROs have a sizable budget—$339 million for the first 2-year cycle—but it is small in proportion to the $100+ *billions* that may be spent by Medicare just for hospital care in the equivalent 2 years. Furthermore, the portion of the PRO budgets directed to quality assurance may also be small because of the large number of other required functions and the uncertainty about the importance that will be placed on quality of care when contract performances are evaluated. If even as much as 25 percent of PRO budgets were spent for quality reviews, a miniscule proportion of the amount spent on inpatient care would be going for quality assurance.

APPROACHES TO EVALUATING THE IMPACTS OF PPS ON THE QUALITY OF CARE

Critical Evaluation Questions

Medicare's PPS for inpatient hospital services clearly has the capacity to alter the quality of care delivered to the elderly in both good and bad ways. Some of the changes are likely to be dramatic, others subtle and difficult to detect. The importance of maintaining an acceptable level of quality of care while reforming the payment system suggests that evaluation of PPS impacts on quality of care should occur on two levels: first, the identification of major negative impacts of PPS on quality of care; and second, a more balanced assessment of the less dramatic changes that are likely to take place in both directions. The first level of evaluation is of the highest priority, but it need not, and perhaps should not, occur earlier than studies in the second category. Because some serious negative consequences of PPS may take years to develop, a plan for evaluating quality impacts must have a long-run perspective.

Evaluation of PPS quality impacts also must consider effects on both the quality of hospital care and the quality of care received in other settings. PPS will have its most immediate impacts in the hospital itself, but over time, as access to care in different settings changes, the impacts on quality will shift to the entire medical care delivery system.

These considerations lead to three critical evaluation questions:

- What, if any, negative effects has PPS had on the quality of hospital care for Medicare beneficiaries?
- What is the net effect of PPS on the quality of hospital care for Medicare beneficiaries?
- How has PPS affected the quality of care in nonhospital settings of care?

Each of these questions is examined in greater detail below.

Evaluating Serious Negative Effects of PPS on the Quality of Hospital Care

Several outcome measures can be used to detect serious negative effects of PPS on the quality of hospital care. Among them are: 1) in-hospital and postdischarge mortality rates; 2) rates of occurrence of complications or iatrogenic events or illnesses; and 3) readmission rates. Most of these data items are reasonably accessible from

Medicare databases, but because they are relatively rare events, large samples will be needed for precise estimation.

In-hospital and postdischarge mortality rates can be measured as total death rates across institutions or for specified types of facilities, rates specific to patient populations (e.g., the very elderly), and rates specific to diagnosis, surgical procedure, or DRG (and combinations thereof). Postdischarge death rates can be measured at various intervals following discharge (such as 1 week or 1 month). Of course, increases in in-hospital and postdischarge mortality rates are to be expected if the less seriously ill patients are shifted to outpatient settings due to PPS incentives or PRO admissions review. Thus, attention needs to be paid to the question of whether elderly patients with given medical conditions or with similar levels of severity of illness are dying in the hospital or shortly after discharge at rates demonstrably above those of the pre-PPS era.

Iatrogenic events are infections, drug reactions, or other mishaps due to treatment in the hospital. These and other preventable problems, sometimes called "sentinel events," can be a signal that quality of care has declined (254). They will help in distinguishing between very bad care and adequate care, so they can serve as useful screening indicators of the direction that inpatient quality of care may be taking. They will not be as useful in distinguishing between satisfactory and excellent inpatient care, and they are not especially pertinent to ambulatory care.

Iatrogenic problems may already be more common than is sometimes recognized; the question is whether the rates of such problems increase as PPS incentives to reduce services and personnel begin to take hold.[6]

Readmissions are defined as admissions to the hospital following a prior hospitalization within a specified period of time (PROs will review any readmission within 7 days of a prior admission). For a variety of reasons, readmissions can reflect a deterioration in the quality of care, so these merit early and close attention. They will occur for several reasons, and care must be taken to attribute to PPS only those that are likely results of the incentives inherent in PPS.

Some patients will require rehospitalization for unrelated problems (e.g., elective surgery followed by admission for an acute problem such as a fracture or a fall). Readmissions can also occur if routine testing or specialized consultations are curtailed, so that unsuspected problems are not detected or confirmed on a first admission. Thus, it is important to determine if PPS incentives for curbing length of stay, routine testing, followup of diagnostic tests, and specialty consults seem to be associated with a rise in readmissions of this sort.

Readmissions can also be prompted by complications arising from surgery. Some complications may be relatively unavoidable, of course, but whereas in the past the patient may have had a long length of stay in a single hospitalization, under PPS the patient may be discharged and later return to the hospital. Other complications may be direct outcomes of poor surgical, medical, or nursing care due to PPS changes in procedures or personnel. Complications may occur for patients who are relatively poor risks for surgery; because PPS incentives favor surgical over medical care for certain types of patients (221,273), this may be an especially difficult area to assess.[7]

Readmission may also occur because of inappropriate care or inadequate recuperation before discharge (without any overt complications). This phenomenon of "premature" discharge is especially hard to detect or evaluate: early discharges may be quite beneficial for some patients, but they do not return to the hospital and are thus not easily incorporated into a balanced evaluation.

Finally, one form of "readmission" arises from sequencing of admissions, one for diagnostic testing and workup and a second for surgery or other definitive therapy. In general, return to the hospital in such circumstances may be undesirable,

---

[6]In one pre-PPS study in a university hospital, 36 percent of 815 consecutive patients on a general medical service had an iatrogenic illness; most of these were related to drugs (278).

[7]Examining changes in the proportions of patients in medical/surgical "pairs" of DRGs may be instructive. Such pairs include DRG #243 (medical back problems) and DRGs #214 and #215 (back and neck procedures) or DRGs #235 and #236 (fractures of the femur, hip, and pelvis treated nonsurgically) and DRGs #209 to #211 (surgical procedures on major joints, hip, and femur).

because of the possible increase in out-of-pocket costs to the patient and the probable rise in anxiety and family disruption. Certainly, the last pattern appears to be less likely to be in the patient's interest than in the hospital's.

In all the areas just mentioned, the crucial evaluation question to be addressed first is whether mortality rates, rates of preventable complications, readmission rates, and the like for patients with similar conditions, are higher in the PPS period than previously, independent of any underlying trends. If they are not, the Nation might be reasonably assured that PPS has not induced provider behaviors *seriously* inimical to the health and well-being of the elderly. If they are, thorough evaluation efforts must be directed at determining and rectifying the cause(s) for apparently harmful effects of PPS.

Evaluating the Net Effect of PPS on the Quality of Hospital Care

An important limitation of mortality rates, readmission rates, or sentinel events is that such rates alone are poor measures of more subtle changes in inpatient care for the elderly. Even if death or readmission rates show little or no change, PPS may have effects in terms of time to full recovery, chronic impairments, or emotional well-being. Moreover, because they are relatively rare events, relying on them to appear in sufficient number to trigger corrective action means that some patients may be harmed.

Examination of the processes of care and "proximate" (i.e., short-term) outcomes of care rendered in the hospital will provide balanced evidence of PPS effects (or lack of them) that is far more convincing to the medical profession, the policymaking community, and the Medicare population than studies based on crude outcome measures. Only medical record audit is likely to provide pre- and post-PPS data with the requisite reliability, validity, and clinical detail.

Such studies would require abstracting medical records (for two time periods, such as 1981 and 1985) for condition-specific process and outcome variables related to medical and nursing care in a nationally representative sample of hospitals within the four census regions (or, better, within the nine census divisions). Important aspects of such studies are that they account for patient complexity (sociodemographic variables such as age and income, level of severity of illness for which the person is hospitalized, and underlying levels of health status and comorbidity). They should cover a range of conditions reflecting medical and surgical reasons for admission. The conditions should be ones for which the medical literature provides consensus on appropriate processes of care and expected patient outcomes, for which information is readily available in the hospital chart, and that account for a large fraction of medical admissions.

Evaluating the Effects of PPS on Quality of Care in Nonhospital Settings

The predicted reductions in lengths of hospital stay, increases in patient transfers, and increases in the use of outpatient care (both for surgery and for postdischarge followup) all argue for study of the quality of care prior to admission and the outcomes of care after discharge. PPS' emphasis on reducing hospital use also calls for special attention to the subset of patients who are never admitted, either because their conditions can be treated adequately on an ambulatory basis or because their poverty or severity of illness makes them "undesirable" patients. With more (and sicker) elderly patients obtaining care in ambulatory settings, from home health and other community agencies, and in long-term care facilities, the need for greater attention to quality of care from those sources is apparent.

The first line of inquiry, of course, is to monitor population-based mortality rates in the elderly population by age, sex, and race. But these measures are likely to be relatively insensitive to the influence of PPS. Hence, they are not likely to provide much insight into this important question. Study of the broader effects of PPS requires longitudinal studies of panels of patients or cohorts of Medicare beneficiaries whose course of diagnosis, treatment, and recovery can be tracked through an entire episode of illness, regardless of whether care was rendered in a physician's office, a freestanding or outpatient surgical clinic, a hospital, a skilled nursing home or intermediate care facility, or the like. Patient outcomes such as physical functioning, emotional well-being, and capacity for independent living, as well as effects on family members, are all critical dimensions of care to be evaluated. These are more amenable to targeted research efforts than to broad statistical analyses based on routine databases.

Data Sources

Data for addressing the critical evaluation questions in the area of PPS impacts on quality of care can be obtained from a variety of sources. The basic sources of information, listed in the order of feasibility and ease of use in evaluation, are: 1) Medicare claims; 2) discharge abstract data sets; 3) medical records; 4) patient surveys; and 5) findings from patient examinations and patient or family interviews and questionnaires.

By and large, data from Medicare claims and discharge abstract data sets tend to be cheaper to obtain and thus available for a larger number of individuals. Information on Medicare program claims, for instance, is essentially automatically available (albeit with a delay of several months from date of service). These data sources tend to suffer more from unreliability (missing data, poor coding of key information such as diagnosis or procedures, inconsistency across sources) and from poor validity (i.e., what they reflect about processes of care may correlate only poorly with patient outcomes). They also tell little about problems related to underservice (needed tests or procedures not performed, drugs not administered) or delay in obtaining care.

Data from patients' medical records, patient surveys, and findings from patient examinations are more expensive to collect, with a corresponding drop in the number of persons who can be studied.[8] They are likely to be both more reliable and more valid. They provide a mechanism for learning about relatively subtle aspects of health status, such as physical functioning or emotional well-being, as well as a means of understanding relationships between process and outcome. Finally, they are a direct way to document the extent and effect on quality of reduced access and underservice.

Table 6-2 summarizes and compares the contents of five national databases on patient characteristics: Medicare Part A and Part B claims, the PRO Hospital Discharge Data Set (PHDDS), the Hospital Discharge Survey (HDS), and Commission on Professional and Hospital Activities (CPHA) data. These and other sources of data that could be used to evaluate PPS impacts on quality of care are described in detail below.

Medicare Claims

Claims filed on behalf of Medicare beneficiaries pertain mainly to inpatient stays in short-stay acute hospitals (Part A) or to care received in ambulatory settings (Part B). Such claims, which are processed and reported to HCFA by fiscal intermediaries and carriers, form the Medicare Statistical System data files. The Part A and Part B files are generally not integrated; linking the inpatient and outpatient files for all individual Medicare patients has been considered until recently a prohibitively difficult task.[9] The Medicare History Sample has demographic and utilization data since 1974 for both Part A and Part B services for a continuing 5-percent sample of beneficiaries (see app. E), but the lag in availability of this file reduces its usefulness for evaluation.

Part A claims-based data on hospital stays are submitted to HCFA by fiscal intermediaries (contractors that administer Part A payments) and are compiled in the Hospital Stay Record. The Stay Record includes the following elements: beneficiary identification number (usually Social Security number); demographic information such as age, sex, and State of residence; hospital where admitted; up to five diagnoses for the admission; up to three procedures performed during the admission; status (alive or not) and destination (e.g., home, nursing home, intermediate care facility, home health care) upon discharge; dates of admission and discharge; days spent in intensive or coronary care units; and aggregate dollar charges

---

[8]For example, abstracting new data directly from patients' medical records could cost as much as $40 per case (188,224). For a study using 1,000 records in each of three conditions, abstracting costs alone would be $120,000.

[9]HCFA has recognized the need to use parts of the Medicare Statistical System simultaneously and is currently trying to develop a sample file that merges Parts A and B data. This file, the "Medicare Automated Data Retrieval System" (MADRS), is described in app. E.

Table 6-2.—Data Elements in Patient-Based National Databases

Major data elements	Medicare claims Part A billing records	Medicare claims Part B billing records	PHDDS	HDS	CPHA
Medicare beneficiary identifier	X		X		
Patient name	X	X	X		X
Date of birth (or age)	X	X	X	X	X
Sex	X	X	X	X	X
Race	X	X	X	X	
Marital status				X	X
Zip code of residence	X		X	X	X
Medical record number	X			X	
Hospital identifier	X		X[a]	X	
HDS number				X	
Date of admission	X		X	X	X
Type of admission (emergency, urgent, elective)	X		X		
Source of admission	X		X		
Date of discharge	X		X	X	X
Disposition of patient (home health care, nursing home, home/self care, etc.)	X		X	X	
Diagnoses:					
Admitting diagnosis	X		X		X
Principal diagnosis	X		X	X	X
Up to four secondary diagnoses	X		X		X
Procedures:					
Principal procedure and date	X		X		X
Up to two secondary procedures and dates	X		X		X
Abnormal tissue indicator					X
Number of days in special care units	X				X
Attending physician	X	X			X
Operating physician	X				
Expected principal source(s) of payment	X		X	X	X
Type of PRO review and action (e.g., preadmission/preprocedure review, admission review, outlier review; approval or denial)			X		
Actual dollars paid	X	X	X		
Current DRG assigned	X		X		
Original DRG assigned	X		X		
Pricer action code	X		X		
Billing and payment dates		X			
Medicare eligibility status (e.g., aged, disabled, end-stage renal disease)		X			
Outpatient psychiatric charges		X			
Reasonable medical (nonpsychiatric) charges		X			
Place of service (e.g., office, home, independent laboratory)		X			
Type of service (e.g., medical care, surgery, diagnostic X-ray)		X			

ABBREVIATIONS: CPHAS = Commission on Professional and Hospital Activities.
HDS = Hospital Discharge Survey
PHDDS = PRO Hospital Discharge Data Set
[a]Recent addition to the national database.

SOURCES: U.S. Department of Health and Human Services, Health Care Financing Administration, *Medicare Statistical Files Manual* (Baltimore, MD: HCFA, September 1983); National Academy of Sciences, Institute of Medicine, *Reliability of National Hospital Discharge Survey Data* (Washington, DC: NAS, 1980); U.S. Department of Health and Human Services, Health Care Financing Administration, "PRO Hospital Discharge Data Set Tape Layout," Baltimore, MD, 1984; and Commission on Professional and Hospital Activities, "PAS Case Abstract" form, Ann Arbor, MI, 1984.

for various hospital services and departments such as pathology, radiology, or physical therapy.

Part B claims-based data are submitted by Medicare carriers (contractors that administer Part B payments) on payment records following their payment of Medicare bills. There are 36 items reported on each Part B payment record, many of them for administrative purposes within HCFA. Data elements from Part B payment records that could be useful in quality of care assessments include the following: patient's name; Medicare status; expense period dates; outpatient psychiatric charges; reimbursement amount; reasonable medical charges (nonpsychiatric); deductible applied; physician or supplier identification code; sex; place of service for the largest charge (e.g., office, home, outpatient hospital, independent laboratory, independent kidney disease treatment center); type of service (e.g., medical care, surgery, consultation, diagnostic X-ray, radiation therapy); physician or supplier specialty code; beneficiary date of birth; and race.

One drawback to using Medicare billing data for quality studies is the lack of comparability and compatibility between the Part A and Part B databases. For instance, the coding systems differ: Part A procedure codes since 1980 have been based on the International Classification of Diseases, 9th Revision, Clinical Modification (ICD-9-CM) (and before 1980 were based on the International Classification of Diseases, Adapted, 8th Revision), whereas Part B procedure codes are based on the Current Procedural Terminology (CPT). Although CPT codes can be classified in the ICD system, the ICD codes cannot be put into CPT. Worse, by the time Part B data reach HCFA, they no longer contain any diagnostic or procedural information, meaning that tracking shifts in the sites of care or changes in the processes of care for specific illnesses is infeasible from these sources alone.

Other major parts of the Medicare database that could be used in quality studies are the Provider of Services File, which gives detailed information about hospitals and nursing homes, and the Health Insurance Master Enrollment File, which is a cumulative file on all individuals ever eligible for Medicare benefits. The latter includes dates of death.

Discharge Abstracts

Most hospitals use some medical records abstracting scheme to process patient care information. Although specific items may vary by abstracting service, the common core of information usually includes items specified for the Uniform Hospital Discharge Data Set (UHDDS) as defined by the U.S. Committee on Vital and Health Statistics: patient identification, date of birth, sex, race and ethnicity, residence, hospital identification, admission and discharge dates, identifiers for admission and operating physician(s), principal diagnosis, procedures and dates done, disposition of patient, and expected source of payment.

PROs compile a more complete version of UHDDS for Medicare known as PHDDS (the PRO Hospital Discharge Data Set), adding data regarding various review activities and more detailed information about the admission (see table 6-2). Some of this information (e.g., patient's name and names of physicians) is never reported to HCFA. PHDDS thus provides a stream of information quite similar to, but completely independent of, the Medicare claims data that are reported to HCFA by the fiscal intermediaries and that constitute the Part A Hospital Stay Record files.[10]

---

[10]In years past, the forerunner to PHDDS, the PSRO Hospital Discharge Data Set, was considered to have much more reliable, valid, and complete data, especially for diagnosis and procedure, than the corresponding Part A files. Unlike the Part A file, however, this data set was not necessarily a full enumeration of Medicare admissions because not all areas of the country had an operational PSRO. Because of the extreme sensitivity of DRG-based payments to diagnostic and procedural information, most observers expect the Part A files now being compiled to be considerably improved compared to the pre-PPS era. These improvements in recording and coding, although clearly welcome, complicate studying changes in medical practice (and quality of care) over time with just HCFA Medicare data.

Exactly how much improvement will be realized, and how quickly, are being monitored. Early in PPS, the HCFA central data processing office was alerted to an unexpectedly high error rate in DRG assignment, and 15 million PPS claims were rerun to check DRG assignments for all Medicare patients under PPS from Oct. 1, 1983 through Dec. 31, 1984. Checking the internal consistency of the data, HCFA found that the error rate dropped from 5.48 percent for the first PPS quarter (October 1983 through December 1983) to 1.59 percent in the fifth PPS quarter (October 1984 through December 1984). This indicates a fairly rapid improvement. At this time, reasons for the errors and whether they are random or systematic are unknown (265).

HDS is a federally supported abstract system begun in 1964 by NCHS and carried out by the Bureau of the Census. HDS is based on a set of hospitals selected from a stratified sample of hospitals; patient records are then systematically sampled within selected hospitals. Most items in the HDS come from the face sheet of the medical record (see table 6-2). Most have been collected consistently over time, although some changes in definitions of certain items mean that trends must be interpreted carefully; this is especially true of principal diagnosis (214).

CPHA administers a private sector abstracting service. CPHA is a voluntary nonprofit organization to which over 1,500 hospitals provide a set of data in return for various interinstitutional comparative analyses and internal medical cost analyses. The data collected by CPHA contain all of the data elements of the UHDDS, as well as indicators for abnormal tissue and the number of days in care units (see table 6-2). A subset of 250 to 300 hospitals provide data on costs and various diagnostic tests. Although data are available over a period of years for a national, representative sample of hospitals, the data are confidential and cannot be linked to identify hospitals, so all analyses must be done by CPHA staff on a contract basis (105).

The Hospital Cost and Utilization Project (HCUP) of the National Center for Health Services Research and Health Care Technology Assessment (NCHSR&HCTA) is another Federal database that contains discharge abstract data. The information for HCUP comes from 12 major discharge abstract services, the American Hospital Association's Annual Survey of Hospitals, and Medicare cost reports. These data files link abstracted clinical information on patients with hospital cost information and community characteristics. Data are available for over 300 short-term, general, non-Federal hospitals for 1970 through 1977. New data are to be collected for 1980 through 1987 from an enlarged sample of about 500 hospitals. Although some of the patient-level charge data are incomplete, HCUP is a potential source of linked quality and cost data (351).

Medical Records and Medical Record Audits

A considerably richer source of quality of care data is the patients' medical records. The content of most hospital medical records in this country reflects standards set forth by the Joint Commission on the Accreditation of Hospitals (JCAH): "The medical record shall contain sufficient information to identify the patient, to support the diagnosis, to justify the treatment, and to document the results accurately." Detailed requirements for the following elements are published by JCAH (155): identification data; medical history of the patient; report of a relevant physical examination; diagnostic and therapeutic orders; evidence of appropriate informed consent; clinical observations, including results of therapy; reports of procedures, tests, and their results; and conclusions at termination of hospitalization or evaluation/treatment.

Medical record data do have some limitations. Some quality-related information will be absent from even the most detailed records, including information relating to postdischarge outpatient care, longer term outcomes such as length of time to full recovery and functioning (or death out of hospital), and patient satisfaction. The reliability and validity of abstract data taken from medical records have been questioned (212,213,214). Finally, collecting evaluation information through medical record abstracting ("audit" or "chart review") tends to be more costly than using insurance claims data.

In general, the accuracy and comprehensiveness of medical record data, especially when collected by trained medical record abstractors, far surpasses that of insurance claims or discharge abstract data. An evaluation of PPS that examines changes in in-hospital processes of care and their relationship to outcomes for the aged would require data collected directly from medical records. Any PPS evaluation that is extended to out-of-hospital impacts, for which almost no adequate claims data exist, would also have to rely in part on medical record data.

Patient Surveys and Direct Data Collection

As noted earlier, measures of patients' health status, often based on self-administered questionnaires, are available to be employed in or adapted for an evaluation of PPS effects on quality of care. No one set of measures will serve the full range of PPS evaluation needs, because some indicators pertain more to outcomes of ambulatory than inpatient care and some are more appropriate for nonelderly populations than for the elderly. Furthermore, these types of indexes or indicators relate more to patient outcomes, such as long-term physical functioning or mental health, than to actual processes of care.

Nonetheless, most of the currently available health status measures would provide adequate bases for devising measures related to what effect PPS may have had on quality of care over the longer run or for more subtle changes of health. Highly reliable and valid measures of patient satisfaction are also readily available.

CONCLUSIONS

Because the issues that can be identified in the area of PPS impacts on quality of care are so numerous and complex, some priorities as to the most critical evaluation questions must be set. This chapter has outlined the following points.

First, unarguably negative effects of PPS on quality must be anticipated by monitoring changes in the following: deaths; postoperative or other complications; "sentinel events" that reflect preventable negative outcomes such as infection or drug reactions; readmissions (including "second" or "sequences of" admissions); and discharge destinations. Often, this monitoring can be accomplished using administrative data such as Medicare insurance claims files and by agencies such as PROs. This type of assessment can be (and some is being) done in the near term.

Second, PPS assessments must examine processes and outcomes of hospital care and their relationships. Critical questions are whether changes in in-hospital processes of care are taking place, whether any such process changes are related to expected patient outcomes, and if so, in what ways patient outcomes are being affected. These types of assessments rely less on administrative data and more on costly direct data collection methods such as medical record audit, patient and family interviews, and health status measurement survey instruments. The advantage of these kinds of evaluations is that they provide stronger evidence of both positive and negative ramifications of prospective payment on quality of care.

Third, PPS can have far-reaching ramifications, especially for long-term care and for outpatient services. Investigating how the outcomes of care are changing in the post-PPS era, with evidence strong enough to link such changes at least provisionally to PPS, will be a third critical evaluation issue before the end of the decade.

Congress recognized the potential threat to quality of care of PPS and built at least two safeguards into relevant legislation. PROs have responsibility for monitoring the quality of care in addition to numerous activities relating to cost containment. And, for the first 4 years, HCFA must report to Congress annually on the broad impacts of PPS, including quality of care (see ch. 10). Yet the question remains whether these arrangements will provide adequate information on the quality impacts of PPS.

PROs are responsible for protecting against certain extreme effects of PPS on inpatient care, but their responsibility stops at the hospital door; severe funding constraints and uncertainty about priorities will restrict PROs' attention to quality of care. They also have cost-containment objectives that, under certain circumstances, could counter the quality assurance efforts.

HCFA has generally been accepted by the Administration as the agency to conduct major PPS evaluations (see ch. 10). As the source of the major routine databases (e.g., Medicare claims and beneficiary history files), this agency is most familiar with the potential strengths and weaknesses of the data. The fact that HCFA is not entirely disinterested in the outcome of such studies, however, may pose questions of bias. External (extramural) research would lessen concerns that any evaluation performed by the agency that has administrative responsibility for PPS will lack full credibility, but congressional oversight of HCFA's role in supporting such evaluations could help protect the integrity of these research efforts. A second problem is that present or contemplated HCFA Office of Research and Demonstrations budgets and staff for PPS research and evaluation, especially in the quality-of-care area, are inadequate (see ch. 10); this is certainly true if longer term patient outcomes are to be monitored or the linkages between processes and outcomes are to be documented and understood.

Other organizations and agencies within DHHS could also carry out substantial parts of the PPS evaluations. Both the Office of the Assistant Secretary for Planning and Evaluation and the NCHSR&HCTA have considerable experience with funding and managing large and lengthy studies of this sort done by outside contractors and grantees. Because they are external agencies with respect to the administration of PPS, questions about credibility and integrity of the research effort would be minimized. Reliance on these agencies, however, would require coordination with and cooperation from HCFA for access to data.

As with HCFA, however, current funding levels for these agencies would not sustain very comprehensive evaluations, almost certainly not ones requiring medical record abstraction or direct data collection from elderly patients or families. Furthermore, any PPS evaluation done by a DHHS agency will be subject to an additional level of control, expense, and delay by the Federal bureaucracy if the Office of Management and Budget requires detailed clearance of data collection materials, questionnaires, medical record audit forms, and the like.

Any evaluation of the effects of PPS on quality of care will be costly, but actual funding requirements will vary depending on the degree to which the evaluation attempts to be comprehensive (i.e., to cover all the critical evaluation questions). The least expensive evaluations will rely nearly exclusively on existing data systems, largely Medicare claims files, but such evaluations will be subject to the limitations and restrictions inherent in those databases.

Selecting ways to assess PPS impacts on quality does not imply choosing one strategy or database to the exclusion of all others; the optimal approach will probably be one that incorporates some work along all the lines discussed. The high cost of in-depth studies reinforces the need for careful specification of process and outcome (health status measures). Allocation of resources to the development of a consensus about the quality measures to be evaluated would be prudent.

# Chapter 7
Access to Health Care

Contents

	Page
Introduction	95
Defining and Measuring Access to Care	95
The Concept of Access	95
A Need-Based Concept of Equitable Access	96
A Market Concept of Equitable Access	96
An Adequate Care Concept of Equitable Access	97
Implications for Measuring Access	97
Potential Impacts of PPS on Access to Care	98
Access to Inpatient Care	98
Access to Other Sites of Care	102
Approaches to Evaluating the Impacts of PPS on Equity of Access	105
Critical Evaluation Questions	105
Data Sources	107
Conclusions	109

Chapter 7
Access to Health Care[1]

INTRODUCTION

Securing access to health care for all Americans was the major goal of American health policy for several decades. Over the past few years, public concern has shifted to the soaring cost of care. Nevertheless, for many Americans, access to care is still far from satisfactory (5). Moreover, many people fear that an overly enthusiastic pursuit of cost containment may jeopardize the substantial gains made in access in previous years.

The impact of Medicare's new prospective payment system (PPS) is of particular importance, since Medicare's eligibility rules are designed to ensure access to care for three especially vulnerable groups: elderly people, disabled people, and sufferers from end-stage renal disease (323). There is concern as to whether these groups, with their special needs, will find their access to care compromised under the new system. Subgroups of the eligible population—defined, for example, by income, place of residence, social or ethnic background, or specific health condition—could also experience special difficulties with access. In addition, since Medicare is such a large part of the market for hospital care, a change in its hospital payment methods affects the entire system. Thus, PPS could, in turn, affect access to care of those outside the system.

The purpose of this chapter is to consider how the effects of Medicare's PPS on access to health care can be evaluated and how the inherent methodological difficulties can be overcome. First, the definitions of access are discussed, and three concepts of equity of access are examined. Second, the potential impact of PPS on equity of access is explored. Then, critical questions for evaluating equity of access are presented, along with a discussion of how they can be answered and data sources.

[1]Parts of this chapter are based on a background paper entitled "Evaluating the Effects of Medicare's Prospective Payment System on Access to Health Care," which was prepared for OTA in December 1984 by Mary Ann Baily.

DEFINING AND MEASURING ACCESS TO CARE

The Concept of Access

The expression "access to health care," like "quality of care," is ambiguous. Consequently, people can unite behind the goal of "assuring access to health care for all Americans" when their views of what access means and how equity of access should be assured are very different.

Access is defined in Webster's dictionary as "permission, liberty, or ability to enter, approach, communicate with, or pass to and from" or "freedom or ability to obtain or make use of" (386). Aday and Anderson provide the most common definition in the health care field, stating "access may be defined as those dimensions which describe the potential and actual entry of a given population group to the health care delivery system" (4).

Note that the expression is access to "health care," not access to "health." This distinction is required, because it is impossible to guarantee that a particular level of health status is achieved or maintained. Of course, when judgments are made about the adequacy of access, differences in access that can be attributed to affecting health outcomes are usually considered of greatest policy importance. Note also that the word of concern is "access" and not "distribution." Even strict egalitarians recognize that the policy goal should not be an equal distribution of health care, given the unequal distribution of health needs.

Another important conceptual distinction is that policymakers who wish to assure "access" often are actually referring to some sort of "*equity* of access." From a policy perspective, measuring changes in access means measuring changes in equity of access, so these terms are often used interchangeably. Either term obscures very important aspects of receiving health care, e.g., how much of the cost people bear themselves and how good the quality of care is compared with other care. Since there is no consensus on the amount of care a person should be able to obtain, how "good" the care should be, or what it should cost (financial and time costs), it may well be convenient to use a term that leaves these questions open. Nevertheless, practical policy dictates that these questions be answered. How changes in equity of access to health care should be measured and evaluated depends on those answers.

A Need-Based Concept of Equitable Access

The traditional health care literature on access emphasizes the relationship between what people get and what they need. In the words of Aday and Andersen (4):

> One of the central issues to be addressed in any evaluation of access to medical care is whether persons who need care are able to obtain it. Equity is said to exist when services are distributed on the basis of need rather than as a result of structural or individual factors such as a family's income level, person's racial characteristics, or the distribution of physicians in an area.

"Need" is a notoriously slippery concept in health care (41,103,395). A technical definition of need emphasizes the relation between health care and health outcomes. A person "needs" the amount of health care that would bring his or her health status as close to normal as possible and keep it there (with some specified probability, since medical outcomes can never be guaranteed). Because health care resources are limited, most people would agree that stopping short of satisfying *all* health care needs is reasonable, even in the narrow technical sense. Need cannot be defined as all care that is of any benefit however small; some attempt must be made to consider the relationship of benefit to cost. How the limit to the satisfaction of needs should be set is debatable. And how this health care should be divided between the provision of technological services and informing and caring is even more difficult to decide.

What is clear is that this approach to equity of access emphasizes comparison of health care utilization rates. It does not say what those rates should be or how much care should be potentially available, and it pays too little attention to the costs and quality of care received as an equity issue in itself rather than merely as a potential barrier to obtaining care. Furthermore, differences among individuals or between groups in utilization for any given health status are considered inequities (4). Labeling all such differences as inequities, however, seems excessive. If health care is bought and sold, and individual incomes and preferences differ, differences in utilization should be expected.

A Market Concept of Equitable Access

A market concept of equity of access is that everyone should be able to buy the health care he or she wants at a cost that reflects the true cost to society of supplying it. If the distribution of income is fair, and if markets for health care and health insurance work well (i.e., are perfectly competitive[2]), then access to care will be equitable. Since preferences and supply costs may vary in different parts of the country or for different groups, there may be differences in the amounts of care available for purchase and the terms on which care is available. As long as these differences represent the outcome of the interaction between consumer tastes and real supply costs, they do not constitute inequities of access.

In contrast to the needs-based approach, differences in ability to pay due to differences in income constitute neither differences nor inequities in access. If the distribution of income is very unequal, poor people may have difficulty obtaining important health care. Under this concept, however, their problem is not one of access to

---

[2]A "perfectly competitive market" is one in which large numbers of buyers and sellers operate independently for a particular product. Other factors are availability of perfect information about the product and easy entry into and exit from the market.

health care but of access to wealth, and this problem should be treated on its own.

Differences caused by imperfectly competitive markets *are* inequities under the market-based concept of access. Health care and health insurance markets are far from competitive. Consumers have inadequate information; providers are licensed; tax subsidies exist for the purchase of insurance. Thus, under this approach access is judged by whether patients with the same health status are charged different prices for the same services, whether artificial barriers exist to location of physicians in underserved areas, whether insurance companies are offering the kinds of policies consumers want to buy, and so on.

The market approach answers the "quantity," "quality," and "costs to patient" questions of access by referring to an unobservable ideal—the result a perfectly competitive market system would yield. More important, this approach fails to incorporate the widely held belief that health care is "special," and ability to pay should play a different role in the distribution of health care than it does in the distribution of other commodities.

An Adequate Care Concept of Equitable Access

An intermediate position between the need-based and market concepts of access holds that equity of access to care means everyone should be able to obtain an "adequate level" (or "decent minimum") of care, without having to bear an "excessive burden" in travel, waiting time, or financial cost (49,234). People who want more than this level of care should be able to purchase it at its unsubsidized supply cost.

The precise content of an adequate level of care and the definition of an excessive burden are value judgments. They depend, first, on society's tradeoffs between health care and other commodities and, second, on tradeoffs among the different kinds of health care.

An adequate level of care also depends on the relationship between health care and health status. Thus, this approach gives highest priority to measuring shortfalls between adequate care for a given health status and actual utilization. The presumption is that people will choose to consume at least the adequate level, whatever their preferences, if no excessive financial burden serves as a barrier. Above the adequate level, however, differences in utilization are to be expected and are equitable if they reflect preferences, incomes, and social costs.

Two approximations of adequacy of care in empirical studies of access are: 1) professionally defined standards of needed care; and 2) the care received by the average middle class American. Neither is fully satisfactory. Standards developed from professional judgments can be overly lavish and biased toward a technical definition of need, and the pattern of care now received by middle class Americans is distorted by a third-party payment system characterized by perverse incentives (234). Thus, although this approach to access is attractive, there are practical difficulties in applying it.

Implications for Measuring Access

As noted earlier, the ultimate purpose of evaluating PPS-related changes in access is to enable judgments to be made about their policy significance—whether the changes have a positive or negative impact on *equity* and to what extent. As the above discussion shows, there is no consensus on what constitutes equity of access, and the three definitions attach very different importance to observed differences in the kinds and amounts of health care obtained or the terms on which it is obtained.

Nevertheless, all three concepts of equity imply that it is changes in the availability and utilization of services that are the important indicators of changes in access for specific groups. Thus, all three concepts point to measures of potential and realized access, although the division is not absolute. Potential access refers to the possibility of obtaining care if the need or desire for it arises. Realized access refers to the actual utilization of care in response to need or desire (4). The concepts also imply that changes in out-of-pocket costs of care to patients may be important indicators of access, but these issues are more fully addressed in chapter 5. Differences among groups in availability or utilization that cannot be explained by differences in health status are particularly suspect.

POTENTIAL IMPACTS OF PPS ON ACCESS TO CARE

PPS will affect access to the full array of health services, because markets for different kinds of health care are interconnected. For example, changes in hospital incentives to admit and discharge elderly patients will affect nursing homes and home health agencies. These effects will probably spread beyond the Medicare population to the non-Medicare population, but perhaps in different directions. Brief discussions of PPS effects on access to other sites of care, including ambulatory and posthospital care, as well as effects on the Medicaid and veteran populations, are included below. The emphasis in this chapter, however, is on PPS effects on equity of access to hospital inpatient care.

Access to Inpatient Care

PPS may affect access to inpatient care in four ways:

- through effects on the number and distribution of hospital beds;
- through effects on the admissions policies of hospitals;
- through effects on the transfer policies of hospitals; and
- through effects on treatment received after admission to the hospital.

The most important aspect of these effects is their differential impacts on different groups of patients, especially vulnerable groups. The groups most often identified as vulnerable include frail elderly patients (especially those over 75), disabled patients, and alcoholic and mentally ill patients. These groups are discussed further below.

Availability of Hospital Beds

PPS may systematically alter the number and the distribution of hospitals and hospital beds by geographic location, size, and type of population served. In the short run, the total amount of Medicare payments going to hospitals will not necessarily decrease very much, and some observers have predicted the amount will actually increase. However, the distribution of Medicare payments to hospitals may change substantially (see ch. 3), and in the long run, the increase in total payments is likely to be slower.

Changes in the patterns of Medicare payments will put serious financial pressure on many hospitals and may affect the *total number of hospital beds*: some hospitals will close; others will reduce bed capacity. Hospital occupancy rates at the moment are low—estimated at 73.4 percent in 1983 for non-Federal, short-term general hospitals (13)—suggesting the existence of excess capacity. Since PPS is intended to encourage efficiency, closures may be desirable if the least efficient or least needed hospitals close. However, the systematic revenue redistributions among hospitals implied by PPS suggests that financial pressure may be tied to factors other than relative efficiency (288,295,369). Furthermore, even the closure of inefficient hospitals or hospital beds may affect access to care for specific vulnerable groups.

In addition to the total number of beds, the *geographic distribution of facilities* may change. When Medicare's PPS system is fully implemented, it will pay the same rate per diagnosis-related groups (DRG) throughout the country, adjusting payment only for whether the hospital is in a rural or urban location.[3] Preliminary simulations by the Congressional Budget Office (CBO) of the impact of PPS on individual hospitals (assuming no change in hospital behavior) indicate that in general, hospitals in the South and Northeast regions will gain substantial revenue under PPS, while those in the West and North Central regions will tend to lose (295). On average, rural hospitals are expected to do worse under PPS than urban hospitals.

The *size distribution* of hospitals also may change. Small hospitals (those with fewer than 75 beds) in rural areas play a special role in access, since they are often the only providers within easy reach of rural populations. Small hospitals could have problems under PPS, because they have

---

[3]A number of observers believe that efforts on behalf of the hospital industry to freeze the implementation of the PPS system to include permanent regional rates may be successful.

higher fluctuations of census, and many serve high proportions of Medicare patients. Moreover, in small hospitals, the cost of administration and the variability of cost of treating patients within a DRG are spread over a small number of patients. However, many of these hospitals will generally not be adversely affected by PPS if they are the "sole providers" in their communities. Such "sole providers" receive help from the provision allowing special exceptions or adjustments to PPS rates.[4]

Hospitals that serve a disproportionate share of low-income patients may have special problems. The burden of providing care to low-income persons is not distributed evenly across hospitals. Certain hospitals, including inner-city and rural public hospitals and university and large city teaching hospitals, have a much greater than average proportion of Medicaid and charity patients in their patient population (180). If these hospitals are "losers" under PPS, the consequences for access to care for the low-income group could be severe. CBO estimates indicate that these hospitals may indeed lose under PPS unless substantial changes in hospital behavior take place (294). The potentially most severely affected disproportionate share providers are those that are *not* major teaching institutions (i.e., those with fewer than 0.25 residents per bed). As a group, urban, Government-owned teaching hospitals that serve poor people are likely to receive increased revenues under PPS (307), primarily because of the adjustment for indirect teaching costs. If this adjustment were reduced to the level that prevailed prior to PPS and treatment patterns remain unchanged, these hospitals would become losers as well.

Admissions Policies of Hospitals

The incentive not to admit patients who cannot pay already exists for hospitals, but to the extent that Medicare's PPS increases the financial pressure on the hospital sector, financial disincentives to provide charity care will increase. Among patients for whom at least some payment is made, the incentive is for the hospital to admit any patient for whom payment exceeds the marginal cost of treatment.[5] In States where Medicaid reimburses hospitals at lower rates than other third-party payers, for example, hospitals have an incentive to avoid Medicaid patients altogether if occupancy rates are high enough without them, or if reimbursement is less than the marginal cost of treatment.

Under PPS, there is a danger that Medicare patients will become less financially attractive as a group than patients covered by payers who reimburse on a more generous basis. Thus, Medicare patients may take the second to last position in the line, just in front of Medicaid patients. However, because DRG rates currently cover marginal costs for most patients within a DRG, and occupancy rates are generally low, Medicare patients as a group are likely to remain attractive to hospitals.

PPS may create financial incentives to hospitals simply to stop treating certain DRGs or certain patients within a given DRG. In the short run, DRG reimbursement rates are probably greater than marginal cost for all DRGs, so there is an incentive to treat all DRGs. In the long run, however, when capacity can be adjusted, specializing in certain DRGs and avoiding others will be advantageous, especially if profitability differs by DRG. To date, no DRGs have been identified as clearly unprofitable for all hospitals in the long run; as cost accounting systems improve, this may change (162). It is especially likely if the system for altering DRG rates is slow to respond to changes in medical technology and input costs.[6]

Although no specific DRGs have been identified as unprofitable, there are several groups of Medicare beneficiaries that can be identified as especially vulnerable to problems with access to hospital care. These groups cut across DRGs and include patients in whom physical illness is accompanied by alcoholism or mental illness, dis-

---

[4] Over 300 hospitals qualify as sole community hospitals at this time (159). A recent study by the National Center for Health Services Research (NCHSR) found that sole community hospitals differed from other rural hospitals by having a greater bed capacity and a greater range of facilities to maintain.

[5] Marginal cost is the additional or variable cost the hospital incurs as a result of accepting the patient over and above what it would otherwise spend.

[6] For example, new advances in lens implants for cataracts provide greater patient benefits but at costs that may make the DRG payment for the procedure unprofitable (see ch. 8) in some hospitals.

abled patients, and very old or frail elderly patients. For example, many elderly patients have multiple medical problems that result in a greater severity of illness than that covered by the DRG payment in many categories. Because "age over 70" or "substantial comorbidities or complications" were the bases for establishing separate DRGs, a number of DRGs have the potential to systematically undercompensate for the frail elderly (30). Box 7-A illustrates some of the problems for alcoholic and mentally ill patients.

Transfer Policies of Hospitals

Transfers, or the change of hospitals after a patient has already been admitted, may present a special access problem, sometimes known as "dumping." "Dumping" refers to the practice of getting rid of unprofitable patients for economic reasons. Once a patient is identified as unprofitable, there is a financial incentive to transfer the patient to another hospital, since the initial hospital receives a per diem payment for the time it has the patient and avoids further losses (the receiving hospital gets the DRG payment for the whole stay). If the receiving hospital is actually a more appropriate source of care for the patient and if the transfer process itself has no adverse consequences, access and quality of care for that patient could be improved. But the hospital has a financial incentive to "dump" patients even when it is not in their best interest.

Patients in the vulnerable groups already identified (e.g., alcoholic and mentally ill patients—see box 7-A) along with racial minorities are particularly vulnerable to "dumping" (133). Veterans Administration (VA) and public hospitals are the likely recipients. Yet these hospitals, along with inner-city teaching hospitals, already provide a substantial amount of undercompensated care. These hospitals may then have more difficulty financing undercompensated care and may have fewer resources to maintain the level of quality that they provide to the rest of their patients.

Transfers and admissions are clinical decisions by doctors; they can be controlled by the hospital administration only to a limited degree. The selective transfer or admission of particular patients also presupposes that unprofitable patients can be readily identified at admission or early in the course of a hospital stay, which generally may not be the case. The hospital administration has more control in decisions about whether or not to stop treating certain DRGs. But on these decisions, there are market constraints. The hospital may need to maintain a full line of services in order to retain its medical staff and its position in the market.

Treatment Policies in Hospitals

The incentives provided by PPS can affect access to care even after patients are admitted to hospitals. One important incentive is for hospitals to specialize in particular DRGs. The other significant incentive is to treat different groups of patients differently. These problems are discussed further below.

If hospitals specialize in particular DRGs, access may be affected either positively or negatively. To the extent that specialization concentrates care for specific DRGs with the most efficient providers, it may reduce costs without impairing quality. For example, open-heart surgery is said to be both cheaper and better when it is done in a hospital that does a high volume of such surgery (189). Concentrating specialized care (including intensive care units, burn units, and other special equipment) in a smaller number of hospitals could, however, increase patient travel time and distance for some patients to an unacceptable degree.

To the extent that specialization in particular DRGs or in particular types of patients within DRGs occurs because unprofitable patients are concentrated in hospitals that are least able to avoid them, the implications for access are more serious. If the DRG rate of payment is too low for a subgroup of patients so that no provider, however efficient, can make a reasonable return on them over the long run, not only will the patients have difficulty finding hospitals that will treat them, but the hospitals they find will be financially pressed as a result.

Differential treatment of patients according to source of reimbursement may be a problem, although there are several constraints to the problem becoming too great. Historically, many hos-

Box 7-A—Access to Hospital Care for Vulnerable Groups: Alcoholic and Mentally Ill Patients

About 9 to 10 percent of the people in the United States are considered to be "problem drinkers," and of these, about half suffer from alcoholism (258). Alcoholics are over-represented in the hospital population. Alcoholism leads directly to diseases such as cirrhosis of the liver; it also raises the probability and increases the severity of other health conditions, such as accidental injuries, cardiovascular problems and cancer (93). From 30 to 50 percent of hospital admissions, excluding obstetrics, are estimated to be for alcoholic patients; most are admitted for disorders other than alcoholism (179,240,258).[1] Among the elderly, the incidence of alcoholism is believed to be somewhat lower than in the general population; however, those who do abuse alcohol are at even greater risk for adverse health effects than younger alcoholics (37).

Even if a DRG is entirely or predominantly composed of alcoholics, if payment reflects the higher cost of treatment of these individuals, then no special problem arises. Indeed, this is true when comorbidities associated with alcoholism qualify as complicating conditions and are thus reflected in the DRG weights. (Some mental disorders are also complicating conditions.) However, alcoholics in DRGs not directly associated with alcoholism or related comorbidities are likely to be unprofitable patients for a number of reasons. They have special physiological problems: For example, they are often malnourished, their infections heal slowly, and they are more likely to experience complications (93,227,258). They may seek care later than other patients and thus may have more advanced disease. Since they are less compliant than other patients (116) and often lack stable home situations, they may have to remain in the hospital longer because they cannot safely be sent home (207). They have multiple health problems and may need workups for more than one condition. Under PPS, multiple workups during the same admission are unprofitable, and the alcoholic patient's noncompliance may make it impractical to schedule another stay.

Alcoholic and mentally ill patients in medical or surgical DRGs are particularly vulnerable to "dumping." (It may also be easy to allow such patients to sign out against medical advice. These patients have been generally found to be uncooperative if special efforts are not made to conciliate them (179).)[2] Moreover, if a particular hospital is known in the community to be insensitive to the needs of alcoholic and mentally ill patients, then such patients may be less likely to select that hospital (207).

Psychiatric disorders other than alcoholism are also associated with physical disorders. For example, one classic study showed a positive and significant correlation between the severity of psychiatric disorder and the number of major physical conditions, such as cardiovascular and respiratory diseases (92). The prevalence of mental disorders in elderly medical and surgical inpatients has been estimated at between 40 and 50 percent (184).

It is more difficult to generalize about the problems of treating mentally ill patients for physical illness, and less is known about the degree to which extra costs are involved. Certain subgroups, such as schizophrenics and patients suffering from dementia, are likely to suffer from malnutrition, lack of regular medical care, noncompliance with therapeutic regimes, and absence of stable home situations which tend to raise the cost of treating them. Patients being treated with psychotropic medications are subject to drug interactions (252).

---

[1]Note the difficulty of arriving at an acceptable definition of alcoholism and the great variability in the estimates of the percentage of alcoholics found in the different studies. Others have pointed out that the diagnosis of alcoholism frequently does not appear on the charts of many patients who have alcohol-related problems (179).

[2]In a study of patients who signed out against medical advice at Peter Bent Brigham Hospital, 42 percent were alcoholics compared with 15 percent in the control group (179).

pitals provided "two-class care" (91); private patients with their own private physicians were treated differently from ward patients. Hospitals are no longer organized in this way, though, and it seems unlikely that there will be an increase in this kind of differential treatment. Two-class care would violate Joint Commission on Accreditation of Hospital standards and Medicare conditions of participation.[7] Most important, it would raise ethical problems for physicians and might expose them and hospitals to malpractice liability.[8] However, it is not necessary for a hospital to have a "two-class" system for differential treatment to occur, particularly with respect to access to specific services. For example, there are strong financial incentives against providing extended hospitalizations requiring intensive care (52) or electrophysiologic testing (198). Those patients who could benefit most from services may not receive them. (See box 7-B for a discussion of rationing of one kind of health service among potential recipients in Great Britain.)

---

[7]Medicare conditions of participation are requirements that a hospital must meet in order to be allowed to receive payments for Medicare patients.

[8]Several cases of two-class care in emergency rooms have recently been reported as results of financial pressures on hospitals. In one case, the Arizona Supreme Court dismissed the case against the physicians because they had been willing to treat the uninsured, indigent patient but held the hospital liable because the patient could not get admitted (73,243,402).

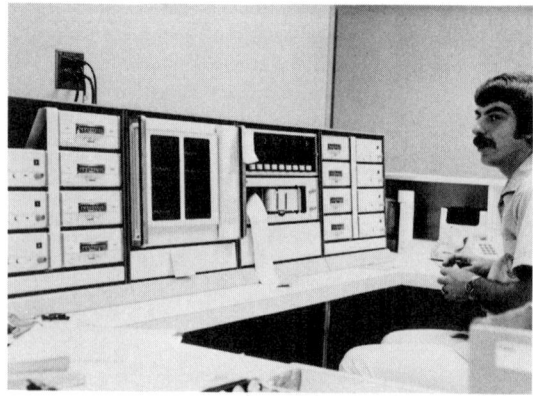

Photo credit: Fairfax Hospital Association

Access to intensive care may be jeopardized by PPS, because of the strong financial incentives against providing extended hospitalizations requiring intensive care.

Access to Other Sites of Care

Although PPS directly affects inpatient care, its incentives reach beyond the hospital stay to other sites in the health care system. Specifically, the incentives of PPS will affect access to ambulatory care, posthospital care (including long-term care and home health care), and VA care. These areas are discussed below. Access for veterans is discussed as a separate section because of the importance of the VA system to the Federal Government.

Access to Ambulatory Care

Ambulatory care is the usual mode of entry into the health care delivery system, so it is of special importance in studies of access to care. Although Medicare's PPS does not cover ambulatory care, PPS incentives may have an indirect effect on equity of access to ambulatory care, both in and out of hospitals for both Medicare and non-Medicare patients. Because of the incentive to reduce the number of services within particular DRGs, for example, many services previously offered only to inpatients (e.g., some diagnostic testing) may be offered at outpatient sites. Some medical technologies, including cataract surgery, have already largely been moved from inpatient to outpatient settings, and others are likely to follow their lead. Access to these services may change, but in unknown ways.

Hospital outpatient care has increased in recent years, partly because hospitals have expanded their services in response to financial pressures and partly because patients have come to expect more types of care from hospitals. The general financial pressure on hospitals will cause them to reexamine the relationship between true costs and returns for outpatient care. There will be an incentive to allocate more costs to outpatient departments, to eliminate any services whose costs cannot be fully covered, to raise charges if demand permits, and to cut back on free or subsidized ambulatory care provided in outpatient departments or emergency rooms. Since low-income persons and persons without insurance are particularly likely to use outpatient departments and emergency rooms as their usual sources of care, the effects of this on their access to ambulatory care could be substantial.

Box 7-B—Access to Specialized Care: The Case of Hemodialysis in Great Britain[1]

One of the technologies that is often used as an example of restricted access to specialized medical care is hemodialysis, the use of a machine to cleanse the blood of a patient whose kidneys have failed. Prior to the inclusion of patients with end-stage renal disease (ESRD) in the Medicare program by the Social Security Amendments of 1972, few machines and expensive dialysis led to varying access for different people in the United States. In some communities, committees decided who would be allowed to receive hemodialysis on their scarce machines. However, since Medicare began to cover patients with ESRD, virtually everyone in the United States, at least currently, has access to some form of dialysis.

The story is different in Great Britain, though, where the National Health Service, with its limited budget, decides who will receive treatment for kidney failure. Most of the patients in Britain who receive hemodialysis have acute kidney failure, not chronic or end-stage renal disease. The United States has about three times the proportion of patients receiving dialysis as in Britain. Kidney transplantation is also a method of overcoming the problem of kidney failure, and it is performed approximately with the same frequency in Britain as in the United States.

What are the criteria for determining who in Great Britain will receive dialysis? There are no official, explicit criteria, but physicians in Britain admit that the following factors influence their hemodialysis decisions: age of the patient (usually those 55 and over do not receive it); vascular complications of diabetes; other medical diseases; physical handicaps; mental illness; and lack of adequate facilities in the home. Rejection criteria vary from dialysis center to dialysis center.

Regional variations in the resources available for dialysis also influence who receives hemodialysis in Britain, although some physicians refuse to admit that some of their decisions are not based on medical criteria. Most local physicians balance their decisionmaking between medical indications and resource realities, thus lessening the disappointment of the patients who might be turned away from a dialysis center to which they had been referred. Patients, for their part, respect the advice of their physicians and usually accept it without complaint.

British physicians, whether or not they admit using resource constraints in their decisionmaking for patients with kidney failure, tend to be more conservative in their criteria. They reportedly do not agree with treating all the patients who are treated in the United States, on philosophical as well as practical bases.

---
[1]Based on a discussion in H. J. Aaron and W. B. Schwartz, *The Painful Prescription* (Washington, DC: The Brookings Institution, 1984).

Access to Posthospital Care[9]

Medicare's PPS gives a financial incentive to hospitals to discharge patients as quickly as possible. As a result, the number of patients who need posthospital care in nursing homes or their own homes is likely to grow, because they are being discharged at an earlier stage in their recovery. In addition, hospitals will be more reluctant to provide care for patients who need only custodial care but cannot obtain immediate nursing home placement. If a hospital, attending physician, or a utilization and quality control peer review organization determines that a patient is no longer in need of acute care, access to post hospital care becomes even more critical. And the existing range of services covered under Medicare's home care and skilled nursing care benefits is so limited that it is likely to cause difficulties for patients discharged earlier and sicker (236). Historically, hospitals have augmented the effective supply of long-term care beds by providing such "back-up" days, largely at Medicare expense (342). Thus, PPS is expected to have a significant impact on the nursing home and home health care industries (201).

---
[9]The General Accounting Office is conducting a study entitled "Information Requirements for Evaluating the Impacts of Medicare Prospective Payment on Posthospital Long-Term-Care Services." One of the key issues identified in a preliminary report is access to services. See ch. 10 for a brief description of this study (297).

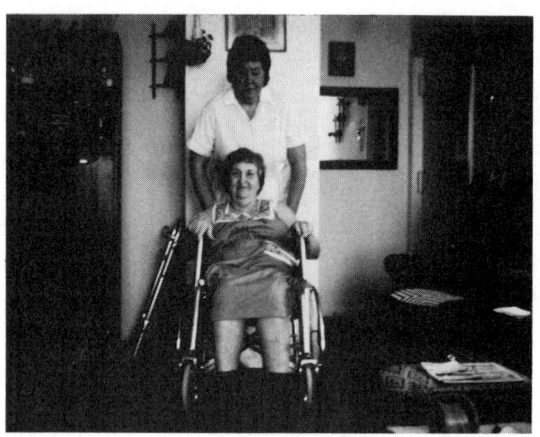

Photo credit: Fairfax Hospital Association

As PPS provides financial incentives to discharge patients at an earlier stage of recovery, access to posthospital care, such as home health care, becomes critical to monitor.

The potential impact of the incentive for earlier discharges raises several issues for evaluation. Are Medicare patients receiving an appropriate level of posthospital care after discharge? Are there adverse effects on access to long-term care of other patients seeking entry into nursing homes, as discharged Medicare patients take the available beds?

Access to nursing home care was a problem in many, but not all, States before the introduction of PPS. Incentives created by the Medicare and Medicaid programs have led to a segmented market, characterized by permanent excess demand for beds. Patients with private funds have no difficulty obtaining beds. Medicaid and Medicare patients do have difficulty, although for different reasons (101,259).

Medicare coverage for skilled nursing care is limited, and the uncertainties of coverage following hospitalization put nursing homes at financial risk. Extra nursing care needs and the requirement of copayment by the beneficiary[10] make many nursing homes reluctant to admit short-stay Medicare patients. Only about 5 percent of skilled nursing facility (SNF) industry revenues are from Medicare.

---

[10]Medicare does not pay for days in intermediate care facilities. Medicare covers 100 percent of the cost of care in skilled nursing facilities (SNFs) for a period of 20 days, and 50 percent of care between the 21st day and the 100th day. Medicare coverage ends after the 100th day. For most illnesses, 100 days is more than sufficient.

In contrast to Medicare coverage, Medicaid coverage is fairly comprehensive and predictable. However, the level of reimbursement is lower; States have chosen to hold down the costs of their Medicaid programs by reimbursing at a level such that the supply of beds is insufficient for the demand. Consequently the queue of Medicaid patients is permanent. This may allow discrimination among patients along dimensions such as race (215) or intensity of care required.

With the increased pressure for early discharge caused by PPS, there is danger of adverse effects on access for discharged Medicare and Medicaid patients. Nursing homes may continue to find short-term Medicare patients unattractive; alternatively, nursing homes may choose to serve the Medicare patients, thereby exacerbating access problems for the Medicaid population.

Access to care will be affected by more than the behavior of the nursing home industry. Most significant will be the potential for an increase in the provision of posthospital care (including nursing home and home health care) by hospitals. There are already indications that many hospitals will decide that the easiest way to handle the discharge problem is to provide such care themselves. Hospitals can also convert acute care beds to "extended care" beds (skilled or intermediate care levels) if they are approved by the State certificate-of-need program. The swing-bed program under Medicare allows small rural hospitals to provide skilled nursing level care to Medicare patients who would otherwise be discharged but have no access to an SNF bed (159). If these responses expand the supply of care sufficiently, access might even improve.

The distribution of cost is another matter for concern. Medicare coverage for nursing home care is significantly more limited than coverage for inpatient hospital care. Thus, substitution may shift costs from Medicare to patients and their families. To the extent that Medicare patients eventually become sufficiently impoverished to go on Medicaid, costs will be shifted to the State Medicaid programs.

Access for Veterans

One group of elderly persons, veterans of military service, has a separate legislated health care system in the VA. The VA provides hospital care and other medical services and supplies with the cost borne wholly by the Federal Government.[11] In 1980, 3 million veterans were over age 65, amounting to 12 percent of the population over age 65 (110). That percent will increase remarkably to 26 percent by the year 2000, before declining later. Under current eligibility rules for VA hospital care, veterans over age 65 do not have to meet criteria of "inability to pay" to qualify for care. Veterans with a service-connected disability have the highest priority for available resources, while other applicants are accepted on a "space available" basis.

Medicare's PPS may shift demand for services to the VA. The potential quantitative importance of such a shift is highlighted by data from a national mail survey of households conducted in 1977 (110). Of the estimated 3.3 million veterans hospitalized in non-VA hospitals, 18 percent were Medicare beneficiaries. These estimated 600,000 hospitalizations with a VA "option" represented about 2 percent of all hospitalizations.

The incentives provided by PPS for non-VA hospitals to cut services within DRGs, to transfer sicker patients to other hospitals, and to avoid admitting certain patients because of severity of illness, DRG classification, or other cost-based reasons is likely to increase the demand for VA hospital care. For example, hospitals that are good at determining the relative costliness of patients before admission would find patients' eligibility for VA care attractive for referral purposes or, after admission, for transfer purposes. Eligibility for VA care gives veterans greater access to some health care services than nonveterans. As long as they can afford it, however, patients will probably continue to prefer non-VA care.

The impact of a PPS-induced shift in the demand for VA care on VA expenditures will depend not only on the extent of the shift and the kinds of patients likely to seek VA care, but also on the response of the VA and Congress to these changes in demand. The VA operates under a national budget appropriation that is allocated by VA's central management among regions, districts, and facilities. If Congress responds to the increased demand for services with higher VA budgets, savings from PPS would be partially eroded. Congress could also change eligibility rules, including the priority ratings.

PPS may be less important to resulting patterns of VA utilization than specific budget legislation and internal policies. Evaluating access, then, must include studying changes in the amount of VA care sought by elderly veterans and the translation of that demand into actual utilization of VA services.

---

[11]The VA operates about 170 inpatient facilities dispersed throughout the nation with a total of nearly 90,000 hospital beds. In addition, ambulatory care, long-term care, drugs, mobility and sensory aids, and other related services are provided at no charge when appropriate and when available.

APPROACHES TO EVALUATING THE IMPACTS OF PPS ON EQUITY OF ACCESS

As noted earlier, equity of access to care cannot be measured directly. Rather, the nature of access must be inferred from measurement of certain indicators of potential (availability) and realized (utilization) access. A great deal of work has been done to define proxy measures of access, and several important empirical studies have attempted to measure access to care in the general population (4). The focus here, however, is on measures that directly relate to the *predicted impacts of PPS* on access to care for *Medicare beneficiaries*.

The remainder of this chapter, discusses the evaluation questions that stem from the predicted impacts of PPS on access. It also analyzes the available data sources for the studies that may provide the answers.

Critical Evaluation Questions

The previous discussion of potential impacts of PPS on access to health care raises the following five critical evaluation questions:

- How has PPS affected the availability of inpatient hospital care?
- How have interhospital transfers of Medicare patients changed since the implementation of PPS?
- Has PPS affected the utilization of inpatient care for vulnerable groups (e.g., alcoholic, mentally ill, disabled, or frail elderly patients)?
- How has PPS affected the availability and utilization of posthospital care for Medicare recipients?
- Has the demand for care in VA hospitals increased, and if so, has the increase resulted in longer waiting lists for medical attention?

Evaluating the Effects of PPS on the Availability of Inpatient Hospital Care

Measuring changes in the availability of inpatient hospital care is straightforward and relatively simple. Interpreting how changes in the availability of inpatient hospital care actually represent changes in access, however, is rather difficult. Nonetheless, studies that compare the availability of care before and after the implementation of Medicare's PPS could signal the possibility that PPS has changed access for specific vulnerable groups. Further studies could then be undertaken to quantify the access changes.

The availability of inpatient care refers both to the number of hospitals and hospital beds and to the number of specialized hospital services. With respect to hospitals and hospital beds, studies could examine the differences pre- and post-PPS in numbers of hospitals or beds by region, State, and county or by urban versus rural location. Because early analyses indicate that hospitals in the South and Northeast will tend to fare better than those in other regions, it is important to know that patients in the other regions will not suffer. Other possible studies include comparisons of the distribution of hospitals by size and by the characteristics of the patients they serve.

Even if there are no undesirable changes in the availability of hospital beds, the availability of specialized, high cost hospital services could change for some patients. Select services, such as burn units, intensive care units, and cardiac catheterization labs, could be studied for pre/post-PPS changes. Any changes discovered, however, could be the result of changes in policy or changes in technology that would have occurred even in the absence of PPS.

Evaluating Changes in Interhospital Transfers of Medicare Patients Under PPS

The incentive that PPS gives hospitals to transfer financially undesirable Medicare patients to other hospitals is strong enough to warrant studies of changes in transfer patterns before and after the inception of PPS. A study of whether the *number* of interhospital transfers has changed, however, provides little information on the *appropriateness* of the transfers: Are patients being transferred to receive better care or to relieve the hospital of financial burden?

The question of the appropriateness of transfers can be answered with most certainty by reviewing the medical records of samples of patients. But prior to such a time-consuming and expensive study, studies are needed to identify patterns of transfers that are likely to be inappropriate. An analysis of the medical, demographic, and socioeconomic characteristics of transferred patients could reveal whether specific groups of patients (e.g., income level, race, or type of illness) were transferred more frequently post-PPS than they were pre-PPS. Studies of the origins and destinations of interhospital transfers by type of hospital (e.g., public/private, teaching/nonteaching, urban/rural) could also provide insight into changes in transfer policies. If hospitals that serve a disproportionate share of indigent patients are constant recipients of transfers, it is likely that access to quality care will be compromised for the transferred patients. Classification of hospitals as "disproportionate share" hospitals is much more difficult than classification as "teaching" or "rural," however.

Evaluating the Effects of PPS on Utilization of Inpatient Care for Vulnerable Groups

As noted throughout this chapter, a particular access concern is the impact of PPS on specific vulnerable groups of patients, including (but not necessarily limited to) alcoholic, mentally ill, disabled, and frail elderly patients. Comparing their utilization of care pre- and post-PPS, as indicated by admission and use of special high cost services, is critical for evaluating the effects of PPS on access.

Although it is relatively easy to measure the admissions and special services used by any particular group, the identification of the members of that group is quite difficult. Some conditions, such as alcoholism or mental illness, carry so much stigma that these conditions are likely to be underreported. Furthermore, despite the importance of studies of known vulnerable populations, it is necessary to be aware that targeting evaluation efforts on groups currently thought to be particularly vulnerable may obscure the identification of other groups for which access problems due to PPS may develop. Problems reported anecdotally may be of some help in identifying any such groups.

Evaluating the Effects of PPS on the Availability and Utilization of Posthospital Care

There are three important types of studies that may measure changes in access to posthospital care. The first is to measure the number of SNF beds actually available to Medicare patients within Medicare-certified facilities. The second is to compare the pre- and post-PPS utilization of SNF days by Medicare beneficiaries, while the third is to compare utilization of home health services.

Interpreting changes in the availability and utilization of posthospital care with respect to changes in access is similar to interpreting changes in interhospital transfers—an increase or a decrease in availability or utilization says little about access to the *appropriate* level of care. In addition, policy changes that promote the use of posthospital care that have occurred independent of PPS make identification of access problems difficult. Patient-based studies of changes in the patterns of use of both hospital and posthospital services will be needed to identify PPS effects with greater accuracy. And, multiple investigator-initiated studies looking at these problems may provide the objectivity and informed judgment needed to interpret observed changes.

Evaluating Post-PPS Changes in the Utilization of Care for Veterans

Since a substantial proportion of veterans who are Medicare beneficiaries are hospitalized in non-VA hospitals, it is important to learn whether Medicare's PPS will increase demand for VA hospital care. The PPS incentives for hospitals to cut services within DRGs and to practice selective admissions are likely to result in decreased access to care for some veterans. Although veterans as a group have more access to some services than other groups, a change in the usual patterns of care may result in decreased access for some veterans. One measure of decreased access is longer VA waiting lists for medical attention. A comparison of pre-PPS waiting lists with post-PPS lists would be relatively easy and would provide the impetus for further investigation. A study of how many elderly veterans have been discharged by each facility in each DRG during the last 4 years —before and after PPS—would also indicate changes in access for veterans. Finally, a study of VA outpatient visits could be used to monitor the volume of care provided to elderly veterans and the mix of outpatient and inpatient care over time (110).

Data Sources

The major databases for the study of access to care fall into four groups: 1) data on the availability and distribution of care (e.g., hospitals and hospital beds, inpatient special services, nursing homes and nursing home beds, home health care agencies); 2) databases on utilization of care (e.g., Medicare program data, VA data, institution-based surveys of utilization); and 3) ongoing and special population-based interview surveys. Many of these are described in appendixes C, D, and E.

At the national level, there are several sources of data on the availability and distribution of health care services (see app. D). The best information on hospital characteristics comes from the American Hospital Association (AHA) Annual Survey of Hospitals. The best sources of data on other facilities, including SNFs and home health agencies, are the Medicare/Medicaid Provider of Services Master File or the national Master Facility Inventory of Hospitals and Institutions. State certificate-of-need databases give information on the numbers and types of facilities and services according to population needs. Of course, the information collected varies from State to State. In addition, periodic special surveys of staffing and equipment in hospitals provide evidence on the distribution of specialized facilities and procedures across hospitals.

The databases on the availability of services are generally excellent indicators of potential access. While the AHA Annual Survey of Hospitals must depend on individual institutions for supplying responses and is not purported to be an official and all-inclusive list of services offered by individual hospitals, it is in fact reasonably accurate and complete. Since data for the AHA survey, the Provider of Services Master File, and the Master Facility Inventory have been collected for a number of years, pre/post-PPS comparisons are possible.

Medicare's Part A claims file is the principal source of detailed information on the utilization of hospital, nursing home, and home health services by Medicare beneficiaries (see app. E). In addition, institution-based surveys conducted under the auspices of AHA and the Commission on Professional and Hospital Activities provide information on limited personal characteristics of patients as well as medical information on diagnoses, surgical procedures, other procedures, and length of stay for different diagnoses. AHA has done a special set of surveys on the relationship between the provision of medical care to the poor and uninsured and hospitals' financial status. It has also conducted a survey of discharge planning designed to provide a baseline before the implementation of PPS.

Data on availability and utilization of VA services are obtainable from the VA's central office as well as from individual facilities. Application forms become part of a patient's medical record at VA hospitals, but only monthly aggregates of some of the application data are available centrally. Currently, the aggregate data available for each VA facility include, among others: total applications; determinations of need for inpatient, ambulatory, or nursing home care; rejected applications; and service-connected disabilities. Unfortunately, age and DRG data are not included, but the samples are 100-percent samples (110).

Waiting list information is also available through the VA central office. The hospital inpatient activity code sheet is a monthly summary provided by each facility for each bed section that indicates the length of waiting lists for applicants, subdivided by service-connected disability and others, and further subdivided by whether they are waiting in another hospital or are waiting outside hospitals. Again, these data are not available by age of applicant (110). The most extensive data on VA hospital discharges are found in the Patient Treatment File. There is also a VA file containing a 20-percent sample of VA outpatient visits. The data in the VA outpatient file are inferior to the data in the Patient Treatment File in diagnostic detail.

Measures of the utilization of care are crude; they have traditionally been limited to simple aggregates of the number of physician visits or hospital bed-days for a group of people, without measures of variation in the intensity of resource use or other dimensions of care. Data on nursing home utilization are especially poor, because they provide no information on patient mix. Furthermore, comparing post-PPS aggregate statistics on Medicare program services utilization for any type of service (e.g., inpatient hospital care, skilled nursing care) with pre-PPS statistics offers little insight into the contribution of PPS due to Medicare policy changes that occurred simultaneously with the inception of PPS.

Population-based interview surveys conducted before and after PPS may be useful to identify some PPS effects with greater accuracy. The data are derived from direct interviews with individuals about their personal characteristics, their insurance coverage, and their use of care during a particular time period. Since they are population-based and periodic, these studies are useful for measuring changes in the amount of hospital care and types of hospitals used by the general population and by key subgroups both before and after PPS.

The most important population-based health care surveys are: 1) the National Survey of Access to Medical Care of the Center for Health

Administration Studies of the University of Chicago; 2) the Health Interview Survey of the National Center for Health Statistics; 3) the National Medical Care Utilization and Expenditure Survey (NMCUES) of the National Center for Health Statistics and HCFA; and 4) the National Medical Care Expenditure Survey (NMCES) of the National Center for Health Services Research (see app. C for a description of these surveys).

Information on the "quality" and "time and money costs" of care has improved considerably in recent years. Traditionally, studies of access emphasized only how much and what kinds of care people obtained, the distance traveled and time waited, and the presence or absence of insurance coverage. In particular, NMCES and NMCUES were important steps toward improving information about the financial burdens of obtaining medical care, although they need to be repeated if results are to be useful.

Overall, the routinely maintained databases on access can show up gross disparities in access to care. But when access becomes more equal, or when interest is focused on the finer points of access for particular high-risk subgroups, or for particular types of care, the routine data become seriously inadequate. Moreover, the need for greater conceptual clarity about what constitutes acceptable access becomes acute.

CONCLUSIONS

Evaluating the impact of PPS on access to health care is particularly important because Medicare's original purpose was to ensure access for its eligible population (100,186). This chapter has shown that PPS incentives could result in hospital behavior that affects access for both Medicare and non-Medicare patients.

Although it is difficult to define "access," clear measures of the volume, geographical distribution, and utilization of many types of health care services in a variety of settings (e.g., hospitals, SNFs) exist. These measures can be used as critical indicators of potential and realized access, but they have to be carefully interpreted. Several types of databases are available for measuring these indicators. Changes in access and equity of access can be evaluated using these data over time and across population groups.

Monitoring changes in access to health care or differences among groups of people in access may identify new equity of access problems or better quantify old ones. Verifying the existence of an access problem may prove easier than determining whether the problem is old or new and, if new, to what extent it may be attributed to PPS. Yet, it may not be as important to know the answer to the latter question as it is to solve equity of access problems. The critical issue becomes whether or not PPS as currently structured can solve the problems, and if not, what changes need to be made.

Chapter 8
Technological Change

Contents

	Page
Introduction	113
Potential Impacts of PPS on Technological Change	113
Potential PPS Impacts on Six Emerging Technologies	113
General Impacts of PPS on Technological Change	120
Impacts of PPS Structure on Technological Change: Updating, Recalibration, and Coding	121
Approaches to Evaluating the Impacts of PPS on Technological Change	124
Critical Evaluation Questions	124
Impact Measures	124
Organizational Arrangements for Evaluating PPS Impacts	125
Conclusions	126

Chapter 8
Technological Change

INTRODUCTION

The effects of Medicare's prospective payment system (PPS) on the three critical aspects of health care previously discussed in this report—cost, quality, and access—depend to a large extent on its effects on the use of medical technologies[1] and, more generally, on the process of technological change in medicine. The decision to develop or use one technology rather than another affects the availability of their benefits to patients and the level of health care costs to payers.

The process of technological change occurs in two stages (27). The first stage—research and development (R&D)—includes three phases:

- *Basic research*—original investigation whose objective is to gain knowledge or understanding of the fundamental aspects of phenomena and of observable facts without specific applications in mind (368).
- *Applied research*—investigation whose objective is to gain knowledge or understanding necessary for determining the means by which a recognized and specific need may be met (368).

[1]Medical technologies, as defined by OTA, are the drugs, devices, medical, and surgical procedures used in medical care, and the organizational and supportive systems in which such care is provided (304).

- *Development*—systematic use of the knowledge or understanding gained from research in the design and development of prototypes and processes (315).

The second stage—the diffusion of a medical technology into the health care system—has two phases: the initial phase in which decisions are made to adopt (or reject) the technology, and a subsequent phase in which decisions are made to use the technology (27). Decisions regarding the *adoption* of a medical technology require that knowledge about the technology be communicated to physicians, hospital administrators, and purchasing departments. *Use* of the technology, once acquired, depends on such factors as medical indications, physician training, concerns about malpractice suits, the organization of medical care, and payment for medical services (27).

Technological change, in health care or in any other field, is influenced by a wide variety of economic, social, and organizational conditions. The individual effects of each are difficult to separate, and the effects of Medicare payment policies are similarly difficult to distinguish. The purpose of this chapter is to discuss strategies for evaluating the effects of Medicare's diagnosis-related group (DRG) based PPS on technological change in medicine.

POTENTIAL IMPACTS OF PPS ON TECHNOLOGICAL CHANGE

Potential PPS Impacts on Six Emerging Technologies

As a prelude to the discussion of the way in which the development, adoption, and use of technologies can affect, and be affected by, Medicare's DRG-based PPS, this section describes six emerging technologies and the manner in which they interact with PPS:

- extracorporeal shock wave lithotripsy (ESWL),
- percutaneous transluminal coronary angioplasty (PTCA),
- implantable infusion pumps,
- intraocular lenses (IOLs),
- therapeutic drug monitoring, and
- thrombolytic therapy for acute myocardial infarction.

These technologies illustrate the variety of ways in which PPS must adapt to the introduction of new technologies and some of the dilemmas the system must face. They also illustrate the potential effect of DRG payment levels and classification methods on the adoption or abandonment of technologies.

Extracorporeal Shock Wave Lithotripsy

ESWL is a recently developed method of breaking up kidney stones through the use of shock waves, without a surgical incision (344). The lithotripter used in this procedure was developed by Dornier Systems of West Germany and is currently manufactured only by this company. Because of its extensive development abroad, this device arrived virtually full-fledged on the American market. It was approved by the Food and Drug Administration (FDA) in December 1984 (343), and Medicare coverage followed shortly thereafter (285). FDA approval of the Dornier lithotripter is only for upper urinary stones, although ESWL has the potential to be used for lower urinary stones and gallstones in the near future. These uses would greatly expand the market for the technology.

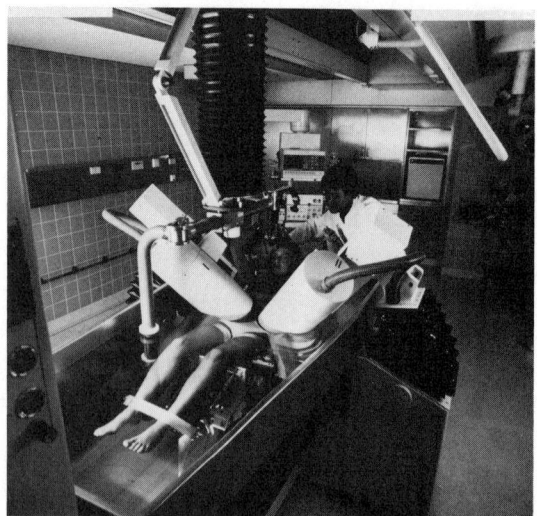

Photo credit: Dornier Medical Systems, Inc., Marietta, GA

The extracorporeal shock wave lithotripter breaks up kidney stones through the use of shock waves, without a surgical incision. Dornier Systems of West Germany developed the device and is currently its only manufacturer.

Because of its noninvasive nature, the Dornier lithotripter is being considered by some hospitals for use on outpatients who can be available for pre- and post-procedure observation and testing. Even for inpatients, the hospitalization time for ESWL is less than that for alternative minor surgery procedures and about one-third that for major kidney stone surgery (6). The Dornier lithotripter is expensive to purchase, but if used to capacity (treating over 1,000 patients per year), it can lower overall hospital costs.

The dilemma that has surrounded ESWL and PPS concerns the manner in which the procedure should be coded into a DRG. Since ESWL is a new technology, there is no procedure code specifically intended for it in the International Classification of Diseases, 9th Revision, Clinical Modification (ICD-9-CM) (see box 8-A). During the brief investigational stage of the technology in the United States, the American Hospital Association (AHA) recommended that hospitals simply choose a code that was agreeable to any third-party payers covering the procedure (65). Now, for the purposes of Medicare reimbursement, hospitals must assign ESWL the same code as ultrasonic lithotripsy (59.95), the only procedure code available in the present ICD-9-CM coding system that represents stone disintegration. This code, when reported without a corresponding code for a surgical incision or other invasive procedure,[2] results in a patient's assignment to DRG #323 or #324, the medical DRGs for urinary stone treatment.

ESWL highlights the problems with using the ICD-9-CM coding system, designed for clinical and statistical purposes, as a basis for payment. It also illustrates the problem with basing the amount of the payment on a distinction between medical and surgical procedures. If ESWL were classified into a surgical rather than a medical DRG, payment for the procedure under PPS would approximately double.[3] If no other decision factors were involved, the low payment level

---

[2] Normally, the code for ultrasonic lithotripsy is used in conjunction with a code for incision, indicating a minor surgical ("percutaneous") procedure in which an ultrasonic lithotripter, a small endoscopic device, is used to fragment the stone before removal. Use of a code for incision as well as lithotripsy results in a higher paying surgical DRG assignment.

[3] A third longer term alternative for ESWL under PPS is the creation of a new code and a new DRG for the procedure.

for ESWL might discourage some hospitals from adopting the technology or from using it for Medicare patients. (Of course, a low level of payment might prevent overpurchase of the lithotripters as well.)

However, the level of DRG payment is only one of several economic factors that will help determine whether the technology is adopted, whether Medicare patients have access to it, and whether outpatient ESWL becomes common. The contemplated incorporation of capital costs into DRG payments and of outpatient services into PPS will be of equal or greater importance, because the main financial impact of the lithotripter is the initial $2 million capital cost of its installation. And in the end, factors such as non-Medicare reimbursement for the procedure and the attractiveness of ESWL to patients may well overshadow all Medicare effects on the diffusion of this technology into the health care system.

Percutaneous Transluminal Coronary Angioplasty[4]

PTCA is a technique developed to mechanically open coronary blood vessels affected by arteriosclerosis, a disease commonly known as "hardening of the arteries." It has excited interest because the only other widely available means of treating this kind of arterial obstruction, aside from medical treatment, has been coronary bypass surgery, an expensive procedure.

PTCA is suitable for only a small subset of patients with coronary artery disease. However, the treatment is successful in restoring blood flow in the arteries of over half the patients that receive it, and success rates rise considerably with appropriate patient selection and increasing experience of the person performing the procedure (124,163,200).

The overwhelming advantage PTCA holds over bypass surgery is its substantially lower cost. A study of 11 institutions across the country found that the average charge for PTCA (and the associated hospital stay) was approximately one-half to one-third that for coronary bypass surgery (153). Another study at a single institution compared long-run charges of the two procedures (242). It found that even considering complications and the need for follow-up procedures (PTCA or surgical) in many of the PTCA patients, total expenditures for angioplasty were 15 percent lower after 1 year than total expenditures for bypass surgery.

Under current coding conventions, PTCA performed as the principal procedure on a patient places that patient in a high-paying surgical DRG, #108. Because this DRG also includes many more costly surgical procedures, it is likely to reward hospitals that perform PTCA. This apparently generous payment for PTCA has led both the Inspector General's Office and the Prospective Payment Assessment Commission (ProPAC) to recommend that the procedure be reclassified into a lower paying surgical DRG, #112 (238). In order for such a reclassification to take place, the computer program used by Medicare intermediaries to assign DRGs must be updated. In the interim, as the Health Care Financing Administration (HCFA) implementation the recommendation, fiscal intermediaries must be instructed to flag the ICD-9-CM code that includes the PTCA procedure; to check with the hospital to see if the procedure performed was actually PTCA; and to assign the lower paying DRG in the event that the procedure was PTCA (238).

Other economic factors besides the level of DRG payment affect incentives to perform PTCA. For instance, if PTCA is unsuccessful, bypass surgery may still be necessary. If the bypass surgery must be performed during the same hospital stay, the hospital will get paid only the DRG rate associated with the surgery. This incentive should generally work in a positive direction, since hospitals that have the highest success rates with PTCA have the greatest incentive to use the technology.

Implantable Infusion Pump[5]

The implantable infusion pump was developed to allow delivery of a drug at a constant flow rate

---

[4]This discussion is based on N.R. Powe, "Percutaneous Transluminal Coronary Angioplasty: Efficacy, Cost, and Effects of Prospective Payment," prepared for the Office of Technology Assessment, U.S. Congress, Washington, DC, July 1985.

[5]This discussion is based on S. Yavner, D. Yavner, and S.N. Finklestein, "Medical Technology and DRGs: The Case of the Implantable Infusion Pump," prepared for the Office of Technology Assessment, U.S. Congress, Washington, DC, December 1984.

The implantable infusion pump allows the constant delivery of a drug to a selected site in the body.

to a selected site in the body. Continuous fixed-rate drug delivery is medically desirable for treating a variety of clinical conditions, including diabetes and cancer. The implantable infusion pump permits stable circulating drug levels, and it allows high concentrations of a drug to be delivered directly to a specific site without harmful effects on other parts of the body. Furthermore, it has the potential to eliminate prolonged hospitalization and problems associated with external pumps and catheterization systems.

One manufacturer, Infusaid, currently has FDA approval for several implantable pump models to be used for infusion of heparin, morphine, and three anticancer drugs. Medicare approved coverage for the implantable pump in September 1984, but coverage is limited to use for cancer chemotherapy (331).

The full cost implications of the implantable pump are still unclear. At present, the pump appears to be cheaper per year than traditional chemotherapy, primarily because users have shorter hospital stays. However, the cost of the initial surgical implantation of the implantable pump is considerable. Thus, despite its potential quality advantages, the implantable pump appears to be more expensive than externally worn infusion pumps.

Since the implantable pump has a variety of current and potential applications, its use may place a patient in any of several DRGs. To further complicate DRG assignment, there is no single code that adequately represents the surgical implantation of the pump, its major cost. And if the primary procedure is coded as "infusion," the patient is placed into a medical DRG with a low payment rate, rather than a surgical DRG with a higher one. There is apparently a great deal of confusion among hospitals about what codes are appropriate at present. Given these ambiguities, PPS cost-minimizing incentives will probably act to inhibit rather than encourage widespread adoption of the implantable pump as standard therapy for its many potential uses.

Intraocular Lenses[6]

IOLs, lenses that are implanted directly in the eye to replace a natural lens, have become the preferred method of restoring sight to patients after cataract surgery. The alternatives, contact lenses or glasses, are considered less desirable for most patients because of inadequate vision correction or difficulty in handling and wearing contact lenses (10).

Although IOLs have been available since the 1970s, improvements in the lenses themselves and in the surgical procedure to implant them have only recently made them the treatment of choice for most cataract patients. The number of IOLs implanted per year nearly tripled between 1980 and 1983 (227), and more than 80 percent of patients now receive IOLs after cataract extraction (238).

IOLs are thus an example of a technology, recently established as a standard procedure, that is both cost-raising and quality-enhancing compared to the alternatives. The current reimbursement for DRG #39 (lens procedures) is based par-

---

[6]This discussion is based on M.E. Farber, "DRG Payment and Medical Technology: DRG 39," prepared for the Office of Technology Assessment, U.S. Congress, Washington, DC, December 1985.

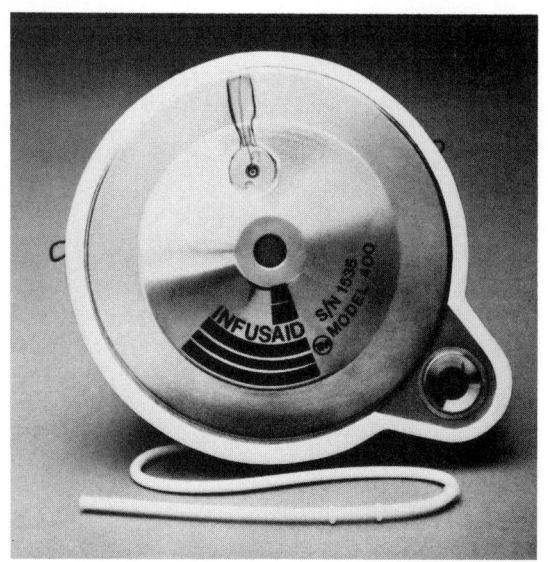

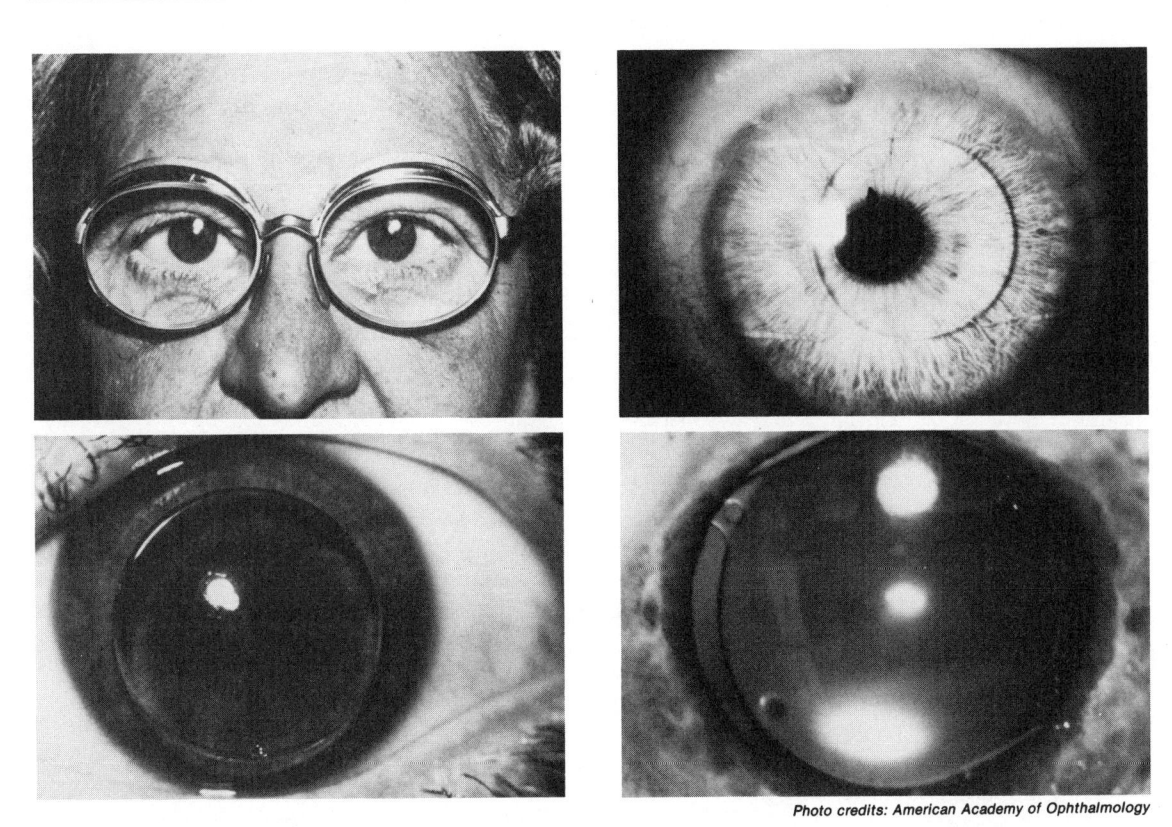

After cataract surgery, sight may be restored by the use of glasses, contact lenses, or intraocular lenses implanted in front of or behind the iris. Since the early 1980s, intraocular lenses have been the preferred method.

Photo credits: American Academy of Ophthalmology

tially on the costs of normal cataract surgery at the time DRGs were created, before IOL implantation became standard procedure. Nonetheless, the benefits of IOLs were well established at the outset of PPS, and the new payment system is unlikely to hinder their diffusion or lead to their abandonment.

Changes in cataract surgery other than an increase in IOL use have also occurred. The most notable from the perspective of PPS are, first, that hospital average length of stay (ALOS) for cataract surgery patients has decreased by nearly one-third since 1981 (238); and second, that there has been a trend from inpatient to hospital outpatient and nonhospital sites as the setting in which cataract surgery is performed (10). Recalibration of DRG weights (see p. 121) will probably serve to account for both the inclusion of IOLs and the shorter ALOS of cataract surgery. However, PPS may well affect the setting in which surgery takes place.

The magnitude of the effect of Medicare policies on the trend away from inpatient cataract surgery depends on three factors: 1) the effect of PPS financial incentives on hospitals; 2) the effect of Medicare outpatient reimbursement incentives on hospitals, physicians, and beneficiaries; and 3) the effectiveness of utilization and quality control peer review organizations (PROs) in monitoring hospital inpatient admissions for cataract surgery.

The effect of PPS financial incentives on hospitals is simple and depends only on whether the hospital's costs of treating a particular inpatient are higher or lower than the DRG payment.

The effect of outpatient reimbursement incentives is more complex. Hospitals that perform cataract surgery on outpatients are reimbursed by Medicare for all reasonable costs of surgery (Public Law 96-499). Thus, whenever inpatient costs for cataract surgery exceed the DRG payment rate, hospitals have an incentive to provide the surgery in an outpatient setting. Physicians who accept assignment[7] are reimbursed by Medicare for 100 percent of their reasonable charges for performing cataract surgery in hospital outpatient or freestanding ambulatory surgical settings, but only 80 percent of charges for cataract surgery performed in hospital inpatient or physician's office settings (47 FR 34082). Thus, many physicians also have an incentive to perform the procedure in outpatient settings (other than the office).

Many PROs are monitoring hospital admissions for cataract surgery. To the extent that it is effective, PRO monitoring may prevent admissions of low-risk cataract patients that would otherwise be DRG "winners" for the hospital.

The magnitude of the net effect of the three factors just discussed depends on how they ultimately balance out. The direction of that effect, however, will almost certainly be to continue the trend to outpatient cataract surgery.

Therapeutic Drug Monitoring[8]

For certain medications, standard drug dosage regimens have different effects in different individuals. Some patients may respond well to the drug, while others receiving the same dosage have a subtherapeutic or a toxic response. One way to minimize such variability in patient response is to monitor the concentration of the drug in the patient's blood serum. This technique is known as therapeutic drug monitoring (TDM).

TDM has become accepted practice for a variety of drugs.[9] The assumption behind the technique is that there is a correlation between the concentration of the drug in the blood and its concentration in the tissue where the drug exerts its therapeutic effect. Combined with supporting clinical signs, too high a drug level in the blood indicates toxicity, while too low a level suggests a subtherapeutic response. The drugs particularly suited to TDM are drugs for which the toxic dose is quite close to the therapeutic dose, whose effect is difficult to detect, or for which there is some other strong reason for desiring rapid, detectable response to the drug (390).

The recent rapid growth in demand for TDM has been a result of both major advances in automated equipment and the growth of the clinical pharmacist profession, which has had a symbiotic relationship with TDM. The technology has aroused interest because of a number of anticipated positive effects on the cost and quality of medical care. These include reduced length of hospital stay; reduced drug-related toxic complications; prevention of hospitalization through outpatient monitoring; and improved outcome in cases where TDM enables the use of more aggressive antibiotic therapy.

PPS has the potential to significantly affect the use of TDM, particularly since the variety of drugs that can be monitored means that a number of DRGs are involved. Some of the effects may encourage use. Cost-containment incentives may encourage greater appropriateness of TDM testing, since such improvements could reduce laboratory costs associated with misleading or unneccesary testing. They could also reduce costs associated with toxicity or subtherapeutic responses due to dosage decisions based on improper samples. To the extent that the cost of improved testing is less than the savings it generates, PPS should encourage more of this kind of testing. It will also probably encourage the trend toward smaller, more efficient, less labor-intensive equipment.

Other effects of PPS may depress TDM use. For instance, the use of TDM does improve outcome in burn patients, but the improvement comes at a financial cost to the institution (40). PPS is unlikely to bring the use of TDM in such cases to a halt, but it may well lead to a decrease in the intensity of its use. It may also discourage the

---

[7]A physician who accepts assignment for a Medicare claim agrees not to bill the beneficiary for any amount over and above the beneficiary's required coinsurance and deductible (where applicable) of the Medicare-determined reasonable charge for that service.

[8]This discussion is based on J.T. Barr, "The Interaction of Therapeutic Drug Monitoring and DRG Payment Levels," prepared for the Office of Technology Assessment, U.S. Congress, Washington, DC, Nov. 16, 1984.

[9]The drugs for which TDM is being used include antiepileptics; cardiac active agents; antibiotics; antiasthmatics; antidepressants; neuroleptics; anticoagulants; immunosuppressants; and antineoplastics.

expansion of TDM methods to new drugs, where instituting drug monitoring is likely to increase overall costs, at least in the first stages of its diffusion.

Thrombolytic Therapy for Acute Myocardial Infarction[10]

An acute myocardial infarction, one form of heart attack, occurs when blood flow to the heart muscles is cut off, causing damage to the heart tissue. This condition occurs most often when a coronary artery is blocked by a thrombus, or blood clot. The development of thrombolytic agents to dissolve these clots has recently received much attention as a way of treating acute myocardial infarction before it has advanced far enough to cause permanent damage to the heart. Restoration of blood flow, of course, does not solve the underlying problem that caused the blockage in the first place. An acute myocardial infarction patient is a likely candidate for procedures such as coronary bypass surgery or PTCA.

Streptokinase, the first thrombolytic agent to be developed, received FDA approval in 1982 (365). Several clinical trials have demonstrated that streptokinase does indeed restore blood flow within a short time. However, it is less well established that restoration of blood flow (which may be temporary) actually decreases overall mortality in patients with myocardial infarction (165, 244), and so far, OHTA has recommended against Medicare coverage (365).

Streptokinase is not the only promising technology for acute myocardial infarction patients. Urokinase (a close relative), acylated streptokinase-plasmin, and prourokinase are all potentially useful thrombolytic agents (172). The alternative arousing the most interest at present, however, is genetically engineered tissue-type plasminogen activator, which acts more specifically on the clot than streptokinase. Early clinical trial results (372) suggest that it has great potential for use as an "easily administered, rapidly effective, and highly specific thrombolytic agent" (172).

There are two possible methods of administration for thrombolytic drugs: intracoronary, in which the drug is injected directly into the coronary artery; and intravenous, in which it is injected into a peripheral vein and carried in the bloodstream to the heart. Intracoronary administration has been shown to be more effective in clinical trials of streptokinase, but because it requires cardiac catheterization the drug cannot usually be administered immediately. Intravenous administration has great advantages in that it can be initiated immediately after the onset of acute myocardial infarction, in an ambulance or even at home, and it costs less because it requires fewer laboratory resources and less highly trained personnel. It can also be used in hospitals that do not have cardiac catheterization facilities. In fact, a primary reason for the excitement about tissue-type plasminogen activatior is that because of its specificity for the clot, it is more effective than streptokinase when administered intravenously (372).

Intracoronary and intravenous methods of administration could result in the same DRG assignment, unless HCFA specifies otherwise when a decision to cover thrombolytic drugs is made in the future. Regardless of the method used, the administration of a thrombolytic drug can logically be coded under ICD-9-CM as 36.0, removal of coronary artery obstruction, and 99.29, injection of a therapeutic substance. The presence of code 36.0 as the principal procedure, in turn, places a patient in DRG #108, a highly weighted surgical DRG. If hospitals anticipate coding all uses of thrombolytic drugs into the same DRG, PPS incentives will favor both use of the lowest cost method of administration and the development of the least costly of the alternative drugs. At the same time, the generous payment that could result from use of thrombolytic therapy would encourage the adoption and use of the technology in general. (If the use of thrombolytic therapy did not "upcode" a patient into a higher paying DRG, PPS incentives to adopt it would depend on whether it lowers costs of treating patients.)

---

[10]This discussion is based on J.B. Perkins, "Streptokinase Treatment for Acute Myocardial Infarction and the DRG Payment System," prepared for the Office of Technology Assessment, U.S. Congress, Washington, DC, Dec. 14, 1984.

General Impacts of PPS on Technological Change

PPS was never intended to affect uniformly the vast range of medical technologies. An expected outcome of per-case payment was to encourage the development and diffusion of cost-saving technologies and to discourage the use of cost-raising ones (305).

Payment effects on R&D are indirect and come about largely through changes in market signals to manufacturers of drugs and devices. To the extent that PPS affects the incentives for purchasers to adopt new technologies, it also affects the incentives of producers to develop them. This is particularly true in the later phases of R&D—applied research and development—when the medical potential of a new technology is becoming realized and its market potential is under investigation. PPS puts pressure on manufacturers to develop products that will be profitable to hospitals under the new set of constraints and opportunities.

Incentives to manufacturers affect not only the subject areas of research and the number of new products developed but also the form those developments take. A change in the number of new technologies produced does not necessarily mean an equal change in productivity. A decrease in the number of new technologies introduced on the market, for instance, could mean that manufacturers are directing their R&D resources toward a few potential "breakthrough" technologies rather than toward many minor modifications of existing ones. Similarly, an apparent increase in new technologies could mean more models of existing equipment rather than more significant innovations.

Hospitals face direct incentives under per-case payment to adopt and use lower cost technologies. All else equal, these incentives act to encourage the adoption and use of technologies in the hospital that:

- decrease per-case operating costs compared to alternative technologies;
- increase hospital admissions for simple procedures in profitable DRGs that otherwise might be done on an outpatient basis;
- are highly visible, attracting patient admissions and filling hospital beds.

All of these generalizations hold true for any particular technology only if the gains are not offset by other costs or by lower payment. If use of a new technology leads to classification of a case into a lower paying DRG, PPS may not encourage its diffusion even if it lowers operating costs.

The incentives regarding the use and adoption of new technology under PPS frequently conflict or produce unanticipated results because of other artifacts of PPS. The Dornier lithotripter, for instance, is very expensive, and its classification into a low-paying DRG may result in little or no profit per case. Yet PPS is unlikely to hinder its diffusion; the lithotripter is immensely attractive to patients, and the current passthrough for capital expenses under PPS means that the major cost of the lithotripter need not enter into per-case decisions.[11]

For experimental technologies, the ultimate effects of PPS on diffusion are particularly hard to determine because judgments about long-term costs and benefits must be made prospectively. For instance, hospitals are likely to be reluctant to adopt an expensive first-generation new technology if a cheaper second-generation model is expected. A technology that has long-run cost saving potential may be discouraged in the early stages of technological diffusion, when costs are higher and benefits less certain (23); costly but quality-enhancing technologies, which tend to be discouraged by PPS in any case, are particularly susceptible to such uncertainties.

Thrombolytic drugs and implantable infusion pumps are two examples of the way PPS may affect experimental technologies. The current coding convention for use of thrombolytic drugs might (once Medicare covered such drugs) result in the assignment of a patient receiving throm-

---

[11]At present (August 1985), capital costs (depreciation and interest) are reimbursed as incurred—a cost "passthrough"—in the same manner as before PPS. Congress has expressed an intention to include payment for capital by 1987 as part of the prospective payment rate and several alternatives have been proposed, but no specific method has yet been selected. The present cost-based method of capital payment is inefficient because hospitals have little incentive to consider the full costs of capital acquisitions (new plant, renovations, and equipment). Of particular concern is the incentive to adopt expensive capital equipment that reduces operating costs but raises total cost per case. Given no change in the current system, hospitals can be expected over time to become too capital-intensive (305).

bolytic therapy to a high-paying DRG, and consequently R&D on these drugs promises to be a highly lucrative investment under per-case payment. The implantable infusion pump, however, has uncertain cost advantages, particularly in its investigational phase. As long as physicians remain ambivalent about the benefits of the pump, PPS may have a depressing effect on its development and adoption, and even on the opportunities to demonstrate its benefits.

Non-PPS incentives compete with PPS incentives to further complicate the picture of PPS effects. Physician preference and belief in the benefits of IOLs, for instance, is strong enough that eyeglasses and contact lenses are unlikely to become the norm again after cataract surgery, despite their cost advantages. On the other hand, it is unclear whether the benefits of TDM to patients are great enough to result in its expansion to new drugs where it may initially increase hospital costs.

Impacts of PPS Structure on Technological Change: Updating, Recalibration, and Coding

The previous discussion illustrates the variety of ways PPS incentives can interact and the difficulty of generalizing about the net effects on any specific technology. It also draws attention to two very strong effects of the structure of PPS on technological change: 1) the impact of pricing changes that take place through updating and recalibration of the PPS base price and DRG weights; and 2) the effect of the coding system used to categorize patients (through the use of technologies) into DRGs.

Since the price paid for a DRG is the primary mechanism through which Medicare's PPS affects the adoption, abandonment, and site of use of technologies within that DRG, the methods of determining that price and of associating it with the use of a particular technology are of critical importance. The impact of the current mechanism for updating and recalibrating the DRG system and the effect of using the IDC-9-CM coding system to classify new drug- and device-embodied procedures are discussed below.

The legislation creating PPS allowed for two methods of changing DRG prices that consider technological change: updating and recalibration. *Updating* consists of an annual increase (or decrease) in all prices by an *update factor* that determines the overall generosity of the system. The update factor has two components. The first component reflects the amount of inflation in the hospital sector. The second component, known as the "discretionary adjustment factor," accounts for cost increases (or decreases)[12] that are not necessarily captured by inflation measures, such as those due to changes in quality of care. This second component can also be used to account for the introduction of new cost-raising technologies in general, but because it raises the levels of payment for all DRGs simultaneously it cannot ensure that any particular new technology will be encouraged relative to its alternatives. The discretionary adjustment factor was originally set at 1 percent per year but was later limited by Congress to 0.25 percent for fiscal years 1985 and 1986. ProPAC has recommended to HCFA a 1-percent decrease, rather than an increase, for the discretionary component of the update factor for 1986, though the Commission did recommend an increase in the update factor overall (236).

The process of adjusting the prices of DRGs relative to each other, through changes in DRG weights,[13] is known as *recalibration*. This adjustment allows the price paid to a hospital for a DRG to stay approximately equal to the average costs of a patient within that DRG. Since the introduction of new technologies can change the costs of treating patients within a particular DRG, this adjustment ensures that those new costs will lead to a new price. The incentives to adopt new technologies, especially cost-raising ones, are strongly affected by the manner in which recalibration takes place.

Recalibration may take a number of forms.[14] Recalibration of all 468 DRGs can be done simultaneously in a statistical and reactive manner, through empirical reestimation of relative DRG

---
[12]In theory, the discretionary adjustment factor, the inflation factor, and the entire update factor could all be negative rather than positive.
[13]The weight assigned a DRG represents its assumed resource use relative to other DRGs. The higher the weight, the larger the Medicare payment is.
[14]ProPAC's definition of "recalibration," in contrast to that given here, includes only the simultaneous adjustment of all DRG weights. The adjustment of only certain DRG weights is called "reweighting" (237).

costs. It can be done as part of a central policy decision to change relative rates, where some DRG weights would be raised (or lowered) relative to the others to encourage (or discourage) use of particular technologies within those DRGs. It can also include mechanisms such as the creation of new DRGs as a way of paying a hospital only if it is using a particular technology (307).

The original PPS legislation required recalibration of DRG weights at least every 4 years (Public Law 98-21), and annual recalibration has been suggested by at least one observer (287). ProPAC is responsible for making recommendations to HCFA regarding updating and recalibration changes and has a charge to pay particular attention to new technologies when undertaking such matters. The ultimate authority for setting DRG prices, however, rests with the Secretary of the Department of Health and Human Services.

Coding issues are somewhat different from updating and recalibration issues because the PPS legislation did not establish any mechanism or specific authority for dealing with them. They were a largely unexpected complication of using the DRG classification system, and they can arbitrarily help or hinder the diffusion of a technology without regard to its actual benefits or detriments. Code assignment affects the incentives for adoption of a technology because the code assigned to a new procedure determines which DRG a patient is placed in when that procedure is used, and thus it determines the final payment level (see box 8-A).

Code assignment is a significant factor in four of the six technologies examined above: ESWL, PTCA, thrombolytic therapy, and the implantable infusion pump. In each of these four cases, a new technology is accompanied by a new procedure for which there is no directly applicable procedure code.

This situation presents two problems. First, until very recently, there has been no established mechanism for creating new codes except during the periodic updating of the coding system, once every 10 years (50 FR 24374). Second, the use of ICD-9-CM as the basis for payment means that interim coding assignments for new technologies must consider not only which code describes the procedure the most closely for statistical purposes, but also which code leads to an appropriate reimbursement level. These two objectives may be inconsistent. In the past, most controversies regarding proper coding for procedures (or diagnoses) have been resolved by experts at AHA, with the support of other professional organizations and the National Center for Health Statistics (NCHS). This arrangement is now complicated by HCFA's direct interest in how procedures are being coded for payment purposes, which may conflict with the interests of both AHA and NCHS.

PTCA provides an interesting example of how this dilemma is being resolved by HCFA. PTCA has been assigned the code that most closely describes it (36.0, "Removal of Coronary Obstruction"). However, the DRG assignment based on this code leads to a payment for the procedure that ProPAC considers inappropriately high, and that Commission has recommended classification of the procedure into a lower paying DRG (237). HCFA agrees with this recommendation and intends to implement it in the upcoming revised GROUPER, the computerized DRG classification system (50 FR 24370). Meanwhile, however, it must instruct Medicare intermediaries to check with the hospital every time that code 36.0 appears to determine whether the code actually represents a PTCA procedure or not. This method could be very cumbersome if many cases or many codes are involved.

ICD-9-CM coding is not the only coding system used in the United States. Physicians' reimbursement under Medicare Part B, for instance, uses a variant of the Current Procedure Terminology, 4th Edition (CPT-4), an annually updated system that codes procedures performed by physicians. CPT-4 is more detailed at coding procedures in most cases than ICD-9, making it possible to "map" one set of codes onto the other for data comparisons. In some cases, however, data from the two coding systems are incompatible.

Box 8-A —ICD-9-CM Codes and DRGs

The diagnosis-related groups used as the patient classification system in Medicare's PPS are based on a coding system known as the International Classification of Diseases, 9th Revision, Clinical Modification (ICD-9-CM). The ICD-9-CM has two parts. The first and largest part is a comprehensive list of diseases with corresponding codes. This is compatible with the World Health Organization's (WHO) list of disease codes, maintained for statistical purposes, and is updated along with the WHO list every 10 years. The second part of ICD-9-CM is a list of procedure codes. These are independent of the disease codes and are not directly based on an international system, although in the past, they have been revised concurrently with the disease codes. The National Center for Health Statistics (NCHS) is the official WHO coding liaison in the United States, but the development and maintenance of the American version of ICD has historically been a cooperative effort of representatives from a variety of Federal agencies and professional organizations (129).

Both the disease and procedure codes in ICD-9-CM are organized according to organ system (circulatory system, digestive system, etc.), with additional sections for subjects such as infectious diseases and accidental injury. Diseases are assigned three-digit codes, with fourth and occasionally fifth digits available to allow more specificity. Thus, for instance, hereditary anemia is code 282; sickle-cell anemia, one type of hereditary anemia, is code 282.6; and the particular form called sickle-cell/Hb-C disease is further specified as code 282.63. The procedure codes are organized in a fashion similar to the disease codes, except that maximum specificity is reached at four digits rather than five.

The process of DRG assignment depends on both the disease and procedure codes. The disease code for the principal diagnosis places the patient in a major diagnostic category and indicates which of several DRGs might be appropriate. The code for the principal procedure (or its absence) is used to determine whether the appropriate DRG is a medical or a surgical one. Surgical DRGs generally have higher reimbursement rates than medical ones. The final choice of DRG then depends on the specific procedure performed, the patient's age, and the presence or absence of coexisting diseases and complications.

The ICD-9-CM coding system, designed for clinical and statistical purposes, presents several problems when used as a basis for payment (129,152,273). First, if inaccurate or inadequate coding was frequent when the DRGs were designed, many hospital cases may have been inaccurately classified; consequently, the DRG weights may be inaccurate themselves. Second, some medical conditions can be described by more than one diagnostic code (152). While any of several diagnoses may be technically correct, their associated codes lead to different DRGs with different weights.

A third major concern regards the procedure codes. Procedures utilizing new technologies may not be appropriately described by any of the current codes, and confusion about which code to use can lead to wide variation in DRG assignment. The code that seems most applicable may lead to an apparently inappropriate DRG; conversely, a DRG with an apparently appropriate payment rate may be based on codes entirely unfitting to the new technology. Coding consultants at the American Hospital Association (AHA) and the Commission on Professional and Hospital Activities (CPHA) help to reduce confusion and promote coding uniformity, but through mid-1985, coding decisions for major problematic technologies have been made by an informal group of representatives from the Health Care Financing Administration (HCFA), NCHS, and several professional groups (notably AHA, CPHA, and the American Medical Records Association). A formal ongoing coding recommendations task force, jointly chaired by NCHS and HCFA, is currently being established (50 FR 24374).

APPROACHES TO EVALUATING THE IMPACTS OF PPS ON TECHNOLOGICAL CHANGE

Critical Evaluation Questions

There are two fundamental questions regarding PPS and technological change. First, how does PPS affect the kinds of technologies available to Medicare patients? And second, how does PPS affect the process of technological development and diffusion?

These can be restated as a number of more specific questions, such as the following:

- How does PPS affect the extent and direction of R&D that underlies technological change?
- How does PPS affect the development and diffusion of technologies that lower total Medicare costs? That lower health system costs?
- How does PPS affect the diffusion of cost-raising but quality-enhancing technologies?
- How does PPS affect the use of technologies that lower quality of health care relative to alternative technologies available?

None of these questions deals with the ultimate benefits and costs of any particular change due to PPS. That question must be addressed in the policy arena because its answer necessarily implies two judgments: one about the value of particular areas of R&D, and the other about the value of technological change in medicine as a whole. A decrease in the rate of technological change, for instance, could be harmful to the extent that it impedes attainable advances in the quality of medical care and the quality of life. It could be beneficial to the extent that it inhibits the adoption of inefficient technologies, or to the extent that it encourages a reallocation of resources to other areas of value. It is impossible to know what costs and benefits have been forgone in a technology that was never developed.

Impact Measures

There is no single measure, or group of measures, that can fully capture the complexity of technological change in medicine and the manner in which it is affected by PPS. The impact measures that do exist are on two levels: 1) aggregate data, in which a small amount of information is collected on a large number of technologies; and 2) focused studies, in which individual technologies or groups of technologies are examined for specific effects.

The aggregate measures available are limited to data on the earliest stages in the existence of emerging technologies. They cannot be used to measure the diffusion (either adoption or use) of technologies; at most, they can be examined as potential measures of the level of activity of R&D and of the changes in that activity. Industrial R&D, it is assumed, is likely to change in magnitude and direction as the market for new technologies shrinks and expands. Federally sponsored R&D is likely to be much less responsive to direct market effects because spending is directly tied to agency budgets.

These potential sources of aggregate measurement can be separated into two parts: the *investment* in R&D activity, and the *outcome* of that activity. Investment is measured in terms of the dollars spent, personnel time, or number of R&D projects. Outcome is measured by the number, type, and value of new products or procedures. For both investment and outcome measures, the areas of interest are changes in the overall level of activity and shifts in activity from one research area to another.

The available sources of data that provide aggregate measures of changes in R&D investment and new products are summarized in appendix F. Unfortunately, they are not very useful for evaluating PPS impacts. Information from R&D databases is unreliable for PPS evaluation purposes because it is not an accurate measure of investment in specific areas of medical R&D; even where these measures can trace changes in the magnitude of activity, they say nothing about changes in its direction. Data on new products, notably patent and FDA data, are also inadequate measures of new technologies. They tend to be incomparable, redundant, or incomplete; and they usually do not measure new techniques, small but important modifications, or new or unconventional ways of using old products. Furthermore, information from these sources is difficult to interpret because counts of new products say nothing about the quality or usefulness of the products, including whether the products are even being marketed or used. Finally, the medical products market shifts in response to numerous factors besides Medicare reimbursement, and attributing any changes in either the magnitude or direction of R&D activity to PPS with any level of statistical significance may be impossible.

Studies of specific technologies can take the form either of individual case studies or of studies of groups of technologies. Individual case studies frequently examine the entire history of development and diffusion of that technology and the influence of public policies on its history. Examples of such case studies are OTA's case studies of magnetic resonance imaging (279) and therapeutic apheresis (173). Group studies more frequently examine and compare the use and acceptance of those technologies in the medical environment. Examples are the studies of the impact of State ratesetting systems on the adoption of new technologies that were described in chapter 3 and studies such as those of Russell (253) and Cromwell, et al. (70), on the impact of cost-reimbursement insurance coverage on the diffusion of certain technologies.

As evidence of the impact of PPS on technological change, technology-specific studies have the advantage of enabling a detailed analysis of policy impacts. They can use statistical techniques to isolate and identify particular impact factors, and they allow an assessment of the actual clinical value of the technology to be considered in the evaluation of PPS effects. However, although studies like those cited above could be mounted to investigate the impact of PPS on technology development and diffusion, such studies inevitably depend on the technologies chosen. Conclusions based on these studies may present very biased views about the effects of the system because the most visible technologies, and thus those most likely to be analyzed, are the ones causing concern to producers and users. Focusing on these technologies can be important when making adjustments to improve the system, but it cannot

allow a balanced evaluation. The difficulty of presenting an unbiased evaluation picture suggests the method of choosing the specific technologies for evaluation is critical.

The conclusions from these studies are also difficult to generalize because the studies tend to concentrate on expensive, capital- and device-embodied technologies rather than procedures, methods, or low-capital technologies (such as many drugs and biologics). One exception to the tendency to focus on device-embodied technologies is Sloane and colleagues' study of a number of surgical procedures (270). Their study found that "although common themes emerge, diffusion of each procedure has its own idiosyncratic features." This dilemma is precisely the one that will complicate studies of technology diffusion under PPS.

Organizational Arrangements for Evaluating PPS Impacts

The only governmental organization that currently has responsibility for evaluating the impact of PPS on technological change in any form is ProPAC (see ch. 10). One of the tasks that ProPAC performs is the examination of specific problematic DRGs, and in order to perform this task, the Commission conducts in-depth studies of individual technologies. The objective of these studies is to arrive at recommendations regarding DRG weights, or new DRGs, that would provide incentives for the appropriate level and use of the technologies while paying an appropriate price. One such study was mandated by the Deficit Reduction Act of 1984 (Public Law 98-369), which singled out pacemakers as needing particular attention under PPS (see ch. 10). Other studies have been encouraged by organizations such as the American Academy of Ophthalmology, which suggested that the Commission review the use of IOLs and the weight of the DRG that includes that procedure (238).[15]

---
[15]As of their first report to the Secretary of Health and Human Services on Apr. 1, 1985, ProPAC had completed in-depth studies of three specific technologies: cardiac pacemakers, cataract extraction and IOL implantation, and PTCA. Other technologies that have undergone preliminary screening analyses are bone marrow transplantation; cochlear implants; ESWL; cyclosporine; magnetic resonance imaging; bilateral hip replacement; and treatments for alcohol dependence, cystic fibrosis, and dermatologic disorders (238).

Two characteristics of ProPAC's method for evaluating specific technologies are important. First, the focus of the technology studies is the impact of particular changes in technology use on DRG classifications and weights, not the impact of PPS on the technologies. Although these effects are interactive, they involve very different concerns. Second, the process used by ProPAC to select technologies for initial study is designed to be receptive to producers and users (Public Law 98-21). Technologies causing the most troublesome financial difficulties under PPS will undoubtedly surface by themselves given this outlet. This process is a much less efficient way of identifying those doing well under the system, however, since producers and users of technologies that are attractive under PPS have an incentive to keep their technologies out of the limelight.

Three organizations other than ProPAC have some responsibility for technology assessment and evaluation in the context of Medicare, but in no case does that responsibility include evaluating the impacts of PPS on technological change. The Office of Health Technology Assessment (OHTA) National Center for Health Services Research and Health Care Technology Assessment (NCHSR&HCTA) evaluates the safety and effectiveness of medical technologies that are being considered for coverage under Medicare and Medicaid. These activities have been recently expanded by Public Law 98-551 to allow examination of cost-effectiveness and medical appropriateness issues as well.

Public Law 98-551 authorized a National Advisory Council on Health Care Technology Assessment at NCHSR&HCTA to "assist the Director [of NCHSR&HCTA] in developing criteria and methods to be used by the Center in making health care technology coverage recommendations." In the past, the selection of technologies for assessment by OHTA was based on requests for information from HCFA regarding coverage deliberations. The Advisory Council will supplement this selection mechanism, though the manner and extent to which it will select technologies for OHTA assessment is not yet clear.

Finally, Public Law 98-551 authorized a separate National Advisory Council on Health Care Technology Assessment at the Institute of Medicine to identify health care technology assessment needs in general and to develop criteria and methods for assessment. This council, not established or funded as of August 1985, is to include both Federal and private sector representatives. It has no direct charge to consider Medicare coverage or reimbursement impacts, though these could conceivably influence the criteria it develops.

CONCLUSIONS

Medicare's PPS may have strong effects on technological change in health care, but the ultimate impact of those effects on the overall benefits and costs of health care will be virtually impossible to analyze. The potential for measuring the impact of PPS on technological change in the aggregate is limited by lack of good operative measures; by poor integration of data; by the difficulty in attributing changes to the influences of PPS; and by the inability to know whether the net value of a change is beneficial, harmful, or neutral. Furthermore, while PPS does set up a framework of incentives for the adoption and use of technologies, these incentives may conflict with each other and with non-PPS incentives in such a way that each technology faces a unique set of impacts.

Although the ultimate impacts of PPS on technological change may never be known, evaluation on a less ambitious level might produce some useful information. Questions for evaluation divide themselves into two categories: 1) questions about the effects of PPS on the magnitude and direction of R&D; and 2) questions about the effects on specific kinds of technologies, such as those that provide an increase in the quality of health care but at some corresponding increase in cost. Consequently, there are two kinds of potential evaluation strategies.

First, current databases on R&D and new products (see app. F) might be enhanced and refined. Surveys such as the National Science Foundation's survey of industrial R&D, for example, might be enhanced to provide an indication of changes in the magnitude of R&D. Although changes in industrial R&D on medical products cannot be tied very well to PPS, they do indicate roughly how investment in new medical products is proceeding relative to other industries. Enhancing databases to the point where they are useful for PPS evaluation purposes, however, would be very costly and is probably impractical.

Second, analysis of the process of development and diffusion of specific technologies or groups of technologies under PPS could be useful. The strength of technology-specific studies is that they can assess the clinical value of a technology and use that assessment in an evaluation of the importance of PPS impacts.

Although databases containing information on new drugs and devices have little use as aggregate measures of technological change, they might be used as one screening mechanism for selecting individual technologies to study. Other possible indentifiers of new technologies are changes in the annually updated CPT codes and surveys of experts in the health care field. A sample of new technologies chosen through one or more of these techniques might be tracked and their potential and real interactions with PPS analyzed. This kind of screening mechanism could allow a relatively unbiased set of technologies to be chosen for analysis.

A focused in-depth analysis of specific technologies based on such a screening mechanism could provide a measure of the impacts of PPS on a level that directly affects patients. In some cases, as with several of the technologies described in this chapter, features of the design of PPS that affect the development and diffusion of specific technologies can be identified. To some extent, the experiences of these technologies may be generalized to similar technologies and can serve as an early warning system for potential future effects. However, this method of monitoring is very sensitive to the technologies chosen for study. In particular, if the technologies chosen for analysis are those whose introduction is discouraged under PPS, the negative effects of PPS will be overemphasized.

Although there are several organizations with some responsibility for analyzing specific technologies in the context of Medicare, none are directly responsible for evaluating the impact of the payment system on specific technologies or on R&D. Furthermore, in at least one case (ProPAC), those activities are part of the PPS structure whose impacts are to be evaluated. This situation does not necessarily preclude ProPAC or other involved organizations from assisting in the evaluation, but it does suggest that the evaluation of PPS impacts on technological change should be functionally separated from other responsibilities of such organizations.

Chapter 9
Clinical Research

Contents

	Page
Introduction	131
Potential Impacts of PPS on Clinical Research	131
Background: Medicare and Funding for Clinical Research	131
Clinical Research Under PPS	133
Approaches to Evaluating the Impacts of PPS on Clinical Research	136
Critical Evaluation Questions	136
Impact Measures	136
Data Sources	137
Conclusions	138

Chapter 9
Clinical Research

INTRODUCTION

Clinical research is research that is conducted on people in a medical setting and is distinguished from nonscientific medical experimentation by the presence of an established research hypothesis and design. It can range in complexity from an elaborate, multicenter randomized clinical trial[1] to a study by a single physician trying a variation of an old procedure in his or her own office; and its focus ranges from basic studies of human metabolism to evaluations of fully developed medical technologies. Clinical research on new medical technologies is an important part of the process of technological change described in the last chapter, bridging the gap between laboratory testing and the accepted use of a technology by physicians. Such research can also be used to determine the value and best use of established medical technologies.

Some observers believe that Medicare's prospective payment system (PPS) for inpatient hospital services is inadvertently decreasing the level of funding for clinical research (241,404). In publicly asserting this, such observers implicitly recognize that Medicare, contrary to its own policy, has been paying for costs associated with experimental technologies. Such payments, to the extent that they have actually been made by Medicare, represent a hidden subsidy of clinical research. Any Medicare payments for experimental technologies have had a multiplier effect on the direct appropriations for clinical research.

In response to concerns that have been raised, the U.S. House of Representatives Committee on Appropriations directed the Health Care Financing Administration (HCFA) and the National Institutes of Health (NIH) to study the impact of PPS on clinical research. This chapter summarizes the evaluation questions applicable to such a study and discusses approaches to the problem.

---

[1]Clinical trials, a subset of clinical research, are the organized testing of new devices, drugs, therapies, or other changes on ill patients, often with control groups for comparison of results. The National Institutes of Health (NIH) *Inventory of Clinical Trials* (320) defines a clinical trial as:

> . . . a scientific research activity undertaken to define prospectively the effect and value of prophylactic/diagnostic/therapeutic agents, devices, regimens, procedures, etc., applied to human subjects. It is essential that the study be prospective, and that the number of cases of patients will depend on the hypothesis being tested, but must be sufficient to permit a definite result to be anticipated. Phase I, feasibility, or pilot studies are excluded.

POTENTIAL IMPACTS OF PPS ON CLINICAL RESEARCH

Background: Medicare and Funding for Clinical Research

In 1983, the total budgeted national support for health research and development (R&D) was estimated at $10.4 billion (362). The Federal Government contributed over half of this ($5.4 billion), including $3.8 billion from NIH; industry spent $4.0 billion on health R&D; private nonprofit organizations spent $0.4 billion, and State and local governments contributed $0.6 billion. The level of health R&D had remained fairly constant, after inflation, in the 5 years prior to 1983 (362).

NIH spends a substantial amount on clinical research, although the precise amount devoted to clinical as opposed to laboratory research is unknown. Some of the research is done in NIH's own clinical center, while other research projects are carried out in general clinical research centers (GCRCs) located in hospitals and funded through NIH's Division of Research Resources. Still other efforts, primarily clinical trials, may take place in any clinical setting. These efforts are funded through grants and contracts sponsored by individual institutes. A 1979 survey of trials indicated that about 5 percent of the NIH health research

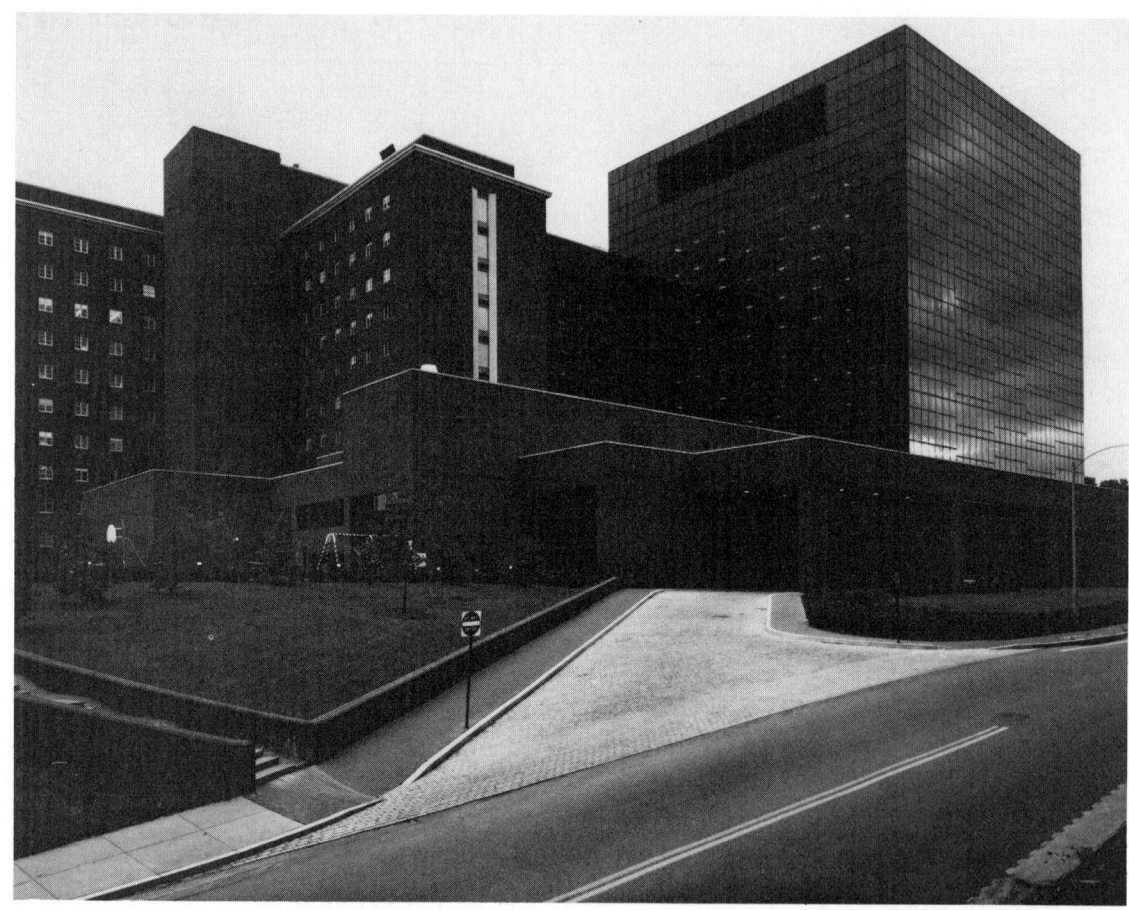

Photo credit: National Institutes of Health

A substantial amount of clinical research is supported by the National Institutes of Health. Some of this research is done in the Warren G. Magnuson Clinical Center, located on the NIH campus in Bethesda, MD.

budget supported clinical trials (306). Other organizations within the Public Health Service, such as the Alcohol, Drug Abuse, and Mental Health Administration (ADAMHA), also spend a significant amount on clinical trials and other clinical research (56).

In addition to receiving budgeted support, clinical research has probably received a great deal of financial support, not explicitly budgeted or openly recognized, from third-party payers of health care costs. One of these payers is Medicare.

Since its inception, Medicare has been prohibited by law from paying for medical services and procedures that are not "reasonable and necessary" (Public Law 89-97). This prohibition, combined with a legislative injunction against cross-subsidization, has been interpreted by HCFA as precluding Medicare payment for clinical research. In accordance with a Federal regulation issued in 1966 (42 CFR 405.422), Medicare policy does not allow reimbursement for research-related costs, including research-related patient care costs, that are over and above "usual" patient care for equivalent patients not on research protocols.

A cost-conscious environment recently resulted in a minor modification by Congress of this stringent restriction on the use of Medicare funds. The Social Security Amendments of 1983 (Public Law

98-21) and the Deficit Reduction Act of 1984 (Public Law 98-369) gave the Department of Health and Human Services (DHHS) (including HCFA) the power to assess "the safety, efficacy, and cost-effectiveness of new and existing medical procedures." Medicare trust funds may be used to pay for patient care costs associated with these assessments if two requirements are met:

- the research is not of the sort that would be undertaken by industry or by NIH, and
- the procedure being investigated "has the potential to be more cost-effective in the treatment of a condition than procedures currently in use with respect to such condition" (Public Law 98-369, sec. 2313(c)(3)).

The same two laws also gave the Prospective Payment Assessment Commission (ProPAC), with the cooperation of the Secretary of Health and Human Services, the power to use Medicare trust funds to conduct clinical research investigating cost-effectiveness. As of August 1985, neither DHHS nor ProPAC had used this authority.

Despite the prohibition against Medicare payment for clinical research, under cost-based reimbursement, Medicare did sometimes pay for hospital costs related to clinical research. Some observers claim that the practice was widespread (160). The method of hospital reporting for Medicare Part A made it nearly impossible for fiscal intermediaries to determine whether an experimental technology was used for any particular patient. When presented with a hospital's bill for services, the intermediary could not easily distinguish between charges that were related to an experimental procedure and those that were not. Intermediaries might sometimes learn from the Part B carrier that an experimental procedure was used in the hospital, but even then, it was difficult to identify the hospital costs or charges associated with the procedure. Moreover, when a patient underwent both established and experimental procedures during a hospital stay, it was difficult to determine what proportion of the cost of care was attributable to the experimental part of the patient's stay.

Thus, under cost-based reimbursement, Medicare intermediaries might have been able to identify admissions that were purely for research reasons or to disallow research costs such as those for data collection, but there was no reliable way to determine what proportions of ancillary tests and patient care costs were attributable to the use of an experimental technology during the hospital stay. A hospital billed Medicare for the services it provided to Medicare patients, and unless the intermediary determined through auditing that a service was associated with research, the hospital was paid.

Virtually all information regarding Medicare payment for experimental procedures under cost-based reimbursement is anecdotal. It is clear that, knowingly or unknowingly, hospitals were reimbursed by Medicare for costs associated with unproven technologies. It is not clear how extensive this reimbursement was because there have been no studies of the subject.

Clinical Research Under PPS

Hospitals' financial incentives regarding clinical research under Medicare's PPS are different from the incentives under cost-based reimbursement. The fear that the incentives of the new payment system will affect hospitals' willingness (or even ability) to maintain clinical research programs has made clinical research under PPS an issue in its own right.

Under PPS, hospitals lose money whenever they treat a Medicare patient with above-average per-case costs and make money whenever they treat one with below-average costs. When research patients are more expensive to care for than nonresearch patients, hospitals have an incentive not to participate in research. This incentive probably operates in the case of most research protocols that require more tests, more patient monitoring and care by staff, or longer hospital stays than the established mode of treatment. In cases in which an experimental technology is costlier than the alternatives, or data collection costs are not entirely covered by research funding, the hospital may have to absorb the extra costs. In any of these cases, PPS would tend to discourage clinical research.[2]

---

[2]The initial diagnosis-related group (DRG) prices were based on estimates of the average costs per DRG in 1981. Whatever research-related costs were reimbursed at that time are included in the DRG prices. This fact does not alter the financial consequences of treat-

(continued next page)

In other cases, however, PPS may encourage clinical research. For example, the existence of a research program enhances a hospital's image in general and can act as a marketing tool to draw admissions. Also, some technologies may actually lower hospital costs during the research phase, because they are cheaper to purchase or because the research protocols themselves are less costly than alternative established treatments (i.e., they require fewer ancillary services or shorter hospital stays).[3] In such cases, hospitals have an incentive to participate in the research as soon as possible. Finally, many technologies may have the potential to lower costs once accepted for widespread use. Producers of these technologies have an incentive to enlist hospitals and physicians to participate in clinical research not only to show safety and effectiveness but also to gather cost information for later use in marketing.

PPS encourages the inclusion of cost-effectiveness studies as part of, or in addition to, the clinical trials of new drugs and devices. The manufacturer of a new technology has a strong selling point, much more so under PPS than under cost-based reimbursement, if it can show cost savings to hospitals from the technology. However, there are important tradeoffs in conducting cost-effectiveness studies simultaneously with clinical trials. The obvious benefit is that doing an economic analysis of a new technology at an early stage is time-saving, cost-saving, and a source of important information for users of the technology—hospitals and physicians. The primary drawbacks are, first, that the clinical trial environment may not present a realistic picture of how the technology will be used and its real cost tradeoffs; and second, that the costs of a technology in its early stages of development and use may be very different from its costs later in the diffusion stage (90).

The examples of possible PPS impacts on clinical cancer research at certain community hospitals (see box 9-A) and on NIH-sponsored GCRCs

---

ing above-average-cost patients, however; it simply makes the average rate of payment higher than it would otherwise have been (assuming that most research raises the cost of diagnosis or treatment). Incorporating past higher-than-average per-case costs into current prices effectively means that past implicit Medicare subsidies of research-related costs now subsidize the provision of patient care in general, although treating expensive research patients is still discouraged.

[3]Surgical staplers, an alternative to manual sutures, are an example of one such technology (36).

(see box 9-B) suggest that the impacts on clinical research may be unevenly distributed. One strong potential difference is between teaching and non-teaching hospitals. Virtually all GCRCs, for instance, are in teaching hospitals. In cancer research, small nonteaching hospitals cannot meet

Box 9-A —PPS and Community Hospital Participation in Cancer Research

More concern has been expressed over the effect of Medicare's PPS on cancer research than on any other research area, and advocates of community hospital participation in cancer research have been particularly vocal (77). The National Cancer Institute's (NCI) Community Clinical Oncology Program is a program specifically for community, nonteaching hospitals that was established to increase the number of patients available to participate in clinical trials and to accelerate the transfer of new cancer treatment technologies to the community hospitals (364). NCI provides funding to cover administrative and data collection costs, without which community hospitals might not be willing to participate in trials. The trials themselves are coordinated by NCI-supported teaching and research hospitals.

With the introduction of PPS, some community hospitals believe that their ability to participate in clinical trials may be endangered if patients participating in research are more costly than those that are not. The Association of Community Cancer Centers has suggested that there be a separate diagnosis-related group (DRG) established for patients participating in research (404), and the National Cancer Advisory Board has suggested that, pending completion of relevant studies,"it may be prudent to continue to fund these patients [participating in NIH clinical trials] on a cost reimbursement basis" (363).

One problem with these approaches is that they require official recognition of Medicare reimbursement for research-related costs. Since DHHS has interpreted the Medicare law as prohibiting payment for most kinds of research, these options are not possible, in the view of DHHS, without regulatory or legislative changes (77). It has not yet been established that PPS is actually posing a barrier to the participation of cancer patients over age 65 in clinical trials, although there are several studies currently being planned or implemented to establish the relative costliness of these patients (see p. 137).

Box 9-B —PPS and General Clinical Research Centers

NIH funds a General Clinical Research Centers (GCRCs) grant program that enables hospitals to designate certain hospital beds for use by patients participating in clinical research. Most GCRCs have facilities that are separate from the rest of the hospital, including their own kitchen, laboratory, and office facilities, as well as their own beds. A GCRC grant may be used for some salaries, renovations, laboratory equipment, and operating costs, including the patient care costs for patients in the hospital solely for research purposes. There are approximately 75 funded GCRCs in teaching and research hospitals in the United States, with a combined total of about 600 hospital beds devoted to research (361). Examples of studies being conducted at GCRCs are studies of the effect of disease and age on drug disposition and action; studies of lecithin treatment for Alzheimer disease; and studies of calcium and phosphorus balance in kidney transplant patients.

Some of the patients using GCRC beds are in the hospital only to participate in research, and the costs of their care are paid for by the GCRC grant. Others, however, would be hospitalized whether or not they were participating in research. Some of these patients' care has been billed to Medicare in the past and has been reimbursed. Under PPS, however, the hospital must absorb any of these patients' costs that exceed the DRG payment. If these patients are more expensive than average to care for, and if the hospital has been reimbursed by Medicare for these costs in the past, part of the GCRC grant must be used to make up the difference unless the hospital is willing to absorb the cost. This in effect reduces the amount of research that the GCRC funds can support.

GCRCs may also be affected by any decreases in hospital occupancy rates that result from PPS incentives to decrease length of stay and emphasize outpatient services. Temporarily unneeded GCRC beds can be used as overflow beds by nonresearch patients, and reimbursement for those patients can help subsidize the costs of maintaining the center. If there are fewer overflow patients and the temporarily unneeded beds lie empty, the hospital's GCRC grant may not be able to support as many research beds, or, consequently, as many research patients (281).

No data on whether PPS is actually affecting GCRCs adversely were available as of August 1985. At centers where most of the patients are in the hospital solely to participate in the research protocol and Medicare has not been relied on extensively as a source of reimbursement, little impact is anticipated. It appears that a particular GCRC is more likely to suffer under PPS if: 1) patient care costs in the GCRC are greater than in the rest of the hospital, due to greater service intensity or longer lengths of stay; 2) research tends to be applied rather than basic research, with many patients in the hospital for necessary therapeutic reasons as well as for research; 3) the hospital has traditionally relied on Medicare and other payers for at least some reimbursement of patient care costs; and 4) overall hospital occupancy declines.

---

the requirements of the cancer centers' exemption to PPS,[4] nor are they eligible for Medicare indirect teaching allowances that might be used to subsidize research.[5]

[4] Public Law 98-21 provides that hospitals fitting the National Cancer Institute's (NCI) definition of a "comprehensive" or "clinical" cancer center can apply for an exemption from PPS. The relevant regulations pursuant to this law specify that to qualify at least 50 percent of all patients discharged from these hospitals must have cancer as the principal diagnosis (49 FR 234). As of July 1985, five hospitals had met these provisions and been granted exemptions (337).

[5] Medicare payments for the indirect costs of medical education, based on the number of interns and residents per hospital bed, were instituted in 1980 when limits on reimbursement for medical care costs were tightened (175). With this extra allotment to teaching hospitals, Medicare may have been shifting some of its subsidy for clinical research from medical care reimbursement payments to indirect medical education payments. The purpose of the adjustment was

PPS may also affect research in different fields more or less strongly. Impacts may be stronger in research fields with a high proportion of diagnostic and therapeutic procedures in the experimental stage; with relatively costly new technologies; or with many Medicare-eligible patients affected. PPS may also have greater effects on diagnostic than on therapeutic procedures, because clinical research on diagnostic procedures often requires more duplicative testing or other services than research on therapeutic procedures.

to accommodate the generally higher costs of teaching hospitals that were not directly tied to teaching (e.g., residents' salaries) but were nonetheless assumed to be unavoidable consequences of having a teaching program. The factors contributing to these costs have not all been identified (175), but the existence of a clinical research program may be one component (160,241).

APPROACHES TO EVALUATING THE IMPACTS OF PPS ON CLINICAL RESEARCH

Critical Evaluation Questions

The introduction of PPS has raised concerns about federally financed clinical research that are somewhat different from the issues discussed in previous chapters. In particular, it has stimulated discussion about whether HCFA has a role in supporting such research. Under Medicare's cost-based reimbursement system, it is likely that HCFA frequently reimbursed hospitals for the patient care costs of patients participating in research protocols, although the extent of such subsidies is unknown. Under PPS, however, there is no extra payment for research-related patient care costs.

The impact and evaluation issues raised in this chapter need to be separated from the policy issues. Quantitative and qualitative studies can assist in answering the question: How is PPS affecting the level and type of clinical research performed, relative to the situation under cost reimbursement? Such studies cannot assist in answering the ultimate policy questions: Should support for any negatively affected areas of clinical research be reinstated, and who (if anyone) should bear the costs of that support?

The potential impact of PPS on clinical research is an evaluation area in which the most fundamental baseline data are lacking. There are no data, even inadequate data, on the size of the past and present Medicare subsidy for such research; on whether research patients cost more to treat than nonresearch patients; on how much more they cost; on what the components of any extra costs are; on whether some kinds of research protocols result in higher marginal costs than others; or on the distribution of these factors across research areas.

The size of the Medicare subsidy for clinical research under cost-based reimbursement has important implications. If the subsidy has been large, then PPS will probably result in a reallocation of resources away from clinical research, resulting in less total research or less research in specific areas or settings, such as community hospital participation in cancer trials. If the subsidy has been low, PPS will have little net overall effect on clinical research, though again it may have more effect in some areas than others.

Impact Measures

Operational measures of the size and distribution of implicit Medicare subsidies for clinical research are difficult to define. The lack of good conceptual measures means that determining the real size and extent of PPS impacts on clinical research will be virtually impossible. Given this, the question becomes one of what proxy measures, however far removed from the desired conceptual measures, are available.

One possible strategy for evaluating PPS impacts on clinical research is to measure changes in the purchasing power of research dollars. NIH, the primary explicit funding source for clinical research, could assimilate data on the number of patients enrolled in clinical trials, manhours funded, and other measures of clinical research activity. If Medicare subsidies are reduced (or increased) by PPS, each NIH dollar spent on research will appear to buy less (or more) research than it did before PPS, even after adjustments for inflation. This change in purchasing power would be independent of the NIH budget (although if the purchasing power of research dollars decreased the total amount of research would also decline unless the NIH budget increased to compensate). An analysis of changes in purchasing power could be conducted across the various research fields to determine which areas are the most affected.

A second possible strategy for evaluating PPS impacts on clinical research is to target areas where effects might be expected. As discussed above, two examples of areas that appear particularly troublesome are cancer research in community hospitals and research in NIH-sponsored GCRCs. On a focused level, it is possible to examine, for instance, the size of community hospital participation in clinical cancer trials; the total research-related costs per patient in those trials;

and the amount of those costs that exceed revenues from NIH, industry, or other research funding sources. While the difficulty in measuring research-related costs and other variables still makes this research design far from ideal, it nevertheless may be adequate for policy decisions.

On a focused level, it may also be possible to examine shifts in the setting of care. PPS may encourage more research in outpatient and home settings, and it has been suggested that the Food and Drug Administration should accept research in nonhospital settings as meeting its requirements where such research is appropriate (39). Conversely, PPS may have particularly adverse effects in research areas such as mental health for which the trend is toward inpatient research (231).

Data Sources

No single database contains information on amounts of clinical research performed in the United States. Information on the level of clinical research funding is available from separate sources—e.g., NIH or ADAMHA—and changes in the amount of research performed largely reflect changes in the research budgets of these organizations. HCFA has been directed by Congress to study jointly with NIH the impact of PPS on clinical research (301) and to report to Congress by the beginning of 1985, but there are currently no data to directly support a comprehensive analysis; as of August 1985, the analysis had not been completed (see ch. 10).

Some information on support for clinical trials has been prepared by NIH in response to a separate congressional request, but this information does not include detailed data on ongoing trials or even data on patients' age (178). Such clinical trial data have not been compiled systematically by NIH since 1979, though some individual institutes have continued clinical trial inventories for their own purposes (306). Observed changes in the total number of trials, number of patients participating in trials, and dollars spent on trials are likely to be due to NIH budget allotment decisions. But it might be possible to extract from this information changes in relative purchasing power for clinical trials. If data were available on the age distribution of patients enrolled in trials, the exposure of specific research areas to PPS could be assessed. Any analysis would still be limited by the difficulty of attributing changes to PPS and the fact that the underlying data would include only clinical trials, but it could serve as a useful indicator of specific areas for further study.

The only research area receiving widespread scrutiny relating to PPS is cancer research. There are currently three efforts to establish the relative costliness of research patients and the impact of DRGs on cancer research:

- The National Center for Health Services Research and Health Care Technology Assessment (NCHSR&HCTA) is conducting a study that compares the hospital costs of patients enrolled in National Cancer Institute (NCI) clinical trials with the costs of nonprotocol cancer patients (351). Data sources for the study are NCI data on patients enrolled in clinical trials and a sample of discharge abstracts and hospital bills drawn from a list of hospitals participating in NCI trials. The study is scheduled for completion in 1986.
- The Eastern Cooperative Oncology Group (ECOG), an affiliation of Eastern U.S. hospitals participating in cooperative cancer research and related activities, is currently analyzing data from a preliminary study on the extent of hospitalization for patients on cancer protocols. If the results suggest that patients over age 65 (about 23 percent of ECOG patients enrolled in clinical trials) undergo significant hospitalization, ECOG plans a further study to address more directly the potential impact of PPS on hospital care for these patients (199).
- The Association of Community Cancer Centers is attempting to estimate the relative costliness of patients participating in research at its member hospitals (206). Preliminary studies of costs in three hospitals (in New Jersey, Oklahoma, and California) supported the hypothesis that research patients have higher costs (404).

These efforts may help shed light on cancer research, but the results cannot be generalized to other medical fields.

CONCLUSIONS

The impact of Medicare's PPS on clinical research raises issues unlike those in other areas of the health care system. In the past, under cost-based reimbursement, third-party payers, including Medicare, implicitly subsidized clinical research. Despite the fact that support for all clinical research (except that involving cost-effectiveness) is and always has been contrary to Medicare policy, in practice, the imposition of per-case payment may significantly affect the amount and type of clinical research performed.

NIH data on an important subset of clinical research, clinical trials might be used to measure changes in research dollar purchasing power as a way of identifying potential areas for further examination. Data on the age of patients enrolled in NIH-funded trials could also be used as a very simple indicator of areas where PPS impacts are likely to be strong. (Of course, these measures would say nothing about what effects prospective payment might have if it were extended to non-Medicare payers, or whether PPS might stifle any efforts to increase enrollment of elderly patients in clinical research.) At present, these data are not collected by the Federal Government on a continuing basis; nor are they supplemented by equivalent data from other funding sources, public or private.

Detailed studies of specific areas of clinical research could also be useful. The selection of areas for study should depend on a careful assessment of the real potential for discouragement of clinical research, such as areas of research in which it is important to enroll elderly inpatients.

The ultimate question regarding PPS and clinical research is one of policy: Should Medicare pay for health care costs associated with experimental technologies? Congress has recently given DHHS limited authority in this direction, by directing that the agency may pay some research-associated costs if the research is intended to determine the cost-effectiveness of a technology (Public Law 98-369). This move represents a break from the previous philosophy that all medical research should be financially and organizationally divorced from payment for medical care. The very fact that the issue of PPS effects on clinical research has arisen argues for a reconsideration of the relationship between funding for clinical research and payment for medical care.

Part Three
Evaluation Strategies

Chapter 10
Current PPS Evaluation Activities

Contents

	Page
Introduction	143
PPS-Related Evaluation Studies by Federal Agencies	143
Mandated PPS Studies by Federal Agencies	144
Nonmandated PPS-Related Studies by Federal Agencies	146
PPS-Related Evaluation Studies by Private Organizations	154
Summary of Issues Pertaining to Current PPS Evaluation Activities	159
Overlaps and Gaps in PPS-Related Research	159
Problems With Data for PPS Evaluation Studies	160
Staffing and Funding for Mandated PPS Studies	160
Conclusions	162

LIST OF TABLES

Table No.	Page
10-1. Studies of the Medicare's PPS Mandated by Congress	145
10-2. ORD-Supported, Nonmandated Studies of Prospective Payment for Hospitals Active in 1985	148
10-3. ORD's Short-, Mid-, and Long-Term Research Priorities Relating to Hospital Payment	149
10-4. HCFA Health Policy Center PPS-Related Assignments	149
10-5. Nonmandated PPS-Related Studies by Public Health Service Agencies	150
10-6. Nonmandated PPS-Related Studies by the DHHS Office of the Assistant Secretary for Planning and Evaluation and by the DHHS Office of the Inspector General	152
10-7. Nonmandated PPS-Related Studies by the General Accounting Office	153
10-8. PPS-Related Evaluation Studies by Private Organizations	155
10-9. HCFA's Funding for Extramural Research and Demonstrations, Fiscal Year 1985 and Proposed Fiscal Year 1986	161

Chapter 10
Current PPS Evaluation Activities

INTRODUCTION

Several Federal Government and private organizations are involved in the evaluation of Medicare's prospective payment system (PPS) established by the Social Security Amendments of 1983 (Public Law 98-21). Organizations sponsoring PPS studies in the Federal Government include the Department of Health and Human Services (DHHS), primarily the Health Care Financing Administration (HCFA); the Prospective Payment Assessment Commission (ProPAC), an independent body established by Congress in the Social Security Amendments of 1983; and congressional agencies such as OTA. Private organizations involved in PPS studies include professional societies, trade associations, and beneficiary groups.

In their research efforts, various agencies and organizations are emphasizing one or more of the impact areas addressed in Part Two of this report: expenditures and costs, quality of care, access to care, technological change, and clinical research. Thus far, HCFA has focused mainly on costs and expenditures under PPS, although the agency has recently initiated a set of research projects pertaining to quality of care. Quality of care issues are also included among the PPS research interests of many private organizations. Within the Federal Government, the potential for addressing access to care rests with the National Center for Health Services Research and Health Care Technology Assessment (NCHSR&HCTA),[1] a Public Health Service (PHS) agency whose domain is health services research. Technological change under PPS is the evaluation focus of the Health Industry Manufacturers' Association and a few other private organizations. No Federal agency has initiated studies of PPS impacts on technological change. The effect of PPS on clinical research is of particular interest to teaching hospitals and groups involved in cancer research.

This chapter examines PPS-related evaluation studies by Federal agencies and a number of private organizations. It also discusses several important issues pertaining to current PPS evaluation efforts, including overlaps and gaps in research, problems with data for evaluation studies, and staffing and funding for congressionally mandated studies of PPS.

---

[1]The name of this agency was formerly the National Center for Health Services Research (NCHSR). The change in its name marked a new emphasis on health care technology assessment and a change in focus on technology assessment issues by the passage of Public Law 98-551 on Oct. 25, 1984.

PPS-RELATED EVALUATION STUDIES BY FEDERAL AGENCIES

Federal activities with respect to the evaluation of PPS fall into two broad categories:

- studies mandated by Congress in legislation or requested in committee report language during the past 3 years, either for the purpose of evaluating PPS or to consider specific issues in the refinement and expansion of PPS; and
- studies funded by Federal agencies as part of their general responsibility to monitor and evaluate their programs or as background to mandated PPS studies.

The following discussion identifies and discusses the congressionally mandated and other PPS-related studies of executive branch agencies, mainly HCFA and other components of DHHS; of ProPAC; and of congressional agencies such as OTA, the Congressional Budget Office (CBO), the Congressional Research Service (CRS), the General Accounting Office (GAO), and OTA.

Mandated PPS Studies of Federal Agencies

A list of PPS studies mandated by legislation or requested in a congressional committee report is provided in table 10-1. Almost all of the congressionally mandated PPS studies were assigned to the Secretary of Health and Human Services and became the responsibility of HCFA. Three studies not assigned to DHHS were assigned to ProPAC.

The Social Security Amendments of 1983 (Public Law 98-21) mandated several reports by DHHS on possible refinements to PPS (see table 10-1). It also directed the Secretary of Health and Human Services to ". . . study and report annually to the Congress at the end of each year (beginning with 1984 and ending with 1987) on the impact, of the payment methodology . . . [on] classes of hospitals, beneficiaries, and other payers for inpatient hospital services, and other providers . . ." Finally, this law directed ProPAC to deliver annual reports to the Secretary of Health and Human Services with recommendations on adjustments to PPS.

The Deficit Reduction Act of 1984 (Public Law 98-369) mandated several additional PPS studies by DHHS (see table 10-1). Most of the studies mandated by this law focus on refinements or adjustments to the new payment system.

The House Appropriations Committee, in its July 1984 report for the 1985 Departments of Labor, HHS, Education and Related Agencies Bill (Report 98-911 on H.R. 6028), called for (though technically did not mandate) three studies pertaining to the impacts of PPS (see table 10-1).

Mandated Studies To Be Undertaken by the Department of Health and Human Services

The preparation of most of the DHHS studies mandated by Congress has been assigned to HCFA (see table 10-1). Only a few of the studies are being managed by other components of DHHS.

Health Care Financing Administration.—As shown in table 10-1, most of the mandated studies under HCFA's direction have been assigned to the agency's Office of Research and Demonstrations (ORD). Several of the mandated studies under HCFA's direction, including the study on incorporating exempted hospitals and exempted hospital units into PPS, pertain to the refinement or expansion of PPS. Other mandated studies reflect congressional anticipation of potential problems under PPS, such as adverse effects on sole community hospitals, uncompensated costs of care, adverse effects on large rural teaching hospitals, underutilized hospitals, wage adjustments, intensity of care, severity of illness, and outlier payments. A report by HCFA due at the end of 1986 will consider the impact of State alternatives to PPS on Medicare, Medicaid, private health expenditures, and tax expenditures. As of August 1985, most of the HCFA-supported, congressionally mandated studies of PPS had yet to be released or had not been completed. All of HCFA's congressionally mandated deadlines for PPS studies had been missed.

Starting in 1984 and ending in 1987, the Secretary's annual PPS impact reports are expected to evaluate the effects of Medicare's new payment system on classes of hospitals, beneficiaries, and other payers for inpatient hospital services, and to evaluate in particular the impact of computing DRG rates by census division rather than nationwide. The Secretary's first report, which is to be largely descriptive, will contain information on the background and objectives of PPS, early findings on the impact of PPS, and descriptions of PPS-related research issues that will be examined as the system develops (336). As of August 15, 1985, the 1984 annual impact report, due December 31, 1984, was in the Secretary's office for clearance.[2]

Other DHHS Agencies.—The National Institutes of Health (NIH) and HCFA are responsible for a mandated study of the effects of PPS on clinical trials (study #31 in table 10-1). An interim report is expected in the fall of 1985. The Office of the Assistant Secretary for Planning and Evalu-

---

[2]Although the first annual report has not been released, a brief oral description was provided to OTA by HCFA staff. The report covers program implementation as well as sections on PPS impacts on: 1) hospitals (by type and region, effects on length of hospital stay, admissions, and case mix); 2) Medicare beneficiaries (providing baseline data for future annual impact reports); 3) quality of care; 4) other providers; 5) Medicare program expenditures (rates of increase over the past 10 years; Part A, Part B, and total); and 6) other payers (brief section) (84).

Table 10-1.—Studies of Medicare's PPS Mandated by Congress

Study topic	Report due date	Agency	Status (as of August 1985)
Reports Mandated by Social Security Amendments of 1983 (Public Law 98-21):			
1983-1984 reports:			
1. Impact of Single Limits on Skilled Nursing Facilities	12/31/84[a]	HCFA-OLP	Complete (1/85)
2. Impact of Hospital PPS on Skilled Nursing Facilities	12/31/84[a]	HCFA-OLP	Complete (1/85)
3. Including U.S. Territory Hospitals	4/1/84	HCFA-BERC	In clearance[b]
4. Incorporating Capital Into PPS	10/14/84	ASPE/HCFA	In clearance
5. Annual PPS Impact Reports, 1984-87	12/31/84-87	HCFA-ORD-OR	In clearance[b]
1985 reports:			
6. Annual Report and Recommendations on PPS to the Secretary of Health and Human Services	Beginning 4/1/85	ProPAC	Complete (4/85)
7. Occupancy of Sole Community Hospitals	4/1/85	HCFA-ORD-OR	In clearance[b]
8. A-B Information Transfers	4/1/85	HCFA-ORD-BPO	In clearance[b]
9. Uncompensated Care Costs	4/1/85	HCFA-ORD-OR	In clearance[b]
10. Cost of Care Information to Patients	4/1/85	HCFA-ORD-OR	Complete (8/85)
11. Large Rural Teaching Hospitals	4/1/85	HCFA-ORD-OR	In clearance[b]
12. Case-Mix Measurement: Refinements of DRGs (including severity of illness, intensity of care, and adequacy of outlier payment)	12/31/85	HCFA-ORD-OR	—
13. Eliminating Rural-Urban Rates	12/31/85	HCFA-ORD-OR	—
14. Exempted Hospitals Report: Long-Term Care Hospitals, Psychiatric Units, Rehabilitation Units, and Pediatric Hospitals	12/31/85	HCFA-ORD-OR	—
15. All-Payer Feasibility, Cost-Shifting	12/31/85	HCFA-ORD-OR	—
16. Impact of Admission, Volume Adjustment	12/31/85	HCFA-ORD-OR	—
17. Physician DRGs—Including Payments for Physicians' Services to Hospital Inpatients in DRG Payment Amounts	7/1/85[c]	HCFA-ORD-OR	Incomplete
1986 reports:			
18. Impact of State Alternatives to PPS on Medicare, Medicaid, Private Health Expenditures, and Tax Expenditures	12/31/86	HCFA-ORD-OR	—
Reports Mandated by the Deficit Reduction Act (Public Law 98-369):			
1984 reports:			
19. Prospective Payment for Skilled Nursing Facilities	8/1/84	HCFA-OLP	Complete (1/85)
20. Prospective Payment System Wage Index Adjustments	8/18/84	HCFA-BERC	Complete (4/85)
21. Options for Prospective Payment for Skilled Nursing Facilities	12/1/84	HCFA-OLP	Complete[d] (1/85)
22. Definition and Identification of "Disproportionate Share" Hospitals	12/31/84	HCFA-BERC	Incomplete
1985 reports:			
23. Urban/Rural Payment Differential	1/18/85	HCFA-ORD-OR	To be included with study #13
24. Advisability and Feasibility of Varying by DRG Proportions of Labor and Nonlabor Components of the Federal Payment Amount	1/18/85	HCFA-BERC	To be included with study #13
25. Pacemaker Payment Review (Part A)	3/1/85	ProPAC	Complete (3/85)
26. Pacemaker Payment Review (Part B)	3/1/85	HCFA-BQC	Incomplete
27. Closure and Conversion of Underutilized Hospital Facilities	3/1/85	HCFA-BERC/ORD	In clearance[b]
28. Certified Registered Nurse Anesthetists	7/1/85	HCFA-BERC/ORD	Incomplete
29. Hospital Specific Variance	9/1/85	HCFA-ORD	To be included with study #13
30. Exceptions to Wage Index Adjustments	—	HCFA-BERC	
Reports Requested by the House Appropriations Committee Report (Report 98-911 on H.R. 6028):			
1985 reports:			
31. Effect of PPS on Clinical Trials	—	NIH/HCFA	Interim report, fall 1985 Completion expected winter 1986
32. Annual Report on Impact of PPS on Blood Banking	—	HCFA	Expected early 1986
33. Effects of PPS on U.S. Health Care System	Beginning 2/86	ProPAC	—

ABBREVIATIONS: ASPE: Assistant Secretary for Planning and Evaluation (DHHS).
HCFA: Health Care Financing Administration
—BERC: Bureau of Eligibility, Reimbursement, and Coverage
—BPO: Bureau of Program Operations
—BQC: Bureau of Quality Control
—OLP: Office of Legislation and Policy
—ORD-OR: Office of Research and Demonstrations, Office of Research
ProPAC: Prospective Payment Assessment Commission

[a]Due date revised from 12/31/83 to 12/31/84.
[b]Report has been completed and is being reviewed within DHHS before being submitted to Congress.
[c]Due date revised from 12/31/85 to 7/1/85.
[d]Report included in larger project, "Study of Skilled Nursing Facilities Benefit Under Medicare."

SOURCES: A. Dobson and W. Sobaski, Office of Research and Demonstrations, Health Care Financing Administration, Department of Health and Human Services, Baltimore, MD, personal communications, May and August 1985; A. Dobson, "Prospective Payment: Current Configuration and Future Direction," presented to the Prospective Payment Assessment Commission, Washington, DC, Feb. 2, 1984.

ation (ASPE), with the support of HCFA, has been the DHHS focus for the congressionally mandated study on how to handle hospital capital spending under PPS (study #4 in table 10-1). This report, due October 14, 1984, was in the Secretary's office for clearance as of August 1985.

Mandated Studies To Be Undertaken by the Prospective Payment Assessment Commission

Medicare's PPS was implemented very soon after the enactment of the Social Security Amendments of 1983. Congress recognized that periodic adjustments to the new system—including the overall amount paid and the way the prices are apportioned among the different diagnosis-related groups (DRGs)—would be needed. Thus, in the same law that established Medicare's PPS, Congress created ProPAC as an independent commission of experts to make recommendations to the Secretary of Health and Human Services and to Congress about these changes. (The Secretary of Health and Human Services is charged with making the actual changes by regulation.)

The Social Security Amendments of 1983 specified that ProPAC Commissioners were to be selected and appointed by the Director of OTA. In addition, the 1983 law gave ProPAC two specific responsibilities:

- to recommend annually to the Secretary of Health and Human Services the appropriate percentage change in Medicare payments for inpatient hospital care (termed "the updating factor") which is to be applied to the previous year's payment rates; and
- to make periodic recommendations to the Secretary of Health and Human Services concerning changes in individual DRG weights and categories, beginning with fiscal year 1986 and at least every 4 years thereafter.

ProPAC's report containing these recommendations (study #6 in table 10-1) is due annually on April 1, and the first such report was delivered April 1, 1985 (237).

The Deficit Reduction Act of 1984 gave ProPAC two additional specific tasks: 1) to review and report on cardiac pacemaker payment under Medicare Part A and the relative weights assigned to those DRGs in which pacemakers are used (study #25 in table 10-1), and 2) to make a recommendation regarding the overall annual rate of increase in allowed routine costs for non-PPS hospitals. The results of ProPAC's study of pacemaker payment under Part A and a recommended update factor for non-PPS hospitals were included in ProPAC's April 1985 report (237).

According to the House Appropriations Committee report language for the fiscal year 1985 Departments of Labor, HHS, Education, and Related Agencies Bill (Report 98-911 on H.R. 6028), "the primary role of the Commission lies in a broader evaluation of the impact of Public Law 98-21 on the American health care system." That report directs ProPAC to submit an annual report to Congress expressing its views on the impact of PPS (study #33 in table 10-1). ProPAC's first report on the impact of PPS on the U.S. health care system is due on February 1, 1986. Although the House report language does not have the force of law, ProPAC intends to comply.

Nonmandated PPS-Related Studies by Federal Agencies

In addition to undertaking the congressionally mandated studies discussed above, DHHS and other Federal agencies are involved in nonmandated research evaluating PPS.

Nonmandated Studies by the Department of Health and Human Services

When PPS was established, several DHHS research and demonstration projects that were to have helped in the design of the new system had not been completed. Some of the DHHS projects that had been started before the passage of the Social Security Amendments of 1983 are being continued in order to address anticipated problems with PPS or with DRGs. In addition, some older projects concerning nonhospital aspects of health care delivery that may be affected by PPS have been extended. And, finally, some new DHHS studies have been undertaken with the purpose of providing background information for congressionally mandated studies. The nonmandated studies of HCFA and other DHHS agencies, especially PHS agencies, are discussed further below.

Health Care Financing Administration.—HCFA conducts or funds intramural and extramural research and demonstrations on a wide range of issues pertaining to Medicare and Medicaid delivery of health services. HCFA's ORD directs more than 300 research, evaluation, and demonstration projects, a substantial number of which focus on hospital payment. ORD projects are split between the Office of Research (OR) and the Office of Demonstrations and Evaluations (ODE) (336).

Table 10-2 provides a comprehensive list of all currently active extramural and intramural, ORD-supported, nonmandated studies of prospective payment for hospitals. Many of these studies will be used as background for the congressionally mandated studies of PPS. As shown in table 10-2, major areas covered by the studies are State alternatives to PPS, evaluation of PPS impacts, and case-mix measurement.

ORD's research priorities relating to hospital payment for the short term (through fiscal year 1986), mid term (fiscal years 1987 to 1989), and long term (fiscal year 1990 and beyond) are shown in table 10-3. Short-term priorities include research on topics such as the refinement and recalibration of DRGs and the development of DRG-type payment systems for nonhospital services such as skilled nursing facilities (SNFs) and for physicians' services provided to inpatients. Mid- and long-term priorities focus on research pertaining to the development of alternative prospective payment systems for other kinds of services or capitation.

HCFA has embarked on two 5-year cooperative agreements for Health Policy Centers with Brandeis University[3] and the Rand Corp./University of California at Los Angeles. The agency has assigned background research related to mandated studies of PPS to these two Health Policy Centers, as shown in table 10-4. Each HCFA Health Policy Center has signed the first year's $975,000 cooperative agreement to do a variety of studies for both OR and ODE. Brandeis is to do 75 percent OR work and 25 percent ODE work, and Rand is to do 75 percent ODE work and 25 percent OR work. However, the first year of the Health Policy Centers' activities have not followed these OR/ODE formulas, probably because demonstrations tend to require more startup time and because of the early congressional deadlines on the mandated OR studies.

Public Health Service (PHS) Agencies.—Shortly after the introduction of PPS, NCHSR&HCTA was designated the focal point for the coordination of prospective payment studies within PHS. Other PHS agencies involved in PPS studies are the Alcohol, Drug Abuse, and Mental Health Administration (ADAMHA); the Health Resources and Services Administration (HRSA); the Centers for Disease Control (CDC); the Office of Health Planning and Evaluation (OHPE); NIH; and the National Center for Health Statistics (NCHS). The nonmandated PPS-related studies of NCHSR&HCTA, ADAMHA, HRSA, CDC, and OHPE are listed in table 10-5.

Most of NCHSR&HCTA's PPS-related work has involved PPS refinement issues, especially patient classification and case-mix measurement (see table 10-5). Indeed, the initial design of DRGs resulted from extramural funding of Yale researchers by NCHSR. NCHSR&HCTA's ongoing study of the impacts of PPS on clinical cancer research (study #6 in table 10-5) directly addresses one of the five important PPS impact areas identified by OTA. In addition, internal staff analyses and special studies, most of which use a unique national database developed for NCHSR&HCTA's Hospital Cost and Utilization Project,[4] have covered PPS-related issues such as patient classification systems, sole community hospitals, and the effectiveness of DRG payment on long-term care.

NCHSR&HCTA regularly supports intramural and extramural studies that seek to enhance understanding of the health care system and which therefore may make evaluation of PPS more feasible. Currently, for example, NCHSR&HCTA is sponsoring studies to refine a predictive model for hospital readmissions (study #9 in table 10-5), to

---

[3]Brandeis subcontracts some of this work to other members of its Health Policy Consortium, which includes The Urban Institute, Boston University Health Care Research Unit, Center for Health Economics Research, and Brandeis.

[4]The Hospital Cost and Utilization Project database is described in app. C.

Table 10-2.—ORD-Supported, Nonmandated Studies of Prospective Payment for Hospitals Active in 1985

Study topic	Period	Funding[a]	Status (as of August 1985)
State Alternatives to PPS:			
1. National Hospital Ratesetting Study	8/78 to 2/85	$5,544,478	Complete
2. Incentive Prospective Payment System for Hospitals Through Fiscal Intermediaries	9/82 to 9/86	Waiver (MA)	—
3. Rochester Area Hospitals' Corp.	1/80 to 12/86	Waiver (NY)	—
4. Finger Lakes Area Hospitals' Corp.	1/81 to 12/85	Waiver (NY)	—
5. Prospective Reimbursement Systems Based on Patient Case Mix for New Jersey Hospitals	12/76 to 12/84	$4,912,802	Complete
6. Proposal of the Development of a Hospital Reimbursement Methodology for New York State for the 1980s	1/83 to 12/85	Waiver (NJ)	—
7. Prospective Payment System for Acute and Chronic Care Hospitals in Maryland	6/80 to 6/84	$2,037,563	Complete
8. Response of Massachusetts Acute Care Hospitals to the Massachusetts Hospital Cost Containment Act	12/84 to 11/87	$ 590,395	—
Evaluation Studies:			
9. Prospective Payment Beneficiary Impact Study	3/84-ongoing	Intramural	In clearance[b]
10. Commission on Professional and Hospital Activities Study (on quality-related process and hospital utilization before and during PPS)	9/84 to 9/88	$ 145,261	—
11. Rand Investigation Into Quality Indicators	9/84 to 12/87	$ 860,679	—
12. Selected Analyses of PPS Impact on Hospital Behavior	7/84 to 1/87	$ 480,423	—
13. Longitudinal Studies of Local Area Hospital Use	7/84 to 7/87	$ 214,290	—
14. Appropriateness of Hospitalization: A Comparative Analysis of Reliability and Validity of the Appropriateness Evaluation Protocol and Standardize Medreview Instrument	7/84 to 1/86	$ 306,342	—
15. Trends in Distribution of Medicare Expenditures	Fall 1985	Intramural	—
16. Relation of Surgical Volume to Mortality After Surgery	Winter 1985	Intramural	Preliminary draft complete
17. Rehospitalization After Surgery Among Medicare Enrollees	Winter 1985	Intramural	—
18. Study of the Relationship Between Cause of Death and Medicare Costs	Spring 1986	Intramural	—
19. National Impact Feasiblity Study (proposed)	2/85 to 9/85	$ 75,000	—
20. Rand Pilot Study (on process and outcome variables available from medical records)	2/85 to 12/85	NA[c]	—
Case-Mix Measurement:			
21. Measuring the Cost of Case Mix Using Patient Management Algorithms	9/78 to 7/84	$1,166,846	Draft submitted
22. Severity of Illness Within DRGs	8/83 to 8/84	$ 87,711	Complete
23. DRGs and Nursing Resources	7/84 to 7/86	$ 427,910	—
24. DRG Refinements for Nursing Care	8/83 to 3/85	$ 349,126	Complete
25. Severity of Illness and DRGs in Selected Cancers	9/84 to 9/87	$ 214,010	—
26. Learning From and Improving DRGs for End-Stage Renal Disease Patients	7/84 to 7/86	$ 187,500	—
27. Children's Hospital Case-Mix Classification System	7/84 to 7/85	$ 395,000	Incomplete
28. Study To Develop and Test Measures of Case Mix, Complexity, Case Mix Severity, and Case Volume for Hospitals	9/78 to 5/84	$ 426,630	Complete
29. Study To Determine Reasons for 7.4% Rise in Overall Case-Mix Index of Hospitals in 1984	1/85 to 3/85	Intramural	Complete
30. Case-Mix and Resource Use in Hospital Emergency Room Settings	3/83 to 9/85	$ 612,785	—
Other:			
31. Prospective Payment in Rehabilitation Hospitals and Programs	10/84 to 9/85	$ 700,000	—
32. Evaluation of National Rural Swing-Bed Program[d]	9/83 to 6/86	$ 722,248	—
33. PRO Quality Objective Report	4/85-ongoing	Intramural	—

[a]Dollar amounts represent extramural funding. Funding levels for intramural projects and projects being conducted with State waivers that permit innovations to financing and delivery of health services under Medicare are not specified.
[b]Report has been completed and is being reviewed within DHHS before being submitted to Congress.
[c]NA = Not available.
[d]HCFA is negotiating with the contractor to extent the scope of the report to address the impact of PPS on the swing-bed program. If approved, the study will be extended until 10/87 and will receive an additional $280,000 (266).

SOURCE: U.S. Department of Health and Human Services, Health Care Financing Administration, *Status Report*, HCFA Pub. No. 03185 (Washington, DC: U.S. Government Printing Office, April 1985); updated by OTA through personal communication with ORD, August 1985.

Table 10-3.—ORD's Short-, Mid-, and Long-Term Research Priorities Relating to Hospital Payment

Short-term: Fiscal years 1984-86

Prospective payment system:
- Refine and recalibrate DRGs
- Develop severity measures for use in PPS
- Study hospitals which are sole providers in their communities and fairness of payments
- Study hospitals not yet involved in the system
- Incorporate factors for capital and graduate medical education into the rates

New developments:
- Develop a DRG-type system that combines payment for acute care and long-term care (skilled nursing facilities)
- Develop a DRG-type system that combines payment for acute care and physician services provided to hospital inpatients
- Study feasibility of hospital outpatient DRGs
- Evaluate impact of Medicare PPS for hospitals with Medicaid programs

Mid-term: Fiscal years 1987-89
- Recalibrate rates for PPS
- Develop, demonstrate, and evaluate an outpatient PPS
- Demonstrate and evaluate systems combining hospital and physician payment
- Demonstrate and evaluate systems combining hospital and skilled nursing facility payments
- Develop competitive-bidding payment models for hospital services
- Demonstrate and evaluate alternative PPS: with disease staging, by patient management category, and with severity of illness adjustments

Long-term: Fiscal year 1990 and beyond
- Demonstrate and evaluate competitive-bidding payment systems for hospital services
- Evaluate the effects of voucher payment systems on hospital efficiency, solvency, accessibility, and capital formation

SOURCE: U.S. Department of Health and Human Services, Health Care Financing Administration, "Selected Activities for Short-Term and Long-Term Agenda," unpublished, Baltimore, MD, 1984.

Table 10-4.—HCFA Health Policy Center PPS-Related Assignments (as of August 1985)

Study topic[a]	HCFA report due date	Center designation
1. Background for Annual Impact Report	9/84-87	Rand/UCLA
2. Sole Community Hospitals' Occupancy	4/1/85	Brandeis
3. Uncompensated Care Costs	4/1/85	Brandeis
4. Large Rural Teaching Hospitals	4/1/85	Brandeis
5. Cost of Care Information to Patients	4/1/85	Rand/UCLA
6. Physician DRGs	7/5/85	Brandeis
7. Case-Mix Measurement Refinements for DRGs (severity of illness, intensity of care, and adequacy of outlier payments)	12/31/85	Rand/UCLA
8. Incorporating "Excepted" Hospitals Into PPS	12/31/85	Brandeis[b]
9. Eliminating Rural-Urban Rates	12/31/85	Brandeis
10. All-Payer Feasiblity, Cost Shifting	12/31/85	Brandeis
11. Impact of Admissions, Volume Adjustment	12/31/85	Rand/UCLA
12. Impact of State Alternative PPS on: Medicare, Medicaid, Private Health Expenditures, Tax Expenditures	12/31/86	Brandeis

[a]These studies directly support one or more of the congressionally mandated studies listed in table 10-1.
[b]The Rand Corp. is taking the lead on rehabilitation hospitals.

SOURCE: U.S. Department of Health and Human Services, Health Care Financing Administration, *Status Report*, HCFA Pub. No. 03185 (Washington, DC: U.S. Government Printing Office, April 1985); updated by OTA staff through personal communication with HCFA, August 1985.

assess factors related to variations in length of hospital stay (study #7 in table 10-5), and to analyze multihospital systems (study #8 in table 10-5).

ADAMHA's PPS-related studies concentrate on the development of patient classification systems (see table 10-5). Psychiatric and alcoholic units and hospitals are currently exempted under PPS. It is widely recognized that a patient classification system that accurately reflects resource use by patients in these facilities is needed if the exemptions are to be eliminated.

HRSA is concentrating on conducting research on the impacts of PPS on health care personnel (see table 10-5). Other PPS-related studies by the agency focus on health care planning.

CDC is planning an intramural study on the effect of DRGs on hospital infection rates, an important quality impact (see table 10-5). CDC's study will determine: 1) the relationship between DRG group and risk of iatrogenic infection, and 2) the proportion of iatrogenic infections that result in additional payment to hospitals. CDC also anticipates that changes in laboratory services will occur as a result of PPS. After developing a forecasting system and predicting trends in laboratory services, CDC hopes to track shifts in sites of services (e.g., from hospital laboratories to ambulatory settings) to monitor the quality of the services and to assist laboratories in maintaining quality.

OHPE is developing an analytic framework and a research agenda to address how the prospective payment system may be affecting access and qual-

Table 10-5.—Nonmandated PPS-Related Studies by Public Health Service Agencies

Study topic	Period	Funding[a]	Status (as of August 1985)
National Center for Health Services Research and Health Care Technology Assessment (NCHSR&HCTA):			
1. Impact of "Per-Case" Versus "Per-Service" Hospital Reimbursement	9/30/79 to 9/29/83	$393,561	Complete
2. Marginal Cost of Hospital Output and Empty Beds	9/1/81 to 5/31/84	$159,235	Complete
3. Measuring Clinical Homogeneity in the Two DRG Systems	7/15/83 to 2/28/85	$111,945	Incomplete
4. Adjustment Artifacts in DRG-Based Medicare Reimbursement	9/1/84 to 8/31/85	$ 21,539	—
5. Trauma Case-Mix Measurement and Hospital Payment	9/30/84 to 9/29/86	$170,588	—
6. Impacts of the Prospective Payment System on Clinical Cancer Research (with NCI)	9/30/84 to 8/31/86	$516,169	—
7. Factors Related to Hospitals' Length of Stay	1/1/81 to 12/31/85	$680,479	—
8. Multihospital Systems' Strategy, Structure, and Performance (Effect of PPS)	9/1/84 to 8/31/86	$202,747	—
9. Prevention of Nonelective Hospital Readmissions	9/30/85 to 9/29/86	$106,159	—
10. Hospital Use Rates in Local Communities in Michigan	4/1/85 to 9/30/88	$ 65,698	—
Alcohol, Drug Abuse, and Mental Health Administration (ADAMHA):			
1. Effects of Prospective Hospital Payment on Acute Inpatient Care for Mental Disorders	1981 to 1983	$ 62,754	Complete
2. Evaluation of the DHHS Proposed DRGs	4/83 to 8/83	$ 9,440	Complete
3. Identification of Resource Determinants for Use in Patient Classification Systems for Prospective Payment	3/1/84 to 8/31/84	$ 10,000	Complete
4. A Comparative Analysis of Functionally Related and Diagnosis-Related Groups	5/10/84 to 3/1/85	$ 9,999	Complete
5. A Study of Patient Classification Systems for Prospective Ratesetting for Medicare Patients in General Hospital Psychiatric Units and Psychiatric Hospitals	6/30/84 to 12/19/85	$665,189	—
6. Selected Data on Psychiatric DRGs From the Commission on Professional and Hospital Activities National Sample Patient File	7/15/84 to 8/31/84	$ 9,950	Complete
7. The Use of Survival Time Analysis as a Method of Patient Classification	9/1/84 to 1/31/85	$ 9,400	Complete
8. Medicare-Medicaid Alcoholism Treatment Demonstration	9/81 to 12/85	$ 60,000	—
9. Secondary Analysis of Drug and Alcohol Followup Data for Relevance to Diagnosis and Classification	7/1/84 to 6/30/85	$ 85,000	—
10. Development of Diagnostic Sourcebook and Minimum Research Criteria	10/1/84 to 9/30/85	$ 68,000	—
11. Utilization of the Severity-of-Illness Index in Psychiatric Diagnosis	1/10/85 to 10/9/85	$ 25,000	—
Health Resources and Services Administration (HRSA):			
1. Experience With the Section 1122 Capital Expenditure Review Program	4/9/84 to 9/30/84	$ 99,957	Complete
2. Implications of the DRG Reimbursement Methodologies on the Health Care System and Impact on Local Health Planning in the Short Term and Over the Long Term	4/84 to 7/85	NA[b]	Complete
3. Compilation and Descriptive Analysis of Major Third-Party Coverages for Health Services as Related to Health Personnel Standards	5/3/84 to 11/2/84	$ 17,614	Complete
4. Assessment of the Impact of DRGs on Changes in the Health Services Administration Function	6/18/84 to 4/17/85	$ 13,047	Incomplete
5. Prospective Payment and DRGs: Impact on the Allied Health Professions	6/29/84 to 8/14/85	$ 13,227	Incomplete
6. Impact of PPS on Medical Records Personnel	Not specified	Intramural	—
7. Evaluation Study To Examine Recent Patterns of Capital Expenditures To Assess Hospital Reaction to DRG Reimbursement	Proposed fiscal year 1985	—	—
8. Evaluation Study To Examine the Impact of DRGs on the Financial Position of the Hospitals in HUD 242 Portfolio	Proposed fiscal year 1985	—	—
9. A Series of Studies To Assess the Effect on Health Professions' Training Costs of the Medicare PPS	Proposed fiscal year 1985	—	—
Centers for Disease Control (CDC):			
1. Effect of DRGs on Hospital Infections	Proposed fiscal year 1985	Intramural	—
2. Impact of DRG System on Diabetes-Related Hospitalizations	10/1/83 to 6/20/84	$ 8,800	Complete
Office of Health Planning and Evaluation (OHPE):			
1. Development of a Research Agenda To Explore Issues of Access and Quality of Care in the Current Health Care Environment	4/10/85 to 6/30/86	$132,000	—

[a]Dollar amounts represent extramural funding. Funding levels for intramural projects and projects being conducted with State waivers that permit innovations in financing and delivery of health services under Medicare are not specified.
[b]NA = Not available.

SOURCE: U.S. Department of Health and Human Services, Public Health Service, National Center for Health Services Research, "Prospective Payment Activity as of April 1985," Rockville, MD, April 1985; updated by OTA staff through personal communication with NCHSR&HCTA, ADAMHA, and HRSA, August 1985.

ity of care. The study will organize the existing data and knowledge base currently available inside and outside DHHS and identify gaps in the database.

NIH has sponsored task forces and workgroups to address PPS issues, especially the effect of PPS on clinical cancer research. A planning group is coordinating efforts to collect data relating to DRGs and to access their impact on biomedical research.

NCHS has been assessing the ability of its databases to provide information relevant to evaluating PPS. In particular, the Hospital Discharge Survey, the National Nursing Home Survey, and the National Ambulatory Medical Care Survey may be used for data purposes. (These surveys are described in app. C.)

Other DHHS Agencies.—Nonmandated PPS-related studies being undertaken in ASPE and the Office of the Inspector General within DHHS are shown in table 10-6. In several cases, the ASPE studies support the Secretary's mandated studies. ASPE's feasibility analysis to determine whether Medicare Parts A and B can be linked at the carrier and intermediary levels (study #4 in table 10-6), for example, follows a HCFA-sponsored study on linking data from Part A and Part B claims at the central database level. The integration of Part A and Part B databases would be an important milestone in the development of prospective payment systems that cover a number of services.

ASPE's project on financing graduate medical education (study #2 in table 10-6) was begun before PPS or the Tax Equity and Fiscal Responsibility Act of 1982 (Public Law 97-248), and it will report on whether teaching hospitals are more expensive than nonteaching hospitals when quality, case mix, and other factors are considered. ASPE is also developing a strategy for studying the impact of hospital prospective payment on long-term care (study #5 in table 10-6).

In March 1984, the DHHS Office of the Inspector General issued a strategy report on its own activities regarding the assessment of PPS (343). Strategies will include the following: 1) monitoring databases for accuracy; 2) examining changes in costs and payments under both Part A and Part B; 3) assessing the effectiveness of utilization and quality control peer review organizations (PROs) and fiscal intermediaries in maintaining the integrity of Medicare; 4) examining the extent of admission, readmission, and transfers for hospitals' financial benefit; 5) ascertaining fraud under PPS; and 6) recommending improvements in the system. Planned activities for fiscal year 1985 reflect this strategy and include assessments of PROs, DRG inspections, and the policy analyses listed in table 10-6.

Studies by Congressional Agencies

In response both to internal priorities and to requests from congressional committees, CBO, CRS, GAO, and OTA have devoted and are continuing to devote substantial resources to the evaluation and monitoring of PPS.

Congressional Budget Office.—CBO is working on a series of four PPS-related studies that will be combined into a single report upon completion. Preliminary papers for two of these studies have been prepared at the request of two Members of Congress: one paper entitled "Impact of Medicare Prospective Payment System on Disproportionate Share Hospitals"[5] and the other "An Analysis of the Impacts of a DRG Specific Price Blending Option for Medicare's Prospective Payment System." The two remaining studies of the series will cover indirect teaching adjustments and the expenditure effects of freezing rates and the transition to national rates. CBO's full report should be available in early summer 1986 (263).

Congressional Research Service.—CRS has completed two studies pertaining to PPS, an "issue brief" on Medicare prospective payment for inpatient hospital services and a paper on graduate medical education under Medicare. Both were prepared for congressional use. CRS is currently preparing a legislative history of the 1983 Social Security Amendments which set up PPS. The

---

[5] As of August 1985, there was no official definition of "disproportionate share hospitals." Section 2315 of the Deficit Reduction Act of 1984 (Public Law 98-369) directed the Secretary of Health and Human Services to "develop and publish a definition of 'hospitals that serve a significantly disproportionate number of patients who have low income or are entitled to benefits under [Medicare] part A'...."

Table 10-6.—Nonmandated PPS-Related Studies by the DHHS Office of the Assistant Secretary for Planning and Evaluation and by the DHHS Office of the Inspector General

Study topic	Period	Funding[a]	Status (as of August 1985)
Office of the Assistant Secretary for Planning and Evaluation (ASPE):			
1. Policy Analysis Needs for Implementation of the Medicare PPS	3/84 to 10/84	$ 253,000	Complete
2. Financing of Graduate Medical Education	10/81 to 9/85	$4,000,000	
3. Hospital Capital Study[b]	1/84 to 9/84	$ 125,000	In clearance[c]
4. Feasibility Analysis To Determine Whether Medicare Parts A and B Can Be Linked at the Carrier and Intermediary Levels[b]	7/84 to 2/85	$ 143,000	Complete
5. Project To Monitor Impact of Hospital Prospective Payment on Long-Term Care[b]	6/84 to 3/85	$ 125,000	Incomplete
6. Analysis of Medical and Hospital Utilization Review in the Private Sector	Proposed fiscal year 1986	$ 350,000 (est.)	—
7. Effects of PPS on Hospital Decisions Regarding Capital Investment	Proposed fiscal year 1987	Intramural	—
Office of the Inspector General (OIG):			
1. The Prospective Payment System and the (DHHS) Office of the Inspector General	3/84	Intramural	Complete
2. Medicare Reimbursement for DRG #469	Ending 11/18/83	Intramural	Complete
3. Overpayment for Lens Procedures	Ending 7/20/84	Intramural	Complete
4. Overpayment for Coronary Procedures	Ending 6/7/84	Intramural	Complete
5. Inappropriate Readmissions and Transfer Practices Under the PPS	Ending 10/23/84	Intramural	Complete
6. Overpayment for Cardiac Arrest	Ending 12/20/84	Intramural	Complete
7. Overpayment for Nail Removals	Ending 1/28/85	Intramural	Complete
8. Review of Peer Review Organizations	Planned fiscal year 1985	Intramural	—
9. DRG Inspections	Planned fiscal year 1985	Intramural	—
a. Vulnerable DRGs (#14, #82, #88, and others that show upcoding potential and significant case-mix changes)	Planned fiscal year 1985	Intramural	—
b. Evaluation of PRO DRG Validations	Planned fiscal year 1985	Intramural	—
c. DRG Validation in Hospitals Selected on a Statistically Valid Basis	Planned fiscal year 1985	Intramural	—
10. Special Policy Analyses	—	Intramural	—
a. Part B Reasonable Charge Levels for Intraocular Lenses	10/84 to 9/85	Intramural	—
b. Assistants at Cataract/Intraocular Lens Implant Surgery at Teaching Hospitals	10/84 to 9/85	Intramural	—
c. Anesthesiology During Intraocular Lens Surgery	10/84 to 9/85	Intramural	—

[a]Dollar amounts represent extramural funding. Funding levels for intramural projects are not specified.
[b]Directly supports one (or more) of the congressionally mandated studies of PPS.
[c]Report has been completed and is being reviewed within DHHS before being submitted to Congress.

SOURCE: K. Means, Office of Assistant Secretary for Planning and Evaluation, U.S. Department of Health and Human Services, Washington, DC, personal communication, March 1985; Prospective Payment Assessment Commission, *Technical Appendixes to the Report and Recommendations to the Secretary, U.S Department of Health and Human Services* (Washington, DC: U.S. Government Printing Office, April 1985); and U.S. Department of Health and Human Services, Office of Inspector General, "The Prospective Payment System and The Office of Inspector General," Washington, DC, Mar. 8, 1984; updated by OTA staff through personal communication with ASPE and OIG, August 1985.

agency is also compiling a database and developing the capacity to model Medicare's PPS system. Plans are being developed for a paper on capital costs under Medicare. In addition, CRS has been providing daily staff assistance to congressional committees and Members of Congress on developing and evaluating PPS legislation in the 99th Congress (167).

General Accounting Office.—During the next 3 to 5 years, GAO plans to review the effectiveness of the mechanisms that were developed to prevent potential problems of PPS. Specifically, the agency will evaluate the adequacy of the databases used to set PPS payment rates, the effectiveness of PROs, and the effectiveness of PPS payment controls to prevent hospitals from maximizing payment.

GAO is engaged in a number of specific PPS-related studies, and more are in the planning and proposal stages (see table 10-7). These studies range from the adequacy of DRG rates in respiratory/inhalation therapy to information require-

Table 10-7.—Nonmandated PPS-Related Studies by the General Accounting Office

Study topic	Due date	Status (as of August 1985)
Ongoing studies:		
1. Evaluation of Utilization Review Efforts for Respiratory/Inhalation Therapy (adequacy of DRG rates)	9/84	Complete
2. Survey of Utilization of Intensive Care Unit Services by Low-Risk Medicare Patients	8/85	—
3. Review of Medicare Reimbursement for Implanting Cardiac Pacemakers	2/85	Complete
4. Information Requirements for Evaluating the Impacts of Medicare Prospective Payment on Post-Hospital Long-Term Care Services	8/15/85	Incomplete
5. Survey of Patient Classification and Utilization Reviews of Nursing Homes	3/85	Complete
6. Evaluation of Medicare's Hospital Admission Monitoring Systems	11/18/85	
7. Survey of Intermediary Audits of Hospital Cost Reports	8/85	Complete
8. Review of Effect on Medicare/Medicaid Costs of Hospital Conversions From Nonprofit to Proprietary Status	1/86	—
9. Survey of Unnecessary Admissions and Premature Discharges	Ongoing	—
Planned studies:		
10. Review of Utilization of Medically Unnecessary Hospital Days of Care by Medicare Patients		
11. Survey of Congressionally Mandated HHS Study of How To Incorporate Capital Costs Into Prospective Reimbursement		
Proposed studies:		
12. Survey of HCFA's Methodology for Calculating the Prospective Rates		
13. Survey To Assure That Medicare Beneficiaries Have Adequate Access to Care		
14. Survey of the Incidence of Unnecessary Surgery		
15. Review of the Accuracy of DRG Classification by Hospitals		
16. Survey of Improperly Allocated Costs		
17. Review of Billing Practices for Hospital-Based Professional Services		
18. Survey of Medicare Reimbursement for Hospital Teaching Costs		
19. Survey of Prospective Payment Plans in States With Medicare Waivers		
20. Survey of States' Compliance With Waiver Criteria for Exemptions Granted After Enactment of Medicare PPS		
21. Survey To Monitor Mandated HHS Studies on Prospective Reimbursement		

SOURCE: U.S. Congress, General Accounting Office, Human Resources Division, "Reviewing the Medicare Prospective Reimbursement System for Hospitals," draft, Washington, DC, February 1984; updated by OTA staff through personal communication with GAO, August 1985.

ments for evaluating the impacts of Medicare PPS on posthospital long-term care services. GAO studies can be generated either internally or by congressional request.

One ongoing GAO study, "Information Requirements for Evaluating the Impacts of Medicare Prospective Payment on Post-Hospital Long-Term-Care Services" (study #4 in table 10-7), will identify Federal information and evaluation requirements for assessing the impact of PPS on posthospital health care (especially nursing home and home health care). A preliminary report has been released on the first stage of the project (297). Key issues were identified as follows:

- Have Medicare patients' posthospital needs changed?
- How are patients' needs being met?
- Are patients having access problems?
- How have long-term care costs been affected?

The second stage of the project will determine whether the questions can and will be addressed by current or planned evaluation studies or data collection efforts. GAO will suggest additional or different studies if such studies are considered necessary to complement ongoing efforts (297).

Office of Technology Assessment.—OTA's Health Program studies and publishes reports on issues of medical technology as requested by Congress. Some of OTA's studies, including the present one, have contained specific references to PPS. The first project to include this issue was the July 1983 OTA technical memorandum "DRGs and the Medicare Program: Implications for Medical Technology" (305). That study was part of a larger OTA assessment "Medical Technology and Costs of the Medicare Program" (307). OTA is also responsible for the oversight of ProPAC, and released its first report to Congress on ProPAC in March 1985 (309).

Studies by the Prospective Payment Assessment Commission

When making its recommendations about the DRG updating factor and changes in individual DRG weights and categories, ProPAC must decide whether PPS is having some undesirable impact on beneficiaries. ProPAC has a statutory responsibility to take into account quality of care (Public Law 98-21). For that reason, ProPAC's research agenda shows a high priority for research on quality of care, which includes assessing current information, developing new databases, and improving quality measures. Specific plans for implementing this research agenda item are being developed.

PPS-related issues are brought to ProPAC's attention from external sources (such as medical specialty societies, the hospital industry, or Congress) and from internal staff or Commissioner analyses. Initial screening analyses are conducted to select technologies for in-depth analyses. The screening guidelines focus primarily on the interaction between quality of care and potential short- or long-term Medicare payment effects. The screening analyses of specific technologies are not evaluations of PPS per se, but the criteria that trigger whether such analyses are undertaken involve evaluation.

PPS-RELATED EVALUATION STUDIES BY PRIVATE ORGANIZATIONS

Many private organizations, including professional societies such as the American Medical Association, trade associations such as the Health Industry Manufacturers' Association, and beneficiary groups such as the American Association of Retired Persons, have an interest in the impacts of PPS and are conducting their own studies, both formal and informal. Because of the lack of timely and comprehensive data needed for their studies, many private organizations are in the process of compiling their own databases to complement or compare with HCFA's databases.

In March 1985, as part of the present study, OTA conducted a survey of over 250 organizations to ascertain the extent of private initiatives in evaluating PPS. Very brief descriptions of studies reported by the more than 70 organizations responding to OTA's survey are provided in table 10-8.

Most of the studies listed in table 10-8 cover more than one area of PPS impact. The majority cover some aspect of quality of care. Access to care and cost of care are topics in almost one-half of the studies. Approximately 20 percent of the studies address issues of PPS effects on health professions education, and about 12 percent deal with technological change. Only one of the groups responding to OTA's survey indicated that it was directly studying the effects of PPS on clinical research.[6]

---

[6]Although the present assessment does not cover PPS effects on employment, it is interesting to note that many of the private organizations listed are conducting employment impact studies. For example, PPS effects on employment in nursing, occupational therapy, and medical records are being monitored by their respective associations.

Table 10-8.—PPS-Related Evaluation Studies by Private Organizations
(based on OTA's March 1985 survey)

Organization/Study topic	Period	Funding	Comments
Provider organizations:			
American Academy of Neurology			
DRG expanded survey to obtain specific data on areas of concern which surfaced in an initial survey on DRGs	3/15/85 to 6/15/85	Internal	
American Academy of Ophthalmology			
Survey to assess impact of DRGs	1985	Uncertain	Council of Medical Specialty Societies (CMSS) is coordinating effort
American Academy of Otolaryngology-Head and Neck Surgery, Inc.			
Request to members to report experiences, both good and bad, especially regarding quality of care	Open-ended, ongoing	None	
American Association for Clinical Chemistry			
AACC Membership Survey on Impact of DRGs	Completed 5/84 and 5/85	Internal	
American Association for Respiratory Therapy			
"Impact of Prospective Payment on Manpower Needs"	1/85 to 12/85	NA[a]	
American College of Cardiology			
1. Decision analysis of DRG payment rates relative to quality care; to determine if DRG payments are adequate to allow appropriate procedures and practices for optimal patient outcome	Ongoing	$20,000/yr.	
2. DRG survey to obtain physicians' perceptions and case reports on PPS effect on quality of care	Ongoing, quarterly until 1987	$ 4,000/yr	
American College of Hospital Administrators			
"Health Care in the 1990s: Trends and Strategies"	Completed 1984	NA	Used the Delphi Method forecasting response to elicit opinions from health care experts in six areas
American College of Physicians			
Two-part questionnaire to members to identify effects of PPS and collect an information base for modifying it regarding quality of care, problematic DRGs, causes and overt manifestations of negative and positive effects of PPS	1985-ongoing	NA	Cooperating with CMSS on a uniform PPS data set for all physician specialties
American College of Preventive Medicine			
Cooperative effort with American Medical Association	Ongoing	NA	
American Hospital Association			
1. Survey on PPS: qualitative survey of hospital chief executive officers' current assessments of problems and opportunities in PPS design and implementation	Quarterly	NA	
2. Annual Medicare financial survey: collects quantitative data summarizing each hospital's experience with TEFRA and PPS in terms of Medicare revenues, costs, and utilization activity	Annual	NA	
3. One-time special surveys on selected PPS issues	As needed	NA	
American Lung Association and medical section of American Thoracic Society			
Pilot survey by questionnaire entitled "Early Impact of the Prospective Payment System on the Pulmonary Community" to compile information on quality of patient care, length of stay, and introduction of new medical technologies	10/84 to 12/84	Internal	
American Medical Association			
1. DRG Monitoring Project: information assessment activity to ascertain current impact of PPS and identify possible problem areas for further study	Continuing. First report available	Internal	
2. Long-term effects of PPS on quality of health care for Medicare beneficiaries	NA	NA	Developing research proposals with Johns Hopkins University
American Medical Record Association			
1. "DRG Variation Analysis Study" to identify discrepancies in coding between medical record departments and PROs	8 mos.—ending mid-1985	$3,000	Results will be published in Journal of American Medical Record Association
2. Survey on the impact of PPS on medical record departments	Published 5/85	NA	
American Nurses' Association			
"DRG Refinement for Nursing Care": variations in nursing care in selected DRGs; appropriateness of refining DRGs to reflect differences in nursing care requirements	9/83 to 3/85	$370,000	Funded by HCFA
American Occupational Therapy Association			
Opinion-based survey on the "Impact of Prospective Payment System on Occupational Therapists"	Completed 1985	$3,500	
American Osteopathic Association			
Collection of anecdotal information resulting from dialogue with affiliates	Ongoing	None	
American Podiatric Medical Association			
Analysis of costs of care provided by podiatrists and other practitioners in 20 hospitals under DRGs and 2 in waivered States (Maryland and New Jersey); description of patterns of foot care provided by podiatrists; development of a database on patients with foot health problems treated by podiatrists	1/85 to 8/85		

Table 10-8.—PPS-Related Evaluation Studies by Private Organizations—Continued
(based on OTA's March 1985 survey)

Organization/Study topic	Period	Funding	Comments
American Psychiatric Association			
The Task Force on Prospective Payment is overseeing a DRG project to: 1) check the heterogeneity of psychiatric DRGs, 2) assess several variables for variance reduction, and 3) compare HCFA database (for MDC-20 and MDC-19).	1984 to 5/85	$150,000	
American Psychological Association			
1. Board of directors special task force on prospective payment which reviews clinical literature and current research and develops position papers	Ongoing	NA	
2. "Survey of PPS Impact on Psychologists" to analyze PPS impact on the provision of hospital services to the mentally disabled, including the use of multidisciplinary treatment teams, use of alternative settings, and particular impact of PPS on the professional services of psychologists	1983-85	NA	
American Society of Clinical Pathologists and the College of American Pathologists			
"PPS/DRG Impact Survey," to collect trend data for hospital laboratories regarding laboratory use, impacts on laboratory personnel, hospital beds, and type of contractual agreements with hospitals	1/84—ongoing	$40,000	Mini opinion-based study 1984
American Society of EEG Technologists, Inc.			
A salary/employment status questionnaire to monitor employment trends and changes and effects of PPS on hospital setting	5/85	NA	
American Society of Internal Medicine			
Questionnaire for incident reporting by members regarding the impact of PPS on quality of care: pressure from hospitals to discharge patients early or underutilize medically necessary tests, etc.; improvements in quality of care through more careful testing, improved communication, increased cost awareness	Ongoing	NA	
American Speech-Language-Hearing Association			
National survey of hospital-based members of association and others on the "Impact of Prospective Payment System on Speech-Language Pathology and Audiology Services in Hospitals"—especially on reduction or elimination of services to inpatients	1985—open ended	NA	Two small sample surveys were conducted at national meetings of the association
Association for the Advancement of Medical Instrumentation			
Survey to evaluate impact of Medicare's prospective payment system on the association's membership and programming	1985 to 1990	$50,000	
Association of American Medical Colleges			
1. Survey on estimated Medicare revenue and expense under TEFRA and PPS, patient mix information, hospital bed capacity, and full-time equivalent residents in training	1985 version planned	Internal	
2. "The Medicare Adjustment for the Indirect Costs of Medical Education: Historical Development and Current Status"	Published in January 1985	NA	Commissioned paper by Judith Lave, Ph.D.
Association of Community Cancer Centers			
"ACCC DRG Research Project" intends to study the following issues: measuring the effect of DRGs on clinical research, conventional cancer patient management, technology diffusion, cancer program development and patient outcomes	1984-1987	$100,000	Will utilize a unique cancer database to gather demographic, clinical, survival, and financial information from more than 100 community and university hospitals
Committee on Allied Health Education and Accreditation of the AMA			
1. Survey on "Impact of Prospective Payment System on Clinical Education for Allied Health Students"—completed	8/84 to 1/85	NA	
2. Survey of program directors, "Perceptions Regarding CAHEA-Accredited Programs and Their Graduates	8/84 to 1/85	NA	
Council of Medical Specialty Societies			
National survey of physician opinions regarding DRGs: information regarding changes under DRG system and their perceived effects on costs and quality of care; addresses physicians' ability to identify specific troublesome DRGs	Pretested 1984; survey to be conducted fall 1985	NA	Multispecialty: 24 member specialty societies
District of Columbia Hospital Association			
"The Inequity of Medicare Prospective Payment in Large Urban Areas," to document the more severe impact of PPS on hospitals in large cities relative to those in suburbs and to recommend changes in PPS to improve equity	Published 9/84	Internal	1981 data used to project impact of PPS in first and fourth years of implementation
Federation of Nurses and Health Professionals			
Planning an opinion-based survey of members regarding quality of care and staffing ratios under PPS	Undecided	NA	Will probably compare 1985 to 1982-84
Florida Hospital Association			
Monitor utilization trends concurrent with introduction of PPS through quarterly hospital utilization surveys	Ongoing quarterly basis	NA	Collect data on: admissions, patient days, Medicare patient days, outpatient visits, Medicare outpatient visits

Table 10-8.—PPS-Related Evaluation Studies by Private Organizations—Continued
(based on OTA's March 1985 survey)

Organization/Study topic	Period	Funding	Comments
Health Industry Manufacturers' Association			
1. "Recalibration and Updating: A Means to Health Care Cost Control and Quality"	Published 2/84	NA	Focus on keeping PPS flexible for incorporating technological change
2. Recalibration case studies for diagnostic technologies	6/85 to 12/85	NA	Contract with Johns Hopkins University; focus on keeping PPS flexible for incorporating technological change
3. Policy analysis of recalibration issues	5/85 to 9/85	NA	Focus on keeping PPS flexible for incorporating technological change
4. "Study and Analysis of DRG Prices: Implications for Manufacturers"	Published 4/84	NA	Focus on keeping PPS flexible for incorporating technological change
Hospital Research and Educational Trust (affiliated with AMA)			
"An Evaluation of the New Medicare Prospective Pricing System as a Cost Containment Strategy" to examine changes in case mix resulting from PPS, conduct an analysis of public general and major teaching hospitals, study changes in the style of care provided, and assess trends in readmissions to acute care hospitals and hospital discharges to nursing homes and home health agencies			
Kansas Hospital Association			
"The State of Rural Kansas Hospitals: A Study of Hospitals in the First Congressional District of Kansas" to determine the early impacts of PPS and other Kansas payment system changes on rural hospitals in Kansas and to form a base for future impact assessments	1980-1984	NA	
Montana Hospital Association			
Financial impact on Montana hospitals of PPS, related to admission patterns and quality of care issues	1/83 to 9/85	$500	
National Coalition of Burn Center Hospitals			
Survey of all hospitals with burn centers to determine the impact of PPS			
New York City Health and Hospitals Corporation			
"Comparison of Resource Utilization: Public and Non-Public Hospital Patients" to identify causes in length-of-stay and cost differences	1981 to 1983	Internal	
Tennessee Hospital Association			
Quarterly utilization surveys	10/83—ongoing	Internal	
Washington Business Group on Health			
Created the Employers Prospective Payment Advisory Committee (EPPAC) to monitor ProPAC and examine impact of PPS	12/83—ongoing	None	Focus on technology assessment, cost shifting incited by DRGs, graduate medical education, coding errors and gaming
Wisconsin Hospital Association			
1. Modeling of the impact of Medicare PPS, including the effect of the 4-year blend, the freeze, and the wage index revision, as requested by member hospitals	Ongoing—as required	NA	
2. Survey on Medicare discharges, days, patient charges/costs, and problem DRGs	Quarterly	NA	
Beneficiary groups and disease-specific foundations:			
American Association of Retired Persons			
Informal reporting by members of experience regarding admissions and discharges	1/85 to 4/85	None	
American Diabetes Association			
Opinion-based study to determine impact of PPS on quality of health care for persons with diabetes	Ending 6/12/85	Internal	The Committee on Government Relations has been charged to report to the National Meeting
American Society for Parenteral and Enteral Nutrition			
"An Evaluation of the Implication and Implementation of the DRG-based Prospective Payment System on Parenteral and Enteral Nutrition Services" to provide society members with practical advice on how to function effectively and to determine if these services are equitably treated under PPS	2/84 to 5/85	$25,000	Also considering development of a proposed change to the ICD-9-CM coding system that would permit identification of parenteral and enteral nutrition cases in hospital and Medicare record systems. Proposing a major data collection effort to detect significant length of stay and cost variations among these patients

Table 10-8.—PPS-Related Evaluation Studies by Private Organizations—Continued
(based on OTA's March 1985 survey)

Organization/Study topic	Period	Funding	Comments
American Spinal Injury Association DRG-related length-of-stay allowance calculations for spinal cord injured persons to attempt to get exemption status for these patients	Completed 9/84	NA	Shared information with ProPAC
Burn Foundation Assessment of the applicability of several case-mix indices to burn care, specifically to improve categorization of burn patients regarding severity level	9/84 to 12/85	$370,000	National study of burn hospitalization at 24 hospitals
Cystic Fibrosis Foundation "Differential Resource Use Study," to study relative resource allocation of treating cystic fibrosis patients compared with caring for other patients in the same DRGs	6/84 to present		Shared information with ProPAC
National Association of Area Agencies on Aging "Effects of Medicare' Prospective Payment System on Community Based Long Term Care" to see if there has been an increased need and/or utilization of home health, chore, home-delivered meals, etc., and to assess if adequate community-based services are available to meet increased needs	Ongoing—5/85	Internal	
National Hemophilia Foundation DRG Data Collection Project	10/84 to 9/85	$46,000/yr.	NHF will report to ProPAC. Preliminary results demonstrate a great disparity between cost of treating hemophiliac patients and other patients classified in the same DRG
General purpose foundations:			
The Commonwealth Fund 1. Task Force on Academic Health Centers Program of Reports to examine conventional wisdom about effects of major public policies (including PPS) on academic health centers including control of size and content of graduate medical education programs, future financing of teaching hospitals, role of academic health centers in caring for the poor, role of teaching hospitals in technological change, and the diversity among academic health centers	11/15/83 to 7/14/85	$530,000	The Johns Hopkins Hospital is the grantee
2. Examining the effects of Medicaid and Medicare financing and delivery innovations to evaluate Arizona's new Medicaid program, California's new Medicaid program, New York's new hospital payment program, and nationwide Medicare cost limits on hospitals as models for future structure of Medicare and Medicaid	12/1/82 to 4/30/85	$325,000	Brandeis University, University Health Policy Consortium, is the grantee
W. K. Kellogg Foundation Study of DRGs to improve quality and cost-effectiveness of inpatient care. The project will include consideration of the differences in levels of nursing care needed, costs for alternative forms of care, use of all hospital resources and the development of educational programs for staff to improve cost-effective care	1984 to 1987	$348,500	Grant awarded to Northwestern Memorial Hospital
The Medical Trust c/o Glenmede (PEW) "State of the Art in Severity of Illness" to determine which severity-of-illness measure best explains the cost differential between teaching and nonteaching hospitals, including costs per case, costs per day, utilization of ancillary services, and average length of stay within the same DRG; which measure is a better predictor of cost rather than ratio of cost to charge	2/85 to 2/87	$310,000	Conducted by New York University Medical Center
Pew Memorial Trust 1. "Planning for the Future of Burn Care Under Prospective Reimbursement"(see Burn Foundation)	9/84 to 12/85	$370,000	
2. "Children's Hospitals' Case-Mix Classification System Project" to determine whether and how DRGs in their present or modified form or some other case-mix system should be incorporated into a prospective payment system for children's hospitals	6/84 to 9/85	$725,000	Conducted by National Association of Children's Hospitals
Robert Wood Johnson Foundation Evaluation of the Impact of New Jersey Reimbursement System on Hospital Operations and Medical Practice	43/83 to 6/86	$700,000	Interviews with key participants, including physicians, nurses, hospital administrators, and State officials

[a]NA = Not available.
SOURCE: Office of Technology Assessment, 1985.

SUMMARY OF ISSUES PERTAINING TO CURRENT PPS EVALUATION ACTIVITIES

Overlaps and Gaps in PPS-Related Research

As suggested in the preceding discussion, thus far, the focus of most of the PPS-related studies supported by Federal agencies has been on issues pertaining to the refinement and expansion of the new payment system. A smaller number of Federal studies address the evaluation of PPS impacts on health expenditures or quality of care. In some cases, the focus of Federal agencies on refinement and expansion issues is a result of congressional mandates for specific studies, but in other cases, Federal agencies chose this focus because of their administrative responsibilities or individual interests. The PPS-related research activities of Federal agencies do not appear to be duplicative.

The focus of most of the PPS-related studies supported by private organizations has been on issues pertaining to the evaluation of PPS impacts, especially identifying negative impacts on quality of care or access to care. Despite their emphasis on PPS impacts, studies by private organizations generally have several limitations. A limitation of most of the studies is that they are either incident- or opinion-based. Another problem is that many of these studies are designed to find only negative impacts on quality and access, and by failing to consider positive impacts, they may give a biased picture. Furthermore, professional associations have neither the resources nor the interest to do more than concentrate on their members' involvement in PPS, so bias is almost inevitable.

OTA found that private organizations have research projects that overlap with some Federal research and with the research of other private organizations (see table 10-8). For several reasons, however, this overlap is probably beneficial. One reason is that although overlapping and duplicative studies cost society more money, they do have a research advantage: If two well-designed studies show approximately the same results, they may validate each other. Credibility is increased by replicability. If two well-designed studies have opposite results, a need for further study is indicated. Another reason that overlap and duplication of effort may be desirable is that most of the organizations involved in evaluating PPS at this time have an interest at stake (including HCFA, because it administers the program); to the extent that duplication counteracts the biases of the different studies that are conducted, it may be used to develop a more balanced evaluation.

The adequacy of Federal efforts to provide a thorough and balanced evaluation of the impacts of PPS on quality and access to care is especially important, because private efforts are geared to finding negative impacts of PPS on quality of care or access to care. The enthusiasm with which interested private organizations have initiated their own studies argues for a commitment on the part of the Federal Government to produce objective and unbiased assessments of the full range of PPS impacts, particularly in the areas of quality and access to care.

OTA found that a major gap in current public and private PPS-related studies is the absence of a comprehensive plan, especially at a level of staffing and funding that would be reasonable, to evaluate the impacts of PPS on the U.S. health care system. A comprehensive evaluation of the impacts of PPS on the health care system would consider all of the dimensions of the impacts discussed in Part Two of this report: namely, expenditures and costs, quality of care, access to care, technological change, and clinical research.

As currently planned, the DHHS Secretary's annual PPS impact reports mandated by the Social Security Amendments of 1983 will not constitute a comprehensive evaluation of PPS impacts. Although the annual impact reports taken together could be planned as a comprehensive evaluation, DHHS' initial plan for the reports is to concentrate on certain dimensions of evaluation in separate years. Also, the Secretary's annual impact reports are required for only 3 more years (through 1987). Many effects that could be attributed to PPS may not be observable until later years.

A second major gap in ongoing and planned PPS-related research is the absence of studies of the quality of data in the databases that are used or expected to be used in the future to evaluate PPS. The few studies that have been done provide enough evidence of poor quality in discharge abstract data pertaining to diagnoses to make analyses of diagnostic trends over time suspect. Under PPS, however, the quality of discharge and other data should improve because of data quality's new relationship to payment and review by PROs (see chs. 5 and 6 and app. G).

Problems With Data for PPS Evaluation Studies

Several distinct problems with data for PPS evaluation studies have been identified by the groups addressing PPS issues. One of these, quality of data, is mentioned above. The other major problem is that, in many cases, the data necessary for particular evaluation questions, such as quality and access measurements, were not systematically collected and analyzed in the past.[7]

A lack of usable baseline data has frustrated many researchers who want to evaluate the impact of PPS on quality of care or access to care. Because there are no good baseline data, trend analyses and comparative studies are infeasible. In some cases, retrospective studies are possible—for example, studies of quality impacts can compare patients' medical records before and since PPS. But such studies, which would require using or abstracting data directly from patients' medical records, are both time-consuming and expensive.

Several professional societies, including the Council of Medical Specialty Societies, are attempting to circumvent the problem of a lack of usable baseline data by surveying physicians or nurses about the change in quality of care. These surveys are soliciting both positive and negative feedback, but will probably reveal fewer positive quality changes because of the visible and emotional nature of negative changes. Furthermore, as noted above, the objectivity of such organizations is questionable. Even so, the findings of these groups will be valuable in identifying particularly deleterious effects that need immediate attention.

Staffing and Funding for Mandated PPS Studies

In the last 3 years, Congress has mandated (or requested in a committee report) PPS-related reports on more than 20 topics by the end of December 1986, giving HCFA and others a large added workload. So far, all of the DHHS deadlines for congressionally mandated PPS studies, including that for DHHS's 1984 annual impact report on PPS, have been missed.[8] Although some of the difficulty in producing the mandated studies may be due to a lack of responsiveness on the part of the Administration, part of the problem appears to result from HCFA's inability to comply with the requirements of mandated studies at its current funding and staffing levels.

This situation brings into question the reasonableness of the original timeframe and the staffing and funding levels for congressionally mandated studies. Given that DHHS received no additional funds or staff with its mandated studies, and given the administrative burdens of the grant and contracting process[9] and the need to develop databases for special analyses, the congressional deadlines appear to have been too tight. Although tight deadlines are understandable given the importance of the change from cost-based reimbursement to PPS and the health care expenditures involved, they appear to be impractical.

---

[7]Under PPS, some data items that were not so important in past studies are taking on new value. For example, discharge disposition of patients (e.g., discharged home for self-care or to a skilled nursing facility), though a relatively unimportant data item on Medicare bills in the past, may become an important indicator to trace the impact of PPS on quality and access to posthospital care.

[8]Although some of the deadlines for mandated studies have been changed—e.g., the deadline for HCFA's study on the impact of single rates for skilled nursing facilities (study #1 in table 10-1) was extended, and the deadline for HCFA's study on including payment for physicians' services to inpatients in DRG rates (study #17 in table 10-1) was moved up—other deadlines have simply not been met. The first annual impact report from DHHS, for example, was due Dec. 31, 1984, and had not been released as of August 1985, purportedly because of delays in the DHHS clearance process. Other mandated studies of PPS are also in DHHS clearance channels and may or may not be released by their due dates.

[9]Because HCFA lacked sufficient intramural staff to handle the large number of mandated studies, HCFA arranged for extramural research on many of the mandated studies. Some of the research may have been slowed by the Federal grant and contracting process, which must be approved by the Office of Management and Budget. Most outside researchers are meeting HCFA's deadlines, but the reports prepared by HCFA staff on the basis of the external research are missing their release dates.

The scope of HCFA's evaluation efforts can be put into perspective by comparing the Federal dollars spent on Medicare's hospital benefits with those spent by HCFA for extramural research and demonstration projects involving hospital payment in general and PPS in particular. In fiscal year 1984, total expenditures for Medicare's hospital benefits were estimated at $43.8 billion (58). HCFA's overall budget for extramural research and demonstration projects supported through ORD in fiscal year 1984 was $32.8 million. An estimated $5.2 million, or about 16 percent, of that amount was for extramural projects involving hospital payment, with about $3.1 million directed to projects pertaining to PPS (45). This $5.2 million represented about 0.01 percent of Medicare's total 1984 hospital expenditures. It is infeasible to accurately estimate HCFA expenditures for intramural research on these topics, but were these expenditures added, the proportions of resources spent on PPS-related research would remain miniscule.

In fiscal year 1985, HCFA's budget for extramural projects involving hospital payment through ORD was about $8.5 million (see table 10-9). For fiscal year 1986, the Administration has proposed a 33-percent reduction in HCFA's overall budget for extramural research and demonstrations supported through ORD—from about $33 million to $22 million (with $6.7 million earmarked for projects on hospital payment) (see table 10-9). Despite the fact that proposed budget reductions have not been passed by Congress in the past, a reasonable assumption is that ORD's fiscal year 1986 research and demonstration budget will not be increased and could be decreased. Any decrease in ORD's funding is likely to further compromise the quality and timeliness of ORD's study reports.

ProPAC is currently evaluating impacts of PPS and its various component parts on the U.S. health care system, as requested by the House Appropriations Committee. The small size of ProPAC's overall budget and staff in relation to its many functions, however, limits the Commission's ability to perform a comprehensive evaluation of the effects of PPS on the health care system in addition to other mandated studies and

Table 10-9.—HCFA's Funding for Extramural Research and Demonstrations, Fiscal Year 1985 and Proposed Fiscal Year 1986 (in thousands)

	Fiscal year 1985	Proposed fiscal year 1986
Hospital payment.............	$ 8,530	$ 6,720
Congressionally mandated......	7,088	6,237
General research	1,442	483
Alternative payment systems....	$ 9,104	$ 5,351
Congressionally mandated......	1,248	1,100
General research	7,856	4,251
Program analysis and evaluation.................	$ 4,692	$ 2,645
Congressionally mandated......	250	200
General research	4,442	2,445
Quality and coverage...........	$ 2,558	$ 1,783
Congressionally mandated......	700	718
General research	1,858	1,065
Other[a]......................	$ 7,758	$ 5,501
Congressionally mandated......	678	1,000
General research	7,080	4,501
Total......................	$32,642	$22,000
Congressionally mandated....	9,964	9,255
General research	22,678	12,745

[a]Includes areas of: physician payment, State programs for long-term care, and beneficiary awareness and prevention.

SOURCE: U.S. Department of Health and Human Services, Health Care Financing Administration, "Research, Demonstration, and Evaluation Spending Plan," Baltimore, MD, April 1985.

functions specified in the Social Security Amendments of 1983.[10] Whenever possible, ProPAC plans to use existing data. Although the Commission does have the authority to initiate research, data collection, and analysis, its budget limits the Commission's potential for generating new data to study PPS impacts on quality or access to care.

This and other chapters of this report have suggested that additional research will be needed if the impact of PPS on Medicare beneficiaries and on the health care delivery system as a whole is to be adequately understood. The requirement that HCFA and other Federal agencies prepare mandated studies of PPS without additional funds or staff positions has imposed a great burden on these agencies. As more groups are affected by PPS, Congress will probably be petitioned to mandate additional studies of PPS. The burden of conducting most of these studies appears to fall

---

[10]ProPAC's budget for fiscal year 1985 is $3.4 million. The Commission has authority for 25 staff, and currently has approximately 23 staff members.

on HCFA, so it is important to recognize that HCFA's present budget and staff for research on and evaluation of PPS is small in relation to Medicare program expenditures and that more definitive study will probably require the allocation of additional resources.

CONCLUSIONS

So far, most of the federally supported studies of PPS have focused on program refinement issues; and most of the privately supported studies of PPS have focused on evaluation issues, especially the evaluation of PPS impacts on quality of care. In some cases, Congress has led Federal agencies to focus on refinement or expansion issues by mandating specific PPS studies, but in other cases, the agencies have selected this focus because of their administrative responsibilities or individual interests.

As of August 1985, DHHS had completed some of the PPS studies mandated by Congress, but had failed to meet any of the deadlines established by Congress. One of the most important mandated studies, the Secretary's annual impact report on PPS due in December 1984, remained in the Secretary's office for clearance. This situation brings into question the reasonableness of the original timeframe and staffing and funding levels for congressionally mandated studies.

In addition to problems with the quality of data, a lack of baseline data has frustrated many researchers who want to evaluate the impact of PPS on, for example, quality of care or access to care. Retrospective data collection from patients' medical records is possible but expensive. PPS itself should have a salutary effect on the quality of data now being collected because of its direct tie to payment and the review by PROs.

PPS studies by Federal agencies do not appear to be duplicative. Although there is some overlap in the efforts of private organizations, both with other private organizations and with Federal agencies, this duplication of effort is probably beneficial. Duplication is important to the credibility of the research results. It will also help to identify areas for further study of discrepancies or gaps in research and evaluation efforts.

Good decisions about refining PPS will require evaluative information. The quality of that information depends on the quality of the studies on which it is based. Good studies will require reliable, accurate, and timely data and sophisticated methods of analysis. Such studies tend to be expensive and labor-intensive. Cutbacks at any point will affect the quality and timeliness of results.

Chapter 11
Strategies for Evaluating PPS Impacts

Contents

	Page
Introduction	165
Content of PPS Evaluation	165
Databases for PPS Evaluation	166
Medicare Databases	167
Non-Medicare Databases	168
Organizational Arrangements for PPS Evaluation	168
Responsibility for Specific Studies	169
Mechanisms for Funding Research	169
Coordination and Oversight of the Evaluation	169
Funding for PPS Evaluation	170

Chapter 11
Strategies for Evaluating PPS Impacts

INTRODUCTION

Part Two of this report (chs. 5 to 9) examined the need for evaluation of Medicare's prospective payment system (PPS) on five separate dimensions of health system performance: expenditures and costs, quality of care, access to care, technological change, and clinical research. Critical evaluation questions in each area and approaches to their study were laid out in Part Two. Many of the PPS evaluation studies suggested in the different chapters involve similar methods of analysis and rely on the same databases.

This chapter discusses the content of evaluation studies required to address the critical questions in the five major areas of PPS impact. Then, it describes the data collection and retrieval systems needed to conduct such studies and compares them to existing ones. The third section of the chapter discusses issues that arise in the organization of the evaluation tasks. The final section lays out the implications of content, data, and organization for funding.

CONTENT OF PPS EVALUATION

The critical PPS evaluation questions identified in Part Two of this report were drawn from OTA's analysis of the financial incentives inherent in the structure of PPS relative to cost-based reimbursement. A shift in incentives can be expected to change the behavior of providers and patients, which in turn can be expected to alter the performance of the U.S. health care system. OTA's analysis of the ways in which the incentives of PPS can affect each of the dimensions of impact allowed specification of critical evaluation questions in each area. Chapter 1 (table 1-2) summarizes these questions for each of the five major PPS impact areas and links each question to the kinds of studies and data sources that can be used to address it. It also provides a rough indication of the relative costs of different kinds of studies in each area.

The range of potential studies of PPS impacts is wide; priorities are therefore required. OTA has identified priority categories through an analysis of the strength of the incentives facing providers and their ability or willingness to act on them, the strength of the relationship between these actions and impacts on quality, access, etc., and the feasibility and cost of measuring these impacts.

The result is a three-tiered approach to the identification of needed studies:

- Category 1: *studies that can identify major undesirable PPS impacts on the health care system as a whole or on vulnerable groups.* These studies are either relatively inexpensive to conduct because they rely on existing databases or are so important that they justify substantial funding.
- Category 2: *studies that provide a balanced and thorough assessment of PPS impacts on the health care system.* These are studies intended to examine both positive and negative results. Their cost is generally (but not always) high because of the need for comprehensiveness and balance.
- Category 3: *studies whose purpose is to develop methods of measuring important PPS impacts.* These are important for the enhancement of capability to monitor PPS impacts. Their cost varies depending on data needs.

Studies in the first two categories are summarized in chapter 1 (table 1-2). Although routinely available data regarding the utilization and organization of health services can be used as the basis for the first line of inquiry into PPS effects, in each critical PPS impact area, more detailed studies requiring more costly data collection strategies are indicated. For example, while Medicare's Part A and Part B data systems are fertile territory for investigation of undesirable impacts on quality (e.g., through examination of age-adjusted mortality rates and other "sentinel events"), they cannot be used for inquiries into more subtle changes in the quality of care. To measure these more subtle changes, studies involving direct data collection from medical records would be needed.

In selecting specific subjects for detailed analysis and in drawing inferences about the contribution of PPS (relative to other factors) to any observed changes in outcome, a great deal of judgment is required. Inappropriately selected subjects or methods of analysis can easily distort summary conclusions about the impacts of PPS. The best insurance against this potential problem would be to have specific issues addressed through multiple investigator-initiated grants selected through peer review. The grants mechanism adds a measure of independence from political interference and at the same time encourages academic or other researchers to develop strong research projects. Success of this funding mechanism would depend, however, on investigators' having knowledge of and access to the full range of databases available for analysis. This would require a commitment on the part of the Health Care Financing Administration (HCFA) and other agencies with pertinent data to maximize the accessibility of data to independent investigators.

The ability to evaluate PPS in the long run may depend on the commitment of resources for category 3 studies. The impact measures that are available in some impact areas are not well developed. In the quality area, for example, not much is known at present about what detectable patterns of utilization suggest a serious problem for quality (see ch. 6). In what cases does a readmission imply that something has gone wrong in the way a patient has been treated? What processes of care during the hospital stay are so strongly linked to outcomes that they can be used as indicators of PPS impact? In the area of cost measurement, cost-finding techniques that more accurately reflect the true costs of treating different kinds of patients are in their infancy (see ch. 5). Good summary measures of technological change simply do not exist (see ch. 8). Finally, measures of patient severity of illness that can be used to analyze the systematic redistribution of surpluses and losses among patients and hospitals need to be refined (see app. H). The importance of having information on the impacts of PPS (or, indeed, of any Medicare policy change) probably justifies additional spending on methods development in these areas.

DATABASES FOR PPS EVALUATION

As table 1-2 in chapter 1 illustrates, data for analyzing critical PPS evaluation questions are available from a variety of sources, ranging from HCFA's routine databases used in the administration of the Medicare program to special surveys of the population conducted as part of evaluation projects. Special data collection exercises, such as population surveys or medical record abstracting, are costly but are sometimes the only feasible way to acquire needed information. This section considers the databases routinely maintained by the Federal Government whose content, accuracy, and structure determine their usefulness for PPS evaluation.

Two questions arise with respect to routinely maintained data systems. First, how adequate are routine data systems as currently structured for evaluating PPS? And, second, what kinds of changes in their content or organization would enhance their usefulness in this regard? Because so many issues for PPS evaluation can be analyzed with Medicare data, these questions are first addressed to Medicare databases. Subsequently, the potential and problems with non-Medicare databases are considered.

Medicare Databases

To administer the Medicare program, HCFA maintains data files in four areas (325):

- beneficiary characteristics;
- provider characteristics;
- provider bills; and
- provider costs.

Data in each of these categories arrive at HCFA through a variety of channels and are processed into specific files,[1] which are further manipulated or merged as the need arises. The basic files are the sources for all derivative files that may be created either to support the operations of the Medicare program or to monitor and evaluate the performance or impact of the system. (App. E provides a detailed description of the files used to administer the Part A Medicare program. Similar files exist for the Part B program.)

The Medicare data files are central to the evaluation of the impacts of PPS. Data on Medicare expenditures, costs, utilization, and mortality have been identified as necessary to address critical evaluation questions. Moreover, these data items need to be available on a disaggregated basis—by diagnosis-related group (DRG), by hospital, by geographic area, and by beneficiary. The sheer size of the data files, particularly the billing files, makes some kinds of analysis based on these data quite costly.[2] Medicare bills are sorted by kind of service (i.e., hospital inpatient, physician, etc.); records of bills for each type of service are maintained in a separate file in chronological order of their arrival. To develop a full history of health care utilization or expenditure for any period across all services for a given beneficiary is an extraordinarily costly data processing task. (Each record in each file would have to be scanned to identify all records for a given beneficiary.) The search could be greatly abbreviated if the individual files were presorted by beneficiary, provider, or geographic area.

HCFA is currently developing a system to presort the Part A and Part B billing files to allow disaggregated analyses based on data integrated from the separate files. This system, referred to as the Medicare Automated Data Retrieval System (MADRS), will organize Medicare billing records by geographic area, provider, and beneficiary (see app. E). When completed, it will enhance the analytic capability for PPS evaluation. The development of MADRS has proceeded slowly. In August 1984, it was estimated that files for the years 1980-82 would be available late in 1984 (181). By August 1985, however, the first files were still unavailable.

The HCFA database also contains the Medicare cost reports, which provide the only universally available and uniform hospital cost data. Between the time a cost report is initially submitted by the hospital and the time it is finally settled by the Medicare intermediary, the cost report goes through numerous changes. Consequently, there are several versions of such reports. The earlier versions are, of course, preliminary and unaudited, but on average, they overstate the final costs by only about 2 percent (72).

At present, Medicare cost reports are not fully accessible in automated form at HCFA. An automated Hospital Cost Report Information System (HCRIS) has been under development for at least 2 years and is designed to hold all versions of the cost reports, including the one submitted by the hospital. As of June 1985, the file for hospitals' fiscal years ending between September 1982 and September 1983 was about 80 percent complete and primarily consisted of settled cost reports (see app. E). HCRIS has not been fully implemented by HCFA; consequently, Medicare cost reports are the only major source of data unavailable in automated form.

---

[1] For the most part, these files are automated and can thus be considered to exist on computer tapes or disks.

[2] In 1984, for example, approximately 12 million inpatient hospital claims, 238 million physician and supplier claims, and 5 million home health claims were filed (376).

Non-Medicare Databases

The Federal Government supports a number of periodic health surveys that can provide useful data for PPS evaluation (see app. C). Several issues arise with respect to these Government-sponsored surveys.

First, because they are generally direct surveys of the population or of patient records, the surveys conducted by the Federal Government are costly. Budgetary constraints have reduced the frequency with which many can be repeated. Once they are conducted, substantial delays often occur before their results are published or tapes are prepared for public use. To illustrate:

- To the National Ambulatory Medical Care Survey (NAMCS), which provides data on utilization of services in physicians' offices, was last conducted in 1981; it was discontinued from 1982 to 1984 for lack of funding. A successor to the annual NAMCS is currently scheduled for a 3-year repeat cycle, with the next survey beginning in 1985. Budgetary constraints have limited more frequent surveys.
- The successor to the National Medical Care Utilization and Expenditure Survey (NMCUES), a 1980 survey which provides a unique database of information obtained from a sample of the noninstitutionalized civilian population on utilization and expenditures for all kinds of medical care, will not be conducted until 1987.

Second, the Government-sponsored health surveys are intended to provide information on a broad range of questions and are not particularly well adapted to the needs of PPS evaluation. For example:

- The Hospital Discharge Survey (HDS), which provides annual national estimates of utilization of non-Federal short-term hospitals, is the only statistically valid sample of hospital discharges for the entire population. Yet the discharges cannot be related to the characteristics of the hospitals in which they occur, because hospitals are classified only in regard to bed size and ownership.
- The sampling designs of most population surveys are not specifically geared to the needs of PPS evaluation. NMCUES, for example, did not base its sample size on the need to observe rare events such as hospitalization in the elderly. And, patients in nursing homes were excluded from the study. Thus, changes in the expenses of Medicare beneficiaries may not be detectable with an adequate level of confidence. The planned successor to NMCUES, the 1987 National Medical Expenditure Survey, will correct some of these problems by including a sample of institutionalized people and sampling a higher proportion of the elderly. The difficulty of making pre/post-PPS comparisons will remain, however.

To remedy these problems will require greater attention on the part of survey designers to the specific needs of PPS evaluation and greater commitment of resources to the maintenance and improvement of the statistical databases that are critical to monitoring the status of the health care system.

ORGANIZATIONAL ARRANGEMENTS FOR PPS EVALUATION

Even more important than specifying particular studies that should be undertaken to evaluate PPS is ensuring that the organization of the evaluative process is adequate. Four factors influence the appropriate organization of PPS evaluation:

- *The complexity of PPS evaluation.* Investigation of the impact of PPS on the important dimensions of health system performance is difficult because of conceptual, methodological, and data problems. Impact measures are difficult to identify in some areas; the ability to attribute observed effects to PPS is limited; and the high cost of research argues for sound judgment in the selection of specific studies.
- *The dual purpose of PPS evaluation.* A principal function of PPS evaluation is to serve as a "warning system" for unacceptable negative consequences—consequences which need to be addressed either through changes in the structure of PPS or through other compensating programs. Beyond this first level

of evaluation, however, a more balanced assessment of its positive as well as negative impacts is necessary.
- *The large number of studies using common data sources.* Reliance on HCFA data for studies of utilization, expenditures, costs, and outcomes of care implies the need for coordination in the development of analysis files from the parent data files.
- *The need for further development of impact measures and databases.* The problems inherent in evaluating PPS highlight the need for better measures of quality, access, cost, and technological change. Basic research studies will be needed if improvements are to be expected.

These factors influence three questions regarding the organization of PPS evaluation efforts:

- What organizations within or outside of the Federal Government should be responsible for conducting what studies?
- What funding mechanisms should be used to carry out the needed research?
- How can the total effort be coordinated?

Responsibility for Specific Studies

With respect to the organizational locus of responsibility for specific studies of PPS impacts, the following criteria are relevant:

- existence of required expertise/experience with the methods and data required for evaluation;
- access to critical databases;
- objectivity with respect to the outcome of the evaluation;
- commitment to evaluation (e.g., personnel, funding); and
- availability of resources to carry out the study.

As discussed in the previous chapter, HCFA has been assigned the leading role in Federal activities to evaluate the impact of PPS. The Secretary of Health and Human Services' annual PPS impact reports mandated through 1987 by Congress are being prepared by HCFA. As the agency with the most detailed knowledge of and access to the critical databases and with the greatest program knowledge, HCFA is most capable of carrying out many such studies.

Nevertheless, HCFA's objectivity with respect to the outcomes of the evaluation must be considered. The slow speed with which HCFA has proceeded with plans for the most critical impact areas (namely, quality and access) and the difficulty it has had in responding to other mandated studies in the allotted time suggests either inadequate resources to carry out the required tasks, inadequate commitment to evaluation, or both.

Mechanisms for Funding Research

The problem of HCFA's potential lack of adequate objectivity can be reduced to some extent by resorting to funding mechanisms that permit independent research on PPS impacts. Extramural projects, preferably funded by peer-reviewed grants, provide the greatest assurance of independence on the part of investigators. The National Center for Health Services Research and Health Care Technology Assessment (NCHSR&HCTA), for example, has a tradition of funding peer-reviewed investigator-initiated grants.

Coordination and Oversight of the Evaluation

The difficulty of ensuring that appropriate studies are undertaken, that available data are used efficiently, that the knowledge of those most qualified and objective is tapped, and that adequate resources are devoted to the effort suggests that a single organization should be responsible for coordination and oversight of the PPS evaluation process. This coordination responsibility needs to be ongoing. Agencies responsible for carrying out studies in specific areas need to be held accountable for the quality and timeliness of the work they produce. The functions of a coordinating organization could include the following:

- assessing the feasibility and cost of alternative studies in relation to their importance;
- developing an annual PPS evaluation agenda;
- recommending an annual PPS evaluation budget;
- identifying the most appropriate organizational sponsors for specific studies;
- recommending the most appropriate funding mechanisms;
- recommending funding levels for individual studies;

- overseeing and coordinating access to needed data;
- overseeing and coordinating changes in data systems to enhance the ability to evaluate PPS;
- reviewing the content of specific studies for their scientific validity; and
- serving as a clearinghouse for both public and private sector studies.

The responsibility for coordinating the PPS evaluation effort could be lodged in any of several Federal agencies. The Office of the Assistant Secretary for Planning and Evaluation within the Department of Health and Human Services (DHHS), for example, has traditionally maintained a coordinating role with respect to evaluation research. Other possible organizations within DHHS would include NCHSR&HCTA, which has extensive experience in supporting intramural and extramural research of this kind and is currently coordinating the PPS-related research of the Public Health Service, and HCFA, which has both program and research expertise. NCHSR&HCTA is low in the DHHS organizational hierarchy, however, and therefore might have difficulty performing the coordinating function. Moreover, if any of the components of DHHS were assigned the coordinating task, attention would have to be paid to their inherent lack of objectivity, since they are part of the implementing Department.

Another alternative is for the Prospective Payment Assessment Commission (ProPAC) to oversee the evaluation. ProPAC has an informal congressional mandate (Report 98-911 on H.R. 6028) to provide a comprehensive evaluation of PPS (309) but has a research budget (approximately $1 million) that cannot begin to meet these expectations. Its legislated function could be altered to include coordination and oversight of PPS evaluation activities throughout the Federal Government. However, as the body with responsibility for recommending relative DRG prices and the annual rate of increase to the Secretary of Health and Human Services, ProPAC may be no less disinterested in the outcome of an evaluation of PPS than is DHHS.

Congressional agencies, such as the Congressional Budget Office, the Congressional Research Service, the General Accounting Office, or OTA, would be capable of providing the oversight that is necessary, particularly if staff with program evaluation skills were assigned the responsibility. The missions of these agencies, however, do not coincide with this oversight function.

Private organizations with experience in health policy research and evaluation are probably not good candidates for the role of coordinator because they would have low access to information and databases held by Federal agencies and inadequate influence over the evaluation process.

FUNDING FOR PPS EVALUATION

Although there are conceptual and methodological limits with respect to what can be known about the effects of PPS on the important dimensions of health system performance, *with adequate funding and personnel*, Federal agencies can do a reasonably good job in tracking changes in expenditures and costs, quality of care, access to care, technology, and clinical research as PPS is implemented and to assess differential impacts on vulnerable groups.

At present, Federal funding of research on PPS does not appear to be adequate to mount detailed studies even in the first category. With each of the major policy research organizations of DHHS facing the possibility of budget cuts for fiscal year 1986, the prospects for adequate funding of PPS evaluation appear to be declining.

The timely and thorough completion of PPS studies mandated by Congress (see ch. 10) appears to exceed the capability of the current resources of HCFA's Office of Research and Demonstrations. In the future, attention needs to be given to the source of funds for the conduct of mandated studies.

Appendixes

Appendix A.—Method of the Study

This assessment was requested as a followup of the 1984 OTA assessment entitled *Medical Technology and Costs of the Medicare Program* and the 1983 OTA technical memorandum entitled *Diagnosis-Related Groups and the Medicare Program: Implications for Medical Technology*. The purpose of the assessment was to consider the needs for evaluation of Medicare's new prospective payment system (PPS) for hospitals established by the Social Security Amendments of 1983 (Public Law 98-21). The question of what data would be necessary for the evaluation of PPS was chosen as a special focus of the study. The assessment began on June 1, 1984.

One of the first tasks in planning an OTA assessment is to choose an advisory panel of experts in various fields. The advisory panel for an OTA assessment suggests source materials, subject areas, and perspectives for staff consideration; assists in interpreting information and points of view assembled by OTA staff; and suggests possible findings and conclusions based on the study. Panel members review staff and contract materials for accuracy and representativeness, discuss policy options of the study, and present arguments for and against the options and conclusions. The final report, however, is the responsibility of the OTA staff.

The advisory panel for this assessment of strategies for evaluating Medicare's PPS consisted of 23 members with expertise in health policy, health care administration, insurance, business, and clinical medicine fields, as well as experience in State and Federal government and academia. John Eisenberg, Associate Professor of Medicine at the Hospital of the University of Pennsylvania, chaired the panel.

The first panel meeting was held on July 16, 1984. OTA staff for the project presented topics and outlines for the panel's discussion of the overall plan for the assessment. Suggestions regarding a workshop on patient classification systems and their relationship to prospective payment were discussed. Major chapter topics selected for the full report were PPS impacts in each of the following areas: costs and expenditures, quality of care, access to care, technological change, and clinical research. Education and manpower issues were deemed beyond the scope of the assessment. OTA project staff agreed to draft a report for the panel's review before the second meeting, tentatively arranged for late December or early January.

OTA held a workshop on inpatient classification systems on September 17, 1984. The purpose of the workshop was to explore strategies for evaluation, refinement, and further development of classification systems. Sixteen experts including researchers, medical records personnel, Federal Government representatives, and others involved in classification systems participated in the all-day meeting. The focus of the discussion was on the reasonableness of evaluation criteria for payment purposes. The contractor who would be writing the background piece on patient classification systems also participated and was asked to incorporate the workshop discussions into his paper.

As the project progressed, an OTA staff memorandum on Medicare databases was requested by the Senate Special Committee on Aging. Since PPS covers Part A of Medicare, the staff memorandum prepared describes and evaluates Part A databases. It was delivered in draft in October 1984 and was delivered in final form in August 1985.

Contracts were let for background papers on a variety of issues for staff use in preparing the assessment. They are listed on p. 174.

Contractor	Subject
Mary Ann Baily Department of Economics The George Washington University	"Impact of PPS on Access to Care"
Judith Barr Associate Dean Northeastern University College of Pharmacy and Allied Health	*"The Interaction of Therapeutic Drug Monitoring and DRG Payment Levels"
Matthew Farber West Virginia University	"DRG Payment and Medical Technology Payment: DRG #39"
Marvin Feuerberg Washington, DC	"Hospital Data Systems and Their Adequacy for Evaluating PPS"
Stanley Finklestein Sloan School of Management Massachusetts Institute of Technology	*"Medical Technology and DRG's: The Case of the Implantable Infusion Pump"
Bernard Friedman Center for Health Services and Policy Research Northwestern University	*"Likely Effect of Medicare's Prospective Payment System on the Veterans Administration"
Kathleen Lohr The Rand Corp. Washington, DC	*"Peer Review Organizations (PROs): Quality Assurance in Medicare"
Peter McMenamin Washington, DC	"Impacts of PPS on Health Service Costs"
Ross Mullner Data Base Development Hospital Data Center American Hospital Association	"Availability of Data Sets To Monitor the Effects of PPS"
Jerri Perkins Perkins & Perkins, Inc. Potomac, MD	"Streptokinase Treatment for Acute Myocardial Infarction and the DRG Payment System"
Neil Powe Robert Wood Johnson Foundation Clinical Scholars Program University of Pennsylvania School of Medicine	*"Percutaneous Transluminal Coronary Angioplasty: Efficacy, Cost, and Effects of Prospective Payment"
Sankey Williams Hospital of the University of Pennsylvania Department of Medicine	"Strategies for Research and Evaluation of Patient Classification Systems"

Background papers with an asterisk (*) are or will be available shortly from the National Technical Information Service (NTIS). In addition, a background paper on extracorporeal shock-wave lithotripsy was prepared by OTA staff. It is available from NTIS.

On January 28, 1985, the advisory panel for the assessment had a second meeting. OTA staff had prepared a preliminary draft of the final report for their consideration. Copies of the contractors' papers were also sent to the panel members prior to this final meeting. Panel members discussed the chapters in depth and made suggestions for improvements.

In February and March of 1985, OTA staff conducted a survey of nongovernmental organizations to ascertain the extent of private initiatives in evaluating PPS. Staff selected over 250 organizations that it felt would be likely to evaluate prospective payment. The types of organizations selected were: 1) provider groups, such as associations of physicians, nurses, other health care professionals, and the 50 State hospital associations; 2) beneficiary groups, such as disease-related interest groups and the American Association of Retired Persons; and 3) foundations known to fund research in the health field. Questionnaires were sent to the directors of these organizations in February, and more than 70 groups had responded by the end of March. Responses were added to chapter 10 of the draft report in tabular form.

After revising the main report to strengthen certain sections and rectify omissions identified by the panel, OTA staff mailed a second draft in April 1985 to more than 140 reviewers. These reviewers represented a broad range of experts in a diversity of settings. Appropriate revisions based on comments received were made by OTA staff, and the report was submitted to the Technology Assessment Board on June 28, 1985.

Appendix B.—Acknowledgments and Health Program Advisory Committee

The development of this report has benefited from the advice and review of a number of people in addition to the Advisory Panel and the Health Program Advisory Committee. OTA staff would like to express its appreciation to the following people for their valuable guidance.

Catherine Abercrombie
Dornier Medical Systems, Inc.

Ralph J. Alfidi
Case Western Reserve University

Laura Allendorf
American Society of Internal Medicine

Dennis P. Andrulis
National Association of Public Hospitals

Richard Averill
Health Systems International

Lawrence Bachorik
Fairfax Hospital Association

Karl Bays
American Hospital Supply Corp.

Dennis Beatrice
Brandeis University

Jill Bernstein
General Accounting Office

Meryl Bloomrosen
Prospective Payment Assessment Commission

Saul Boyarski
Washington University

William Broglie
Health Care Financing Administration

Robert Brook
The Rand Corp.

Joan Buchanan
The Rand Corp.

Paul Campbell
Health Industry Manufacturers' Association

Rosanna Coffey
National Center for Health Services Research & Health Care Technology Assessment

Catherine Cohen
American Society of Clinical Pathologists

Dennis Cotter
Prospective Payment Assessment Commission

Carol Cronin
Washington, DC

Carolyne Davis
Health Care Financing Administration

Allen Dobson
Health Care Financing Administration

George Drach
University of Arizona

Paul Eggers
Health Care Financing Administration

Suanne Estabrook
Intermedics, Infusaid Inc.

Robert Flinn
Peoria, IL

Deborah Freund
University of North Carolina

Jan Garfinkle
Advanced Cardiovascular Systems

Benjamin Gerson
New England Deaconess Hospital

Paul Gertman
Health Data Institute and Boston University

Paul Ginsburg
The Rand Corp.

Phyllis Giovannetti
University of Alberta

Peter Goldschmidt
U.S. Veterans Administration
Washington, DC

Joseph Gonnella
Jefferson Medical College

Mark Goodhart
American Hospital Association

Thomas Granneman
Mathematica Policy Research

John Griffith
University of Michigan

Paul Grimaldi
Coopers & Lybrand

Ann Haendel
National Center for Health Services Research & Health Care Technology Assessment

Frank Holden
U.S. Veterans Administration
Boston, MA

Charles Hollingsworth
National Institutes of Health

Susan D. Horn
The Johns Hopkins Medical Institutions

Lisa Iezzoni
Boston University

Stephen Jencks
Health Care Financing Administration

Janet Kline
Congressional Research Service

Doris Konicki
American Medical Association

Ephraim Levin
National Institutes of Health

Rachael Levinson
National Institutes of Health

Janet Lundy
Congressional Research Service

Max Magner
E.I. du Pont de Nemours & Co.

Linda Magno
Health Care Financing Administration

Susan Marcus
Veterans' Administration
Perry Pt., MD

John E. Marshall
National Center for Health Services Research & Health Care Technology Assessment

David McCallum
Georgetown University Medical Center

Stephanie Mensh
American Academy of Ophthalmology

Frederick C. Miller
Georgetown University Medical Center

Dianne Milstead
Health Care Financing Administration

R. Curtis Morris
University of California at San Francisco

Steven Morris
Health Care Financing Administration

Lee Mortenson
Association of Community Cancer Centers

Philip Nathanson
Health Care Financing Administration

William Nicholls
Health Care Financing Administration

James F. O'Donnell
National Institutes of Health

Joseph Onek
Onek, Klein, & Farr

Julian Pettingill
Congressional Research Service

Harold Pincus
National Institute of Mental Health

Lisa Potetz
Prospective Payment Assessment Commission

Ellen Pryga
American Hospital Association

Deena Puskin
Prospective Payment Assessment Commission

Guy S. Reeder
Mayo Clinic

Martin Resnick
Case Western Reserve University

Jamie Reuter
Congressional Research Service

William Robinson
Bureau of Health Professions

Wayne Roe
Health Industry Manufacturers' Association

Elizabeth S. Rolph
The Rand Corp.

Donald Sickora
Health Care Financing Administration

Herbert Silverman
Health Care Financing Administration

Brenda Sims
Delaware Review Organization

Helen Smits
University of Connecticut Health Center

William Sobaski
Health Care Financing Administration

Barbara Starfield
Johns Hopkins School of Hygiene and Public Health

Bruce Steinwald
Prospective Payment Assessment Commission

Roger Straw
General Accounting Office

Bruce Stuart
Pennsylvania State University

Susanne Stoiber
National Institutes of Health

Sherry Terrell
Health Care Financing Administration

Boyd Thompson
American Medical Care Review Association

Michael Vaida
California Hospital Association

Susan Van Gelder
General Accounting Office

Douglas Wagner
George Washington University

Peter Welch
Office of Management and Budget

Norman Welford
U.S. Food and Drug Administration

Richard Wild
Health Care Financing Administration

Mary Kay Willian
Prospective Payment Assessment Commission

Patricia Willis
Health Care Financing Administration

Jerome Yates
National Institutes of Health

Donald Young
Prospective Payment Assessment Commission

Wanda W. Young
Blue Cross of Western Pennsylvania

Gerald Zelinger
Health Care Financing Administration

HEALTH PROGRAM ADVISORY COMMITTEE

Sidney S. Lee, *Committee Chair*
President, Milbank Memorial Fund
New York, NY

H. David Banta
WHO Consultant and Director of
  Project on Future Health Technologies
The Netherlands

Rashi Fein
Professor
Department of Social Medicine and Health Policy
Harvard Medical School
Boston, MA

Harvey V. Fineberg
Dean
School of Public Health
Harvard University
Boston, MA

Melvin Glasser*
Director
Health Security Action Council
Washington, DC

Patricia King
Professor
Georgetown Law Center
Washington, DC

Joyce C. Lashof
Dean
School of Public Health
University of California-Berkeley
Berkeley, CA

Alexander Leaf
Professor of Medicine
Harvard Medical School
Massachusetts General Hospital
Boston, MA

Frederick Mosteller
Professor and Chair
Department of Health Policy and Management
School of Public Health
Harvard University
Boston, MA

Norton Nelson
Professor
Department of Environmental Medicine
New York University Medical School
New York, NY

Robert Oseasohn
Associate Dean
University of Texas-San Antonio
San Antonio, TX

Nora Piore
Senior Fellow and Advisor to the President
United Hospital Fund of New York
New York, NY

Dorothy P. Rice
Regents Lecturer
Department of Social and Behavioral Sciences
School of Nursing
University of California-San Francisco
San Francisco, CA

Richard K. Riegelman
Associate Professor
George Washington University
  School of Medicine
Washington, DC

Walter L. Robb
Vice President and General Manager
Medical Systems Operations
General Electric Co.
Milwaukee, WI

Frederick C. Robbins
President
Institute of Medicine
Washington, DC

Rosemary Stevens
Professor
Department of History and Sociology of Science
University of Pennsylvania
Philadelphia, PA

---
*Until October 1983.

Appendix C.—Major Population-Based Health Care Surveys

Introduction

The need to monitor health care costs and expenditures, utilization of services, and health status of the population is heightened by the changes in Medicare's prospective payment system (PPS). This appendix describes the major Federal and private population-based health surveys that are available for this purpose. The surveys described in this appendix are of two general types:
- surveys of the general population, and
- surveys of special populations.

Surveys of patients in long-term care institutions are also included, but surveys conducted only in years prior to 1977 are not. Information is provided on sample design (e.g., probability sample), type of population surveyed, and size of sample. If the sampling involved more extensive methods than a probability sample of the general population, then more detailed information about the sample design is included.

The primary sponsor of the Federal surveys has been the National Center for Health Statistics (NCHS), although other agencies such as the Bureau of the Census have played an essential role in the design and conduct of the surveys. Certain studies planned for the future will be cosponsored by various Federal health agencies and will draw on the information and expertise obtained in the past.

In the private sector, the American Hospital Association (AHA) conducts surveys of public opinion on health issues. The Center for Health Administration Studies (CHAS) at the University of Chicago has been important in conducting household surveys pertaining to access to medical care. This appendix summarizes private surveys, but it does not include every private survey conducted.

Federal Health Surveys

Table C-1 summarizes some salient characteristics of Federal population-based health surveys, including their sponsoring agencies, the frequency with which they are conducted, survey dates, and their availability. Table C-2 summarizes data elements of each survey. Data tapes for all the Federal surveys described below are available for purchase by the public.

Federal Surveys of the General Population

Health Interview Survey (HIS).—HIS, initiated by NCHS in 1957, has been conducted annually through 1984. This survey is designed to collect information on the social, economic, and demographic characteristics of sampled individuals, as well as on their health status and utilization of medical services.

HIS data are obtained from an annual sample of the noninstitutionalized population of the United States. Continuous sampling of the population is used for HIS, and each week a sample of the target population is interviewed. In 1981, 41,000 households containing approximately 110,000 persons were sampled.

From each person interviewed, HIS collects data on the following categories (352):
- social, economic, and demographic characteristics;
- illness and injury recall;
- description of health conditions and related disabilities;
- limitation of activity;
- hospitalization;
- accidents resulting in injury;
- physician visits; and
- limitation of mobility.

The health items in HIS are defined in terms of the impact they have on the lives of individuals rather than on medical criteria. Periodically, usually every 2 to 5 years, HIS has collected data on health-related items other than those listed above. These "rotating items" include measures such as mobility limitation, dental care, and insurance coverage.

Also, most questionnaires have included one or more special supplements. These supplements have usually been planned for a 1-year collection period, but some have been included periodically according to a planned schedule. Others, originally intended as one-time items, became rotating supplements when their timeliness and importance indicated a need for trend data. Examples of the rotating supplements are health insurance coverage, hearing impairment, loss of income, nursing care/special aids, personal health expenses, prescribed and nonprescribed medicines, smoking habits, vision impairment and use of corrective lenses, and X-ray visits. The combination of rotating items and supplements provides greater coverage of information and allows HIS to respond to changing needs (352). HIS data are available in the form of standardized microdata tapes, and special tabulations can also be obtained for public use from NCHS. The latest data available are from 1981.

Health and Nutrition Examination Survey (HANES).—HANES is a modification and expansion of the Health Examination Survey (HES) and has been conducted two times by NCHS since 1971.

Table C-1.—Major Federal Population-Based Health Care Surveys

Survey	Sponsoring agency	Frequency	Survey year	Next expected survey	Time lag	Cost
Surveys of the general population:						
Health Interview Survey (HIS)	NCHS	Annual	1969-84	1985	1-2 yrs.	$425/tape
Health and Nutrition Examination Survey (HANES)	NCHS	Cyclical (5 yrs.)	1971-75, 1976-80	1988	1-2 yrs.	$125-$305/tape
National Medical Care Expenditure Survey (NMCES)	NCHSR	One time	1977	1987	NA[a]	To be determined
National Medical Care Utilization and Expenditure Survey (NMCUES)	NCHS, HCFA	One time	1980	1987	3 yrs.	To be determined
National Survey of Personal Health Practices and Consequences (NSPHPC)	NCHS	Twice	1979, 1980	—	1-2 yrs.	$125/tape
Survey of Disability and Work (SDW)	SSA	One time	1978	1988	1 yr.	$255/tape
Surveys of special populations:						
Hospital Discharge Survey (HDS)	NCHS	Annual	1965-84	1985	1-2 yrs.	$125/tape
National Ambulatory Medical Care Survey (NAMCS)	NCHS	Annual	1973-81	1985	1-2 yrs.	$125/tape
National Long-Term Care Survey (NLTCS)	ASPE, HCFA	Twice	1982, 1984	—	2 yrs.	To be determined
National Nursing Home Survey (NNHS)	NCHS	Irregular	1969, 1973, 1974, 1977	1985	2 yrs.	$185-$305/tape
Survey of Institutionalized Persons (SIP)	ASPE	One time	1976	—	2 yrs.	NA

ABBREVIATIONS: ASPE = Assistant Secretary for Planning and Evaluation.
HCFA = Health Care Financing Administration.
NCHS = National Center for Health Statistics.
NCHSR = National Center for Health Services Research.
SSA = Social Security Administration.

[a]NA = Not available.

SOURCES: R. Mullner, "An Inventory of U.S. Health Care Data Bases," *A Review of Public Data Use* 11(2):85-192, June 1983; and L. A. Aday, R. Anderson, and G. V. Fleming, *Health Care in the U.S.: Equitable for Whom?* (Beverly Hills, CA: Sage Publications, Inc., 1980).

Through direct physical examination and clinical tests, HANES gathers data on such measures as the prevalence of medically defined illnesses, population distributions of blood pressure, visual acuity, serum cholesterol levels, etc. Medical history, demographic, and socioeconomic data are also collected. HANES also collects nutritional status information, which is used for monitoring changes over time (319).

HANES I, which began in 1971 and ended in 1974, consisted of a detailed health examination given to persons 25 to 74 years of age; the nutrition component of HANES I was directed to individuals from 1 to 74 years of age. HANES II, which began in 1976 and ended in 1980, collected nutrition and health status information from individuals aged 6 months to 74 years. These data will be used as a way of monitoring changes in nutritional status. Besides a medical history questionnaire, HANES II used two dietary questionnaires (including a food frequency interview), medications and vitamin usage, dietary supplement interview, and a behavior questionnaire. Physical examinations were conducted, as well as special clinical procedures, X-rays, urine and blood samples. Both HANES I and II had sample sizes of approximately 21,000 examined individuals. HANES III is being planned for 1987 (356).

National Medical Care Expenditure Survey (NMCES). —NMCES was conducted by the National Center for Health Services Research (NCHSR) in 1977-78. This survey was designed to assess the costs of health care, the utilization of services, and the costs of illness for

Table C-2.—Data Items Represented in Major Federal Population-Based Health Care Surveys

Survey characteristics	Surveys of the general population							Surveys of special populations			
	HIS	HANES[b]	NMCES	NMCUES	NSPHPC	SDW	NAMCS	HDS	NNHS	NLTCS	SIP
Health care costs:											
Hospital		X	X	X	X				X		
Physician		X	X	X					X		
Long-term care			X	X				X	X	X	
Other health care costs			X	X					X		
Source of payment			X	X	X				X	X	X
Utilization of services:											
Hospitalization	X		X	X	X			X	X		
Outpatient or emergency	X			X					X		
Physician visits	X		X	X	X			X	X		X
Diagnostic services		X	X	X	X			X	X		
Medication therapy		X	X	X	X				X		
Long-term care										X	
Discharge summary							X				X
Health status:											
Age/sex	X	X	X	X	X	X	X	X	X	X	X
Description of conditions (principal diagnosis)	X	X	X	X	X	X	X	X	X	X	X
Medical history	X	X	X								
General well-being (self-perceived health status)	X	X	X		X						
Limitation of activity/function	X			X		X			X	X	X
Access to care	X		X								

ABBREVIATIONS: HANES = Health and Nutrition Examination Survey
HDS = Hospital Discharge Survey
HIS = Health Interview Survey
NAMCS = National Ambulatory Medical Care Survey
NLTCS = National Long-Term Care Survey
NMCES = National Medical Care Expenditure Survey
NMCUES = National Medical Care Utilization and Expenditure Survey
NNHS = National Nursing Home Survey
NSPHPC = National Survey of Personal Health Practices and Consequences
SDW = Survey of Disability and Work
SIP = Survey of Institutionalized Persons

SOURCES: **HIS**: U.S. Department of Health and Human Services, Public Health Service, National Center for Health Statistics, *Current Estimates Health Interview Survey*, DHHS Pub. No. (PHS) 80-1551 (Washington, DC: U.S. Government Printing Office, November 1979).
HANES: U.S. Department of Health, Education, and Welfare, Public Health Service, National Center for Health Statistics, *Plan and Operation of HANES 1 Augmentation*, DHHS Pub. No. (PHS) 78-1314 (Washington, DC: U.S. Government Printing Office, June 1978).
NMCES: U.S. Department of Health and Human Services, Public Health Service, National Center for Health Statistics, *NMCES Household Interview Instruments*, DHHS Pub. No. (PHS) 81-3280 (Washington, DC: U.S. Government Printing Office, April 1981).
NMCUES: U.S. Department of Health and Human Services, Public Health Service, National Center for Health Statistics, *Procedures and Questionnaires of the National Medical Care Utilization and Expenditure Survey*, DHHS Pub. No. 83-20001 (Washington, DC: U.S. Government Printing Office, March 1983).
NSPHPC: U.S. Department of Health and Human Services, National Center for Health Statistics, *Highlights From Wave 1 of the National Survey of Personal Health Practices and Consequences, U.S. 1979*, DHHS Pub. No. (PHS) 81-1162 (Washington, DC: U.S. Government Printing Office, June 1981).
SDW: U.S. Department of Health and Human Services, Social Security Administration, *1978 Survey of Disability and Work*, Pub. No. 13-11745 (Washington, DC: U.S. Government Printing Office, January 1982).
NAMCS: U.S. Department of Health and Human Services, Public Health Service, National Center for Health Statistics, *Public Use Data Tape Documentation, National Ambulatory Medical Care Survey* (Washington, DC: U.S. Government Printing Office, April 1981).
HDS: U.S. Department of Health, Education and Welfare, Public Health Service, National Center for Health Statistics, *Development of the Design of the NCHS Hospital Discharge Survey* (Washington, DC: U.S. Government Printing Office, September 1970).
NNHS: U.S. Department of Health and Human Services, Public Health Service, National Center for Health Statistics, *Nursing and Related Care Homes*, DHHS Pub. No. (PHS) 84-1824 (Washington, DC: U.S. Government Printing Office, December 1983).
NLTCS: U.S. Department of Health and Human Services, Public Health Service, National Center for Health Statistics, "Long-Term Care Survey," OMB Pub. No. 0990-0077, Form LTC-3 (Washington, DC: U.S. Government Printing Office, April 1982).
SIP: U.S. Department of Commerce, Bureau of Census, *1976 Survey of Institutionalized Persons: Methods and Procedures* (Washington, DC: U.S. Government Printing Office, June 1978).

different diagnostic categories. The effects of Medicare and Medicaid on use and costs of personal health care was also a focus of the survey.

The primary source of information for NMCES was a household survey. Eligible persons in sampled households were questioned about the use of health services, expenditures, and insurance coverage. Approximately 13,500 households were interviewed six times during an 18-month period. Throughout the year, supplementary questionnaires were also distributed. The two other sources of information for NMCES were interviews with insurance companies and employers responsible for insurance coverage of the household respondents and interviews with the medical providers of 50 percent of the household respondents.

The NMCES sampling design was a stratified multistage area probability design from two independently drawn national area samples. The sample for the household survey consisted of the civilian, noninstitutionalized population of the United States.

NMCES collected the following data items on each sampled individual (348):
- health care expenditures;
- insurance coverage;
- source of payment;
- tax treatment;
- medical services used;
- X-rays, tests, and supplies;
- accessibility;
- self-perceived health status;
- disability days;
- limitations;
- health or medical conditions;
- age;
- sex;
- race and ethnicity;
- marital status;
- family composition;
- education;
- income; and
- employment.

National Medical Care Utilization and Expenditure Survey (NMCUES).—NMCUES, sponsored jointly by NCHS and the Health Care Financing Administration (HCFA), was first performed in 1980; a second cycle is planned for 1987.

The 1980 NMCUES consisted of two household surveys. One was a national survey that obtained data from a probability sample of the civilian, noninstitutionalized U.S. population. Repeat interviews were conducted with 6,600 households at 12-week intervals. The second survey was a household survey that obtained information from 4,000 Medicaid-eligible households in four States. Information was obtained in these surveys about health status, patterns of health care utilization, charges for health care services received, and methods of payment. Individual and family social, economic, and demographic data were also collected. The household survey data were augmented by information from the Medicare administrative records for persons identified as Medicare beneficiaries.

Specific data items in NMCUES included the following (357):
- conditions and illness,
- disability days,
- emergency room visit,
- hospital outpatient department visit,
- medical provider visit,
- hospital stay,
- prescribed medicine,
- other medical expenses,
- limitations,
- access to health care,
- background information, and
- health care charge and source of payment.

The NMCUES Public Use Files contain respondent data from the national household survey only (357).

A joint survey between NCHS, the National Center for Health Services Research and Health Care Technology Assessment (NCHSR&HCTA) and HCFA is being planned for 1987, as a followup to NMCES and NMCUES. The survey, the National Medical Expenditure Survey, will consist of four components: household, records, institutional, and disease panel. The household component (approximately 13,000 households) will draw its sample from HIS. This innovation will allow oversampling of groups of particular policy interest, such as the elderly, the poor, and persons with functional limitations. Since reliance on household data alone often results in problems of missing data, record checks to supplement respondent information will be important. The institutional component will be used in order to produce an accurate picture of public program expenditures. The Institutional Population Component will survey approximately 10,000 persons in nursing homes, psychiatric institutions, and facilities for the mentally retarded. The disease panel component of the survey will possibly contain up to three "disease panels" of approximately 1,000 individuals each, followed for at least 5 years. HIS would be used as the sampling frame, from which persons with certain conditions can be identified. Besides the core questions of the survey, supplemental disease-specific questions will be administered to these individuals (359).

National Survey of Personal Health Practices and Consequences (NSPHPC).—This survey was initially conducted by NCHS in 1979. One goal of the survey was to examine the relation between "personal health practices and physical health status." Information was collected from a 30-minute telephone survey of individuals sampled from the population aged 20 to 64 residing in the United States. The "second wave" or followup of the survey was performed in the spring of 1980 and included measures of change in the aggregate population and in individuals between the first and second survey. Thus, it was possible to determine if health practices were stable over time. Self-perceived health status and the utilization of health services were also determined. An attempt was made to learn the "extent to which failure to practice health maintenance leads to illness, and the extent to which illness inhibits the practice of good health habits" (355).

Survey of Disability and Work (SDW).—SDW was conducted in 1978 by the Social Security Administration (SSA). The survey was designed to provide statistics on the number and characteristics of the disabled, to establish national disability rates for various age groups, and to estimate the prevalence of health problems among the population.[1] These data were useful in establishing levels of medical severity. SDW also collected data on work limitations and mode of adjustment; the public's knowledge of Government programs in the area of disability; work incentives; socioeconomic, attitudinal, and psychological factors; and financial status of the individual (i.e., proportion of disabled who were below the poverty level).

To evaluate the adequacy of the SSA program for noninstitutionalized disabled persons and to provide estimates on the number of potential beneficiaries, SDW observed both disabled beneficiaries and disabled nonbeneficiaries. To compare the closeness of the disabled nonbeneficiary population to the beneficiary population and to analyze different characteristics among nondisabled persons, disabled nonbeneficiaries, and beneficiaries, SDW used a two-frame sampling approach. The first frame was a general population frame of noninstitutionalized persons. The 1976 HIS provided data on this general population (120,000 persons). The second frame consisted of recent Social Security disabled beneficiaries and recently denied applicants (also noninstitutionalized). These data were provided by the SSA's Master Beneficiary Record of 1.8 million persons.

The individuals represented in the first frame were classified in one of five categories ranging from nondisabled to severely disabled. Information was obtained from data items reporting "chronic conditions and activity limitation, usage of medical services, and employment status." Individuals in the second frame were also classified in five categories: one stratum for nonbeneficiaries and four age group strata for beneficiaries. In order to obtain enough working beneficiaries to support the planned analyses, SDW oversampled younger beneficiaries. SDW interviewed a total of 5,652 persons from HIS and 4,886 from SSA to yield an overall total of 9,859 individuals. Care must be taken in using SDW data because of the many problems in sampling design and procedures (see 366).

SDW collected data on the following categories (366):
- family background,
- work experience,
- health conditions,
- attitudinal data,
- work limitations,
- job training,
- income,
- job satisfaction,
- disability benefits, and
- knowledge of Government programs.

Federal Surveys of Special Populations

Hospital Cost and Utilization Project (HCUP).— HCUP is conducted by NCHSR&HCTA. The overall purpose of the project is to identify and explain variations in hospital behavior, use, and costs over time and place.

HCUP data files link hospital, patient, and county information for 384 short-term, general, non-Federal hospitals from 1970 to 1977. (Information on general characteristics of physicians that can be linked to patient abstracts has been obtained for a subset of 160 hospitals.) Twelve major discharge abstract services provide clinical information on the use of inpatient services in sample hospitals. The AHA Annual Survey of Hospitals and the Medicare cost reports provides data on hospital characteristics. Data on community characteristics are obtained primarily from the Area Resource File (see app. D) and from the Bureau of the Census.

Following the implementation of Medicare's PPS in 1983, NCHSR decided to extend the HCUP data to include information for 1980-87 and to enlarge the sample size to 500 hospitals. Sample weighting of the universe of short-term, general, non-Federal hospitals will provide national estimates. By extending the period of data collection, it will be possible to analyze data from three periods: 1) the decade prior to changes in Medicare's reimbursement policy; 2) the years when the Tax Equity and Fiscal Responsibility Act of 1982 was in effect; and 3) the period during which Medicare's PPS was implemented (61).

---

[1]Disability was described in the study as "a limitation in the kind or amount of work or housework a person can do resulting from a chronic health condition or impairment lasting 3 months or longer, and may range from the inability to perform any kind of work to secondary limitations in the kind or amount of work performed" (366).

Currently, NCHSR&HCTA is recruiting hospitals for the study, and completion dates of data files will depend on the sources of data and the efforts required to produce uniform records. Patient and hospital files for 1980-84 are expected to be compiled by summer 1986. The lowest predicted time lag between data collection and release of information is 14 months for hospitals and 16 months for patients. Generally, county data from the Area Resource File is available with a 2- to 3-year time lag.

The following represent examples of data items in HCUP files:
- hospital characteristics:
  —size,
  —ownership,
  —scope of services,
  —revenues,
  —costs;
- patient characteristics:
  —diagnostic information;
- community characteristics:
  —population demographics,
  —socioeconomic factors,
  —availability of health resources; and
- physician characteristics:
  —specialty,
  —board certification,
  —age,
  —years in practice.

All information remains confidential, so that no individual or institution can be identified separately. According to NCHSR statutes, the HCUP database can be used for research purposes only. The confidentiality ruling does place limitations on what can be studied. No information was collected on patients' complete residence by zip code, city, or county (consistent patient location data are available on a national basis for Medicare patients only). No information is available on patient income, health history, health beliefs, occupation, household size, use of services prior to hospital admission or after discharge, or breadth of health insurance coverage. Despite these limitations, the HCUP database represents a very extensive set of files on hospital utilization (349).

Hospital Discharge Survey (HDS).—HDS, designed by NCHS as a national ongoing survey to monitor the admissions and discharge of patients to and from hospitals, began in 1965. Data for the survey are obtained from a sample of medical records of inpatients discharged from a national sample of short-stay general and specialty hospitals in the United States. The sample for the 1980 HDS included approximately 224,000 medical records from 420 hospitals participating in the study.

HDS provides detailed information on the characteristics of patients (age, sex, race, date of birth, and marital status), diagnosis, surgical operations or procedures, and lengths of stay. Information is also available on patterns of use of care in different size hospitals in the four major geographical regions.

HDS uses a two-stage stratified sampling design. First, a sample of 10 percent of short-stay hospitals is selected from the Master Facility Inventory of Hospitals and Institutions (see app. D). All hospitals containing at least 1,000 beds are selected with certainty; hospitals with fewer than 1,000 beds are stratified according to size and geographic location. Probabilities for selection vary from certainty (for hospitals with at least 1,000 beds) to 1 in 40 (for the smallest hospitals) (26). Second, discharges are sampled from selected hospitals according to a probability sample such that the overall probability of selecting a discharge from each hospital size class is approximately equal.

National Ambulatory Medical Care Survey (NAMCS). —NAMCS is conducted by NCHS and provides annual data from patient records selected from a national sample of office-based physicians. The survey was conducted annually from 1973 to 1981; it was discontinued from 1982 to 1984 for lack of funding. Future surveys are planned for every 3 years beginning in 1985. In the future, the survey may encompass neighborhood health clinics and hospital outpatient facilities as well as office visits. Data tapes and documentation from NAMCS are available to the public and can be obtained from NCHS.

The basic sampling unit for NAMCS is the physician-patient office visit. The sampling frame is composed of all physicians who are listed in the master files of the American Medical Association or the American Osteopathic Association, but physicians who are federally employed and who specialize in anesthesiology, pathology, or radiology are considered ineligible for the survey. The 1981 sample included 2,846 physicians (2,725 M.D.s and 121 O.D.s). Of 2,333 eligible physicians, 1,807 (77.5 percent) participated in the study.

The 1981 NAMCS was a three-stage probability sample of primary sampling units, physician practices, and patient visits. The primary sampling unit is the first level of sampling and consists of a mutually exclusive and exhaustive set of 1,900 distinct geographic areas (counties, groups of counties, and Standard Metropolitan Statistical Areas). A sample of 87 primary sampling units was created by the National Opinion Research Center.

Within each sampled primary sampling unit, eligible physicians were classified into nine specialty groups: general and family practice, internal medicine, pediatrics, other medical specialties, general surgery, obstetrics and gynecology, other surgical specialties, psychiatry, and other specialties. A sample of physicians was then drawn such that the overall probability of selecting any one physician was approximately equal.

The third sample stage, the selection of patient visits, involved: 1) dividing the total physician sample into 52 random subsamples of equal size and assigning each subsample to 1 week in the year; and 2) selecting a systematic random sample of visits by the physician during the assigned week. The sampling rate for patient visits varied from a 100-percent sample for very small practices to a 20-percent sample for very large practices.

Approximately 30 Patient Records were completed during the assigned week. These procedures minimized the data collection workload and maintained approximate equal reporting levels among sample physicians regardless of practice size. Actual data collection was performed by the physician and his or her office staff.

The 1981 NAMCS contains the following data items on each visit (354):
- patient age and sex;
- patient race and ethnicity;
- physician specialty and type of practice;
- principal reason for visit expressed by patient;
- major reason for visit, prior visit status, and referral status;
- diagnostic services ordered or provided;
- principal diagnosis rendered by the physician;
- medication therapy ordered or provided;
- nonmedication therapy; and
- disposition and duration of visit.

National Long-Term Care Survey (NLTCS).—NLTCS was administered in 1982 and 1984 by the Bureau of the Census and was sponsored jointly by the Office of the Assistant Secretary for Planning and Evaluation (ASPE) and HCFA.

The 1982 NLTCS was designed to identify the over-65 Medicare population who need assistance with one or more "activities of daily living." This survey obtained data to assess the following (312):
- the number and characteristics of noninstitutionalized aged persons with varying degrees of impairment,
- the kind and amount of purchased and nonpurchased services received by impaired aged persons,
- the out-of-pocket costs for services and the ability of individuals to pay,
- the number and characteristics of impaired persons not receiving services, and
- the relationship between the degree of impairment of the individual and the services received.

The 1982 NLTCS was conducted in two stages. The first stage obtained a sample of approximately 36,000 persons from the Medicare rolls (HCFA's December 1981 and March 1982 Health Insurance Skeleton Eligibility Write Off files). These individuals were screened with a telephone interview to determine whether they experienced problems with normal daily activities persisting for at least 3 months. In the second stage of the survey, persons in the noninstitutionalized population who were found to have some long-term difficulties (6,400 persons) were interviewed by personal visit. The informal caregivers of those with dependencies were also interviewed (66).

The 1982 NLTCS collected specific data in the following categories (312):
- diseases,
- impairments and health conditions,
- "activities of daily living" and "instrumental activities of daily living" dependent activities,
- level of dependency,
- medical supports,
- social service supports,
- informal supports,
- sources of payment for medical services,
- income,
- assets,
- family structure,
- living arrangements,
- social interaction, and
- mental status.

A second NLTCS was implemented in 1984. This survey included approximately 35,018 participants who were sampled in 1982 and approximately 4,800 selected from Medicare enrollees who turned 65 after April 1, 1982. The 1984 NLTCS made five types of estimates (156):
- longitudinal characteristics for those persons who were impaired in 1982,
- longitudinal characteristics for persons who were not impaired in 1982,
- longitudinal characteristics for persons who were institutionalized in 1982,
- cross-sectional estimates for persons impaired in 1984, and
- cross-sectional estimates for persons in institutions in 1984.

Data tapes, descriptive analyses, and documentation from the 1982 NLTCS are available.

National Nursing Home Survey (NNHS).—NNHS was first conducted by NCHS in 1973-74, and a second survey was completed in 1977. Beginning in 1984, NCHS plans to conduct the survey at regular 6-year intervals.

NNHS collects data on nursing homes, services provided, patients, and staff. Utilization, charges for care, and cost of care can be assessed, as can nursing homes' certification status for participation in Medicare and Medicaid. The 1977 survey also collected information from residents who had been discharged from nursing homes. The 1977 sample, which included all homes that provided some level of nursing care, was expanded from the 1973-74 sample, which did not include homes providing only personal or domiciliary care.

In 1977, 1,698 facilities drawn from the Master Facility Inventory of Hospitals and Institutions (see app. D) were sampled. A sample of residents, discharges, and staff in these facilities was selected for further data collection and interviews.

NNHS provides national and regional estimates of utilization, expenses, and services of facilities; demographic characteristics; health status; services received; charges of residents; and staff. The resident and discharge surveys have data on the following (358):
- demographic characteristics,
- health status,
- functional status,
- participation in social activities,
- monthly charge, and
- source of payment.

The following additions were tested for the 1984 version: brief physical examination; psychiatric evaluation of patient; history of nursing home care; costs of care; and reason for admission (358).

Survey of Institutionalized Persons (SIP).—SIP was conducted by the Bureau of the Census in 1976. Residents of institutions, their families, and institution administrators were interviewed about the services and resources of long-term care facilities. The residents included persons with chronic conditions (diseases or handicaps), the mentally retarded, and those in nursing homes or homes for the aged.

SIP was designed to provide insights into the process of institutionalization; its impact on individuals and society; and the characteristics of institutions, their resident populations, and the residents' families. The survey included questions regarding social and employment activities, medical needs, care received, and financial status. Specific concerns included the appropriateness of admission, quality of life provided, legal rights, type of care provided, cost and source of payment, and effect of Government programs.

Institutions were sampled in 18 strata: 6 types of institutions (psychiatric, physically handicapped, mentally handicapped, children, nursing homes, other facilities) and 3 facility size categories. The 1973 Master Facility Inventory of Hospitals and Institutions (see app. D) was used as the basic frame for selecting sample institutions. SIP interviewed a total of 9,337 residents over the age of 14, who were mentally and physically able, from the 822 institutions that participated.

Data items collected by SIP included the following (311):
- background information;
- age, sex, education, employment;
- treatment services;
- social activities;
- reason for choice of institution;
- discharge expectations;
- financial status;
- source of payment;
- physician services;
- nursing services;
- counseling and therapy services;
- limitations (activity and function); and
- medication therapy.

The families of residents answered similar inquiries, in addition to ones regarding previous history, discharge expectations, and the effects (including financial) of institutionalization on the family (311).

Private Health Surveys

Private Surveys of the General Population

American Hospital Association (AHA) National Opinion Study.—In 1982, AHA conducted an interview survey of 1,800 heads of household over 18 years of age nationwide. Funded jointly by AHA and the Council on Allied Hospital Associations, the project was intended to provide national data and a common survey instrument that may be used by others to provide comparable local data. The purpose of the survey was to assess public perceptions about health care quality, access, costs, changes in health insurance, and ethical issues. This information will be useful in providing baseline data to measure changes in public opinion over the next few years.

Specific questions were asked in regard to hospitalization, rating of area and nationwide hospitals, health care expenditures, Government regulation of health care, and accessibility of health care. Survey results have been published by AHA (255).

Center for Health Administration Studies (CHAS) National Survey of Access to Medical Care.—In 1975-76, CHAS and the National Opinion Research Center at the University of Chicago conducted a household survey of the U.S. population that addressed issues of access to health care and problems in obtaining care when needed. Previous surveys conducted by CHAS (1953, 1958, 1964, and 1971) emphasized total health care experiences and costs. However, there are many comparable items available from the five surveys which permit trends in some key indicators of access to be measured over time. In 1982, a followup telephone survey was conducted by Louis Harris and Associates in conjunction with CHAS (2).

The initial purpose of the 1976 survey was to provide baseline national indicators of access for an evaluation of a program of hospital-based primary care group practices funded by the Robert Wood Johnson Foundation in Princeton, New Jersey. The access framework and questionnaire designed for the survey were developed to provide empirical indicators in order to improve access for the population in areas served by the groups.

Interviews for the 1976 survey were conducted in 5,432 households representing the noninstitutionalized population of the United States. The investigators selected a random sample of an adult and child under 17 years of age from each household, yielding a sample of 7,787 individuals in the 1976 survey. The overall response rate was 85 percent. In addition to the sample of the noninstitutionalized U.S. population, special oversamples of persons experiencing episodes of illness, non-Standard Metropolitan Statistical Area Southern blacks, and persons of Spanish heritage living in the Southwest were drawn.

The following specific data items were collected in the 1975-76 CHAS survey (4):

- characteristics of health delivery systems:
  —availability,
  —number of personnel and facilities,
  —distribution of personnel and facilities,
  —convenience of regular source of medical care,
  —selection of regular source of medical care,
  —sources of medical care used by those with no regular source,
  —sources of regular medical care,
  —type and extent of third-party coverage;
- characteristics of population-at-risk:
  —general health care beliefs and attitudes,
  —knowledge of health care information,
  —education,
  —occupation,
  —age,
  —sex,
  —race and ethnicity,
  —length of time in the community,
  —perceived need,
  —evaluated need;
- utilization of health services:
  —type of provider—physician, hospital, dentist,
  —site of visit,
  —purpose—preventive or illness-related,
  —time interval; and
- consumer satisfaction.

The Equitable Healthcare Survey.—The Equitable Healthcare Survey, designed by Louis Harris and Associates, was sponsored by the Equitable Life Assurance Society of the United States in 1982. Besides obtaining opinions from the general public (1,501 adults), the survey questioned 100 physicians who lead medical societies, 100 hospital administrators, 50 senior health insurance executives, 250 corporate benefits officers, and a national sample of 26 union leaders responsible for health care benefits. The survey explored topics including general attitudes toward the U.S. health care system, utilization of medical services, escalation of health care costs, and cost-containment policies (98).

Hospital Care in America.—Hospital Care in America was a survey of consumers, government officials, and members of the health care community conducted in 1978 by Louis Harris and Associates. The survey was designed to provide an analysis of attitudes toward health and hospital care. The sample consisted of the adult civilian population of the continental United States. Items in the survey included: general attitudes toward health care; preventive medicine; perceptions of health care in the United States; attitudes toward types of hospitals; hospital costs; administration of hospitals; national health insurance; and hospitals and the future (144).

Physician and Public Opinion on Health Care Issues.—The American Medical Association has commissioned a series of surveys since 1972 to measure attitudes on health care issues. The sample consists of 1,503 randomly selected respondents residing in the United States. The interviews were conducted by telephone by a consulting firm. Specific questions included attitudes toward problems facing health care, national priorities for spending, public image of physicians, Medicare issues, and the voluntary physician fee freeze (17).

Private Surveys of Special Populations

Commission on Professional and Hospital Activities (CPHA) Files.—CPHA maintains one of the largest abstracting services in the United States. Over 1,500 hospitals submit patient discharge information to CPHA, whose master files contain clinical and demographic data on 25 percent of all patients treated in U.S. short-term, general, non-Federal hospitals. This sample is *not* random, but depends on member hospitals' data. The National Master Sample Research File is selected from these master files to provide annually 2 million patient records that are nationally representative of short-term general hospitals. The "2 million" file is drawn in quarterly increments of 500,000.

The data collected contain all of the data elements of the Uniform Hospital Discharge Data Set (see ch. 6), as well as additional indicators such as the number of days in care units. The following items represent specific data (64):

- patient identification;

- date of birth;
- race and sex;
- date of admission;
- type of admission (emergency, from SNF, etc.);
- date of discharge and disposition of patient (home or self-care, SNF, intermediate care facility, short-term hospital, etc.);
- diagnosis (principal and six additional);
- procedures;
- attending physician;
- operating physician;
- expected principal source(s) of payment;
- patient care data (laboratory tests, drugs, vital signs, etc.); and
- stay summary (acute days used, days awaiting SNF or intermediate care facility, etc.) (64).

University of Chicago Access Impact Study of Community Hospital Program.—The purpose of the University of Chicago Access Impact Study, sponsored by the Robert Wood Johnson Foundation, was to evaluate the success of the Community Hospital Program groups in improving access to medical care in the communities they served. Community Hospital Programs tended to attract people who had no previous regular source of care or who used hospital outpatient and emergency rooms. Twelve of the fifty-three Community Hospital Programs were surveyed. Community surveys were conducted in 1978-79 and 2 years later. Randomly selected adults and children were selected for intensive interviewing. Personal interviews were the primary method of data collection, and the questionnaire was modeled after the 1976 National Survey of Access to Medical Care conducted by CHAS and the National Opinion Research Center at the University of Chicago. Respondents were questioned regarding regular source of medical care, convenience (evening, weekend coverage, home visits), utilization, and satisfaction (5).

Appendix D.—Major Databases Covering the Availability of Health Care Services

Introduction

This appendix discusses the major databases containing information on the availability and services of U.S. health care facilities (e.g., number, geographic location, bed size, and capacity). The primary sources of information are the American Hospital Association's (AHA) Annual Survey of Hospitals, the Master Facility Inventory of Hospitals and Institutions (MFI), and the Medicare/Medicaid Automated Certification System (MMACS). Additional sources of data include the Area Resource File (ARF), State certificate-of-need (CON) databases, and ambulatory care surveys.

AHA's Annual Survey of Hospitals

The Annual Survey of Hospitals conducted by AHA is a basic source of data on the characteristics of U.S. hospitals. The survey has been conducted since 1946, and its results are published in the fall of each year. Data are collected for the survey through a questionnaire mailed to all hospitals in AHA files (approximately 7,000 hospitals), which include nonmember as well as member hospitals in the United States and associated areas. AHA depends on the American Osteopathic Hospital Association for a list of osteopathic hospitals and on the Joint Commission on Accreditation of Hospitals for a list of long-term care facilities.

The Annual Survey of Hospitals collects data on more than 500 items, including information on facilities and services, utilization patterns, hospital expenses, and staffing patterns. Examples of specific items are as follows (12):
- geographic location (by county and zip code);
- classification (type of ownership);
- major type of service (e.g., short-term);
- facilities and services (general medical, surgical, and selected ancillary services);
- beds and utilization by inpatient service;
- total facility beds and utilization;
  - —licensed bed capacity,
  - —newborn nursery,
  - —surgical operations,
  - —outpatient utilization,
  - —adult pediatric and neonatal beds,
  - —Medicare and Medicaid utilization (discharges, visits),
  - —65 and older utilization;
- financial data:
  - —revenue,
  - —expenses,
  - —unrestricted funds,
  - —restricted funds,
  - —capital expenditures;
- personnel; and
- medical staff.

Data from the Annual Survey of Hospitals are available on data tapes (1969 to present) and customized computer printouts (in the form of tables, listings, or labels). To the users of AHA's recently acquired National Data Network, annual survey data from 1978 are also available online. Users of the Data Network System can also maintain their own databases on the system and can merge them with the AHA databases (12).

Since data for the AHA Annual Survey are collected via a mailed questionnaire, individual hospitals must take responsibility for supplying complete and accurate responses. For nonreporting hospitals or those that submit incomplete survey questionnaires, data are estimated. The survey provides information on some services provided by the hospitals, but it does not provide an exhaustive list of all services. According to AHA, "the intent is *not* to serve as an official and all inclusive list of services offered by individual hospitals" (12).

Master Facility Inventory of Hospitals and Institutions (MFI)

MFI, which is maintained by the National Center for Health Statistics (NCHS), is the most comprehensive file of inpatient health facilities available in the United States. The file includes data from 33,000 facilities that provide either medical, nursing, or custodial care. Because it provides statistics on the number, type, and geographic distribution of facilities, MFI often serves as a source of data for probability samples used in conducting other national surveys (e.g., the National Nursing Home Survey described in app. C). Facilities are categorized in MFI into three types:
1. hospitals (short- and long-term);
2. nursing and related care homes; and
3. custodial or remedial care facilities (resident treatment centers for alcohol and drug abusers; homes for the mentally retarded, blind, deaf, emotionally disturbed, and physically handicapped; orphanages; and homes for unwed mothers).

MFI began in 1962-63 with the files of four Federal agencies containing the names and addresses of facilities, the directories of national associations, and State licensure files. Every 2 years, NCHS conducts a series of mail surveys to all facilities except hospitals. These surveys are intended to ensure that information about the basic characteristics of the facilities is accurate. In addition, State licensure agencies, national voluntary associations, and other sources periodically submit their most recent directories or lists of new facilities.

In order to gather information on hospitals, NCHS cooperated with AHA in a joint survey from 1969-78. AHA collected data for its member hospitals, while NCHS surveyed the 400 nonmember hospitals. Since 1978, AHA has been surveying all hospitals as part of its annual survey described above, and NCHS has purchased hospital data tapes from AHA.

The following types of data are contained in the MFI files (353):

- Hospitals:
  —data items available from AHA tapes (see above);
- Nursing homes:
  —location,
  —ownership,
  —major type of service,
  —licensed and staffed beds,
  —beds certified for Medicare and Medicaid,
  —admission policy with regard to age, sex, and conditions,
  —patient census by age and sex,
  —inpatient days of care,
  —number of admissions, discharges, and deaths,
  —staffing,
  —number of patients receiving nursing care,
  —services routinely performed,
  —basic monthly charge,
  —operating expenses;
- Other facilities:
  —location,
  —ownership,
  —major type of service,
  —licensed and staffed beds,
  —beds certified as intermediate-care beds,
  —admission policy regarding age and sex,
  —patient census by age and sex,
  —inpatient days of care,
  —number of admissions,
  —discharges and deaths,
  —staffing,
  —basic monthly charge,
  —operating expenses.

In conducting a survey as large as MFI, it is very difficult to obtain replies from all respondents or to verify each one's existence. Many facilities either do not respond to several inquiries or are found to be beyond MFI's scope (do not meet definitional criteria or minimum bed size), and some questionnaires are returned as undeliverable (317). Also, MFI does not include hospital-based skilled nursing facilities (SNFs) and intermediate-care facilities (ICFs) (67).

Final data and methodology from MFI are released to the public in biennial editions of *Health Resources Statistics*. Special tabulations of data tapes may also be available (353).

Medicare/Medicaid Automated Certification System (MMACS)

To participate in Medicare or Medicaid, institutions (including SNFs and ICFs) must be certified. The purpose of the certification process is to ensure that each participating institution provides safe and effective care to the beneficiaries of these programs. After initial certification, the institution is periodically reviewed. The review is conducted first at the State level, with final approval given by the Health Care Financing Administration (HCFA).

MMACS has two parts: 1) the Survey Report Form, and 2) the Provider of Services (POS) File. The Survey Report Form contains the criteria that measure an institution's ability to provide acceptable care and the decisions of the State agency regarding certification. Data from certification applications and surveys are then used as the basis for the POS File.

The POS File is the source of information on provider characteristics for the Medicare Part A data systems. This file includes information on the characteristics of the institutions, such as bed size, services, and staffing.

The POS File is updated daily, and recertifications replace the associated earlier certifications (which are placed in a separate history file). Approximately 7,000 hospitals, 5,200 SNFs, 3,000 home health agencies, 3,500 independent laboratories, and 1,600 other Medicare-participating facilities are included in this file.

The following data items are available in the POS File:

- type of facility;
- location of facility (city, State, county, Standard Metropolitan Statistical Area, HCFA region);
- type of control (voluntary, proprietary, etc.);
- number of beds (total and certified);
- services offered; and
- number of employees (salaried physicians, nurses, pharmacists, social workers, occupational therapists, speech therapists, physical therapists, and other employees).

Data from the POS File are used to support the Directory of Medical Facilities, which is a compendium of participating and nonparticipating medical care institutions. This directory is used by Medicare intermediaries for admission approval.

Data tabulations and analyses based on information from the POS File are published annually. Other divisions of HCFA, Congress, and private organizations may request various listings and tabulations from this data (325).

MMACS currently records a great deal of duplicative information. For instance, if one facility maintains both SNF and ICF beds, these are recorded as two facilities. However, HCFA is conducting a project to eliminate duplications in the 1984 and 1985 data, and duplications among data from 1981 have recently been eliminated. Some information deficits also occur, because many institutions are not Medicare/Medicaid certified. In order to determine the number of nursing homes in existence, both the POS File and MFI must be cross checked (in 1981, 161 facilities found in MFI were not listed on the MMACS file) (67).

Area Resource File (ARF)

ARF is a health resource database maintained by the Office of Data Analysis and Management of the Bureau of Health Professions, Health Resources and Services Administration (HRSA). The ARF System has three major parts that integrate data from a number of sources; it combines information on health resources with areawide demographic and socioeconomic variables. The purpose of ARF is to provide a data file for analysis of the geographic distribution of resources. The information that ARF contains is derived from 75 source files.

The core of the overall ARF System, the county-specific record, has expanded since 1971 to include more than 7,000 variables at the county level. The information can be divided into eight categories:
- health facilities,
- health professions,
- measures of resource scarcity,
- health status,
- economic activity,
- health training programs,
- socioeconomic characteristics, and
- environmental characteristics for each county.

The health facilities category contains data on hospitals obtained from the AHA Annual Hospital Survey. Data in the health facilities category can be integrated with data from the other categories. The health facilities category also contains information on the number and the enrollment of health maintenance organizations as well as limited data on nursing homes. The nursing home data are obtained from the MFI, the National Nursing Home Survey, and the AHA Annual Survey of Hospitals. Only data that are reported on a county level are used.

The advantage of ARF is that the use of the county as the basic geographic unit permits aggregation of data in various ways. The following geographic areas have been defined in the system that allow linking ARF with other data files:
- Standard Metropolitan Statistical Areas,
- Primary Metropolitan Statistical Areas,
- Area Health Education Centers,
- State Economic Areas and Economic Subregions,
- Veterans Administration Service Area Codes,
- Bureau of Economic Analysis Areas,
- Federal Regions,
- Health Service Areas,
- Peer Review Organization Areas, and
- Medicare Prevailing Charges Locality Codes.

The second part of the ARF System is the State/National Timeseries Database. This database contains data on education and the medical professions obtained from the basic county-specific ARF and other sources. Specific information consists of characteristics of the professions' training systems, size and characteristics of the supply of each profession, population and demographic characteristics, health care expenditures and financing, and health services utilization.

The third part of the ARF System contains four internal components, which expand the capabilities of the system: 1) detailed hospital files; 2) detailed support files on various disciplines; 3) a data dictionary/directory system; and 4) a graphics/mapping capability. The hospital files include both facility- and county-level information. The facility-level hospital file contains one record per hospital. The county-level hospital file consists of facility data aggregated to the county level for hospitals that responded to the AHA Annual Survey of Hospitals (345).

Certificate-of-Need (CON) Databases

In 1974, Congress passed the National Health Planning and Resources Development Act (Public Law 93-641). This law requires that State planning agencies review and approve development of new health care facilities and other major capital expenditures. Each facility must file a CON application, which is reviewed by the local and State planning agencies. State planning agencies have the responsibility of determining the numbers and types of facilities and services needed by their populations (308). The Department of Health and Human Services (DHHS) (through HRSA) and private organizations, such as Hospital Research Associates, Inc., have maintained databases of all new institutional health care facilities as reported on CON applications.

HRSA collects the following State and national data on the number and dollar volume of CON applications (total, approved, and disapproved) for (347):
- hospitals;
- nursing homes;
- health maintenance organizations;
- ambulatory facilities; and
- other facilities (i.e., SNFs, kidney disease treatment centers, rehabilitation hospitals).

If DHHS discontinues maintenance of CON data, private organizations will play a larger role as data sources. Hospital Research Associates, a private company, has been tracking CON data since 1977 and lists projects, sorted by State, in 230 categories. Over 75,000 projects are included. The CON program categorized projects into four areas: capital construction, medical equipment, services, and bed changes. Hospital Research Associates maintains data on total number of applications in each area as well as the application cost. Each facility is categorized in the following ways (145):
- new facility,
- renovation,
- expansion,
- conversion/relocation,
- change of ownership,
- replacement,
- addition/deletion of beds, and
- replacement of beds.

Until recently, States that failed to comply with the law risked losing their Federal planning money. Even so, one State (Louisiana) never passed CON laws. Furthermore, since 1982, the Federal planning program has been funded on continuing resolutions that have specified that noncomplying States not be penalized. As a result, some States (e.g., Minnesota, Idaho, New Mexico, and California) have discontinued CON applications. This situation will greatly affect the future use of CON data. If the Federal planning program is discontinued, States may still collect CON applications voluntarily, but DHHS will not continue maintaining a database (29). The use of CON data as a comprehensive measure of new facilities and equipment is also undermined by the fact that States have very different expenditure limits above which CON approval is necessary.

Ambulatory Care Center Surveys

The National Association for Ambulatory Care Centers (NAFAC), formerly the National Association of Freestanding Emergency Care Centers, has completed two surveys of freestanding emergency centers to obtain data on environmental factors (e.g., health care costs, demographic changes, and competitive forces) and characteristics of the centers (e.g., number, location, ownership, scope of services, patient volumes, etc.). NAFAC defines ambulatory care centers as "those physicians' offices which are open extended hours, offer expanded treatment capabilities, treat patients on a non-scheduled basis, utilize advertising and marketing principles and are most sensitive to the laws of supply and demand" (216).

The first survey was completed and available for sale in February 1983. The second survey was available for distribution in June 1985.

For the second survey, "The FEC Factor II: The Second Comprehensive National Study of Freestanding Emergency and Urgent Care Centers" the following data items were collected:
- identification information (location);
- facility ownership;
- facility characteristics;
- area characteristics;
- services provided, volumes, and types of conditions seen;
- patient characteristics;
- number of personnel;
- equipment;
- supplies used;
- drugs most frequently prescribed; and
- reimbursement and finances.

Data for the FEC II survey were collected until October 1984, and NAFAC obtained a 20-percent response rate from an estimated 1,200 facilities. (As of May 1985, NAFAC estimated that there were 2,500 ambulatory care centers.)

It is difficult to determine the exact number of ambulatory care centers for a number of reasons. Without any licensing or regulation of the industry, there is no comprehensive central list of centers. Also, many ambulatory care centers can be established at a capital cost substantially below the CON level. Other difficulties arise from the number of different definitions of ambulatory care centers. The Federal Government, for example, estimates that there are currently 1,800 "immediate care centers." DHHS identifies three types of immediate care centers: 1) facilities that are open continuously, provide episodic care for many types of illnesses and injuries, and are staffed by emergency physicians; 2) facilities similar to physicians' offices and offering evening care; and 3) facilities that provide episodic care for minor emergencies and are open 12 to 16 hours a day, 7 days a week (147). Until all ambulatory care centers are licensed or regulated, it will be difficult to maintain adequate availability data.

Appendix E.—Medicare Part A Data Systems

Introduction

The Medicare Part A (Hospital Insurance) data systems were developed and designed for their use in the administration of the Medicare program. Hence, the administrative requirements of the past have governed their content, quality, and timeliness. The Part A data systems provide a record of reimbursement-related actions and the information on which those actions were taken. Although they also provide an information base for program and policy analyses and research, these functions have been secondary. Public use tapes exist for only two of the files discussed in this appendix, a situation that limits the ability of outside researchers to pursue independent research. Nevertheless, the Part A data systems provide a rich base, often the only database, for evaluating some of the important impacts of Medicare's prospective payment system (PPS).

Basic Data Files

Medicare Part A data systems contain data in four major categories:
- *Beneficiary enrollment and eligibility status*—the characteristics of and benefits available to the Medicare enrolled population. The records containing these data elements originate in the Social Security Administration (SSA).
- *Inpatient hospital claims*—characteristics of the patient, the services rendered, and the charges billed during a hospital stay. These data originate in hospital bills.
- *Hospital costs*—capital and operating costs of Medicare-certified hospitals. These data are submitted each year directly by hospitals to intermediaries on Medicare cost reports.
- *Provider characteristics*—attributes of the institutions and kinds of services they provide to Medicare patients. Data on hospital characteristics are available from both the Medicare cost reports and the process of certifying hospitals for treatment of Medicare patients.

The data elements in these categories arrive at the Health Care Financing Administration (HCFA) through a variety of channels and are processed into specific files[1] including:
- the Health Insurance Master Enrollment Record File (referred to as the HIM File), which contains up-to-date information on each Medicare beneficiary;
- the Hospital Stay Record File, which contains a record of each inpatient hospital stay;
- the Hospital Cost Report Information System (HCRIS), which contains data extracted from the Medicare cost reports; and
- the Provider of Services (POS) File, which contains data items pertaining to the Medicare hospital certification process.

These files, which can be further manipulated or merged as the need arises, are the basic sources for all derivative files that may be created either to support the operations of the health insurance programs or to monitor and evaluate the performance or impact of the system. Each of these data files is described in greater detail below.

Health Insurance Master Enrollment Record (HIM) File

The HIM File contains information supplied to HCFA by SSA. It includes basic identifying and demographic information about Medicare Part A beneficiaries and also indicates whether the beneficiary is covered under Part B of Medicare (Supplementary Medical Insurance), the extent to which certain limited benefits are still available to the beneficiary, and the beneficiary's current status regarding deductible and coinsurance.

The HIM File is updated frequently to reflect changes in beneficiaries' eligibility for benefits. All hospital claims arriving at HCFA are passed against the appropriate beneficiary's record within a few days, and in that process, some information about the beneficiary is also appended to claims records for use in the claims files. The HIM File also contains current information on Medicare inpatient admissions, because with each admission the hospital makes a "query" to HCFA through the fiscal intermediary to confirm the patient's eligibility for Medicare coverage. This query is answered by checking the HIM File, and in that process, the beneficiary's record is flagged as a current hospitalization.

Hospital Stay Record File

Prior to October 1983, the Hospital Stay Record File aggregated individual bills pertaining to a hospital stay for a 20-percent sample of Medicare beneficiaries (340). Diagnostic and surgical information were coded (using the ICD-9-CM[2] classification) from narratives for this 20-percent sample.

---

[1] For the most part, these files are automated and can thus be considered to exist on computer tapes or disks.

[2] ICD-9-CM, the International Classification of Diseases, 9th Revision, Clinical Modification, is designed for the classification of morbidity and mortality information for statistical purposes, and for the indexing of hospital records by disease and operations, for data storage and retrieval (322).

In October 1983, hospitals were required to provide diagnostic and procedural data for all Medicare bills, and under PPS, the hospital will submit only one bill per hospital stay. Since October 1983, the Hospital Stay Record File has included diagnostic and procedural information as well as provider and beneficiary demographic data for 100 percent of Medicare hospital stays. Data on diagnoses, DRG assignment, enrollee demographic data, major procedures performed, and patient charges by department are taken from the HIM File and patient billing data supplied by the fiscal intermediaries (contractors authorized by HCFA to make Part A payments to hospitals). The file is updated quarterly.

The procedures for reporting diagnostic information included in the Hospital Stay Record have changed substantially since these data became a reporting requirement. Beginning in 1977, fiscal intermediaries were required to report the first 45 characters of diagnostic information and the first 41 characters of surgical information reported on the provider bill for the 20-percent sample on which diagnostic information was reported. HCFA used an automated system to code the narratives. When codes could not be established using the automated process, they were coded manually.

In 1981, HCFA began to allow institutional providers to report coded ICD-9-CM information rather than narrative. In October 1983, the reporting of this information using ICD-9-CM cases became a requirement rather than an option. Also in October 1983, HCFA began to require that hospitals report up to four additional diagnostic and two additional surgical procedure codes in addition to the principal diagnostic and surgical codes that had been previously required.[3]

The currency of the Hospital Stay Record File depends largely on the timeliness of bill submission by hospitals and processing HCFA and SSA. The vast majority of bills are submitted within 1 month of discharge, but some bills are submitted up to 18 months later. The average time is about 1 month, and one-half of all bills are submitted within 17 days (394). Intermediaries take between a week and 10 days to put bill data on magnetic tape, edit the data for consistency and completeness, and send them to HCFA. Thus, at least 50 percent of the bills are processed within 2 months, but a small proportion are subject to delays that are much longer. Transit and batching time at HCFA takes an average of 2 to 3 weeks (394).

Hospital Cost Report Information System (HCRIS)

HCRIS is a new automated database of selected information extracted from Medicare cost reports. The cost report is submitted annually by each hospital within 4 months of the end of its fiscal year to the fiscal intermediary. Until the advent of PPS, the Medicare cost report was the primary document on which hospital payment was based.[4]

The cost report form has changed frequently and become more complex in response to changes in law and regulations pertaining to hospital reimbursement. For the most part, the changes in the cost report form have represented the addition of more detailed data or reorganization of existing data. Several important kinds of data have been consistently available over the lifetime of the Medicare cost reports.[5]

The cost report consists of a number of worksheets (analogous to income tax forms) which require the hospital both to provide statistical and financial data and to perform calculations to arrive at a level of reimbursement. The data items included in HCRIS are those identified by HCFA as necessary to meet the most often used and highest priority data needs. The Medicare cost reports include the following basic elements:

- hospital statistics—selected characteristics of the hospital, including:
  —type of ownership or control,
  —number of beds available,
  —inpatient days,
  —average number of employees on payroll,
  —number of admissions;
- operating expenses by hospital cost center;[6]

---

[3]As a consequence of these changes, Medicare has adopted a new billing form, the UB-82, which provides room for the additional diagnostic and procedural data as well as more detailed charge data by revenue-producing cost centers. The UB-82 is currently being phased in and is expected to be universal by the end of this year (119).

[4]The cost report is still necessary for computing hospitals' payments both because of the 3-year transition period and the exclusion of certain costs (e.g., outpatient, capital, medical education) from DRG payment. HCFA is required to keep hospital cost reports until Sept. 30, 1988 (Public Law 98-21), but the form of those reports may change.

[5]The most recent cost report form, HCFA-2552-84, is to be used by hospitals reporting on fiscal years beginning on or after Oct. 1, 1983. This form, reporting on the first year of the PPS, is as extensive as its predecessors. It consists of a total of 112 pages of forms and worksheets, although not all of the data items are applicable to any given hospital. The changes from the previous form (HCFA-2552-83), e.g., items pertaining to paramedical expenditures, appear to be relatively minor additions as required by PPS. HCFA's latest proposed form, HCFA-2552-85, for fiscal years beginning on or after Oct. 1, 1983, is currently being circulated outside of HCFA for comments (117).

[6]While specific cost centers are defined on the cost report, hospitals, may, with the approval of the intermediary, combine or break down additional cost centers as they desire. Hospital cost centers include revenue-producing units such as radiology or pharmacy as well as non-revenue-producing units such as housekeeping or laundry. They also include outpatient cost centers as separate entities.

- depreciation expenses by type (e.g., movable equipment, buildings and fixtures);
- capital expenditure data by project;
- total charges by cost center;
- Medicare charges by cost center;
- routine inpatient nursing salary costs;
- malpractice costs; and
- standard financial statement information—assets, liabilities, income, etc.

Hospitals must submit a cost report to their fiscal intermediary within 3 months of the close of their fiscal year; they routinely receive a 30-day extension. The fiscal intermediary then has up to 1 year to review, audit, and finally settle on the amount due to the hospital. In this process, some data items on the cost report as submitted may be challenged and changed by the fiscal intermediary. Thus, the final settled cost report data present a more accurate picture of allowed hospital costs than do the submitted reports, but they also involve a substantial lag time (one additional year). The difference between the "as submitted" and "as settled" cost reports for fiscal year 1982 was estimated to be $700 million, or about 2 percent of total Medicare hospital payments (72).

On paper, HCRIS is a powerful addition to the Medicare data systems. Prior to its implementation in 1982, HCFA had no automated files for Medicare cost reports. When cost reports were required for some aspect of program operation or analysis, hard copies would have to be obtained from the intermediaries. For example, in computing the first weights for diagnosis-related groups, HCFA actually entered data from the most recent copy of each hospital's report which were obtained directly from the fiscal intermediaries (229). There is also a shortened public use version of this data file, the HCRIS-180.

As of June 1985, the HCRIS file of cost reports for hospitals' fiscal years ending on or before January 1, 1982, was reasonably complete and consisted primarily of "as submitted" reports. The file for fiscal years ending between January 2, 1982 and September 29, 1983, was about 80 percent complete and primarily consisted of settled reports. The file of cost reports for fiscal years ending between September 30, 1983 and September 29, 1984, data reflecting the first year of regulations under the Tax Equity and Fiscal Responsibility Act of 1982 (Public Law 97-248), was about 15 percent complete and primarily consisted of settled cost reports (377).

About 90 percent of the data in the HCRIS database is received by HCFA in automated form from fiscal intermediaries; the remainder (largely from those hospitals with low Medicare utilization or an all inclusive/no charge structure) is received in hard copy.

Although HCRIS is intended to contain data from the cost reports submitted by hospitals prior to settlement as well as the final settled cost reports, HCFA has temporarily suspended the transmission of "as submitted" cost reports, purportedly because of the fiscal intermediaries' workload problems (340). HCFA's Bureau of Data Management and Strategy has recommended the transmission of the "as submitted" cost reports for the first year of PPS, hospitals' fiscal years ending between September 30, 1983, and September 29, 1984.[7] If this recommendation is approved, the "as submitted" file for fiscal year 1984 could be about 80 percent complete by April 1986 (377).

The expected timeframe for the completion of the HCRIS file for final settled cost reports is at least 17 months from the end of the hospital's fiscal year: 4 months for hospitals to submit, 12 months for the fiscal intermediaries to settle, and 1 month for the fiscal intermediaries to transmit (340). Since the file for any given fiscal year includes 200 to 300 hospitals whose fiscal year ends August 31 (11 months after the September 30 fiscal year end for many other hospitals), the whole reporting cycle takes approximately 28 months if these hospitals are included in the file for the same fiscal year (170). To this time lag must be added any delays in the issuance of the reporting forms, as is the case currently. Of course, this time lag could be shortened by the utilization of "as submitted" cost reports, but this involves some loss of accuracy and, in any event, there is no "as submitted" cost report data on the HCRIS file at present.

Provider of Services (POS) File

The POS File contains information on approximately 7,000 hospitals, 5,200 skilled nursing facilities (SNFs), 3,000 home health agencies, 3,500 independent laboratories, and 1,600 other Medicare participating facilities. Data from Medicare certification applications and surveys form the basis for this file, which is updated on a daily basis with new certification/recertification information (325). Recertification information replaces preexisting information, which is then placed in a history file.

The POS record varies with each kind of facility and includes some data specific to the particular provider type. Among the data included are:
- facility location (i.e., city, State, county, Stand-

---

[7]HCFA-2552-84 was recently approved by HCFA and distributed to the fiscal intermediaries and hospitals by mid-April and the end of April, respectively. Fiscal year 1984 cost reports are due within 60 days after the forms and instructions are received. Obviously, this will cause additional delay for the completion of the HCRIS file for the first year of PPS.

ard Metropolitan Statistical Area, HCFA region, responsible professional standards review organizations);
- facility type;
- type of control;
- total number of beds;
- number of certified beds;
- services offered; and
- number of registered nurses, licensed practical nurses, pharmacists, social workers, occupational therapists, speech therapists, physical therapists, and other employees.

The data for each facility in this file are identified by the same provider number used in billing and claims records, making it possible to link these data to the provider records.

Derivative Files

The basic files described above are large, either because they contain many records, many data entries on each record, or both. Derivative files are often created to extract a smaller number of records or selected data items, thus reducing the data processing burden. Derivative files are also often created when data from two or more basic files need to be linked together for the sake of analysis. Medicare's Part A data systems contain three such derivative files:
- the Medicare Provider Analysis and Review (MEDPAR) File;
- the Medicare History Sample File; and
- the Medicare Automated Data Retrieval System (MADRS).

Each of these files is described below.

Medicare Provider Analysis and Review (MEDPAR) File

Records in the MEDPAR File are created by merging data on the hospital's characteristics and costs with a shortened version of the Hospital Stay Record File. The MEDPAR records include the data on diagnoses, procedures, and departmental charges that are contained in the Hospital Stay Record. Although the Hospital Stay Record File since October 1983 has included data on 100 percent of hospital stays, MEDPAR will continue to report on a 20-percent sample of beneficiaries. The 1984 MEDPAR File, like the Hospital Stay Record File for that year, will record up to four diagnoses and two procedure codes in addition to the principal diagnostic and surgical codes. There is also a public use version of this file.

The MEDPAR File is created on a quarterly basis. The most current full year is the 1983 MEDPAR File.

In June 1985, HCFA was still working on the completion of the fiscal year 1984 MEDPAR File, and the file was 82 to 83 percent complete. Normally, the fiscal year 1985 MEDPAR File would have been expected to be 94 to 95 percent complete by April 1985. The delay is apparently due to the transition to the PPS and data processing problems by the fiscal intermediaries caused by the transition to UB-82 (119). In the future, HCFA expects the file for any fiscal year will be available within 3 to 6 months of the end of that fiscal year. Because the time taken to submit bills is to a large extent outside of HCFA's control, it is expected that the MEDPAR file will be only 90 to 95 percent complete within this timeframe.

Medicare History Sample (MHS) File

The Medicare History Sample File is based on a 5-percent sample of Medicare enrollees for 1974 and later and provides a history of the utilization of Medicare services for enrollees included in the sample. Selected enrollee characteristics are obtained from active and inactive HIM files. Utilization data for each year are obtained from inpatient hospital, SNF, home health agency, and physician office and outpatient bills processed by Medicare intermediaries and carriers.

A single record for each Medicare beneficiary is updated on an ongoing basis with utilization data from the billing records as well as characteristics data from the HIM records. Once a beneficiary is included in the Medicare History Sample, that person remains on the file regardless of utilization activity or death. A 5-percent sample of new Medicare enrollees is added each year.

One section of the Medicare History Sample record identifies the demographic characteristics of the enrollee, the basis for entitlement, and where applicable, date and reason for termination from Parts A and B of the program. This section is created when the enrollee is first added to the Medicare History Sample file.

Annual additions to the demographic records include data that may change over time, such as whether the enrollee is entitled under Part B and/or Part A, whether coverage under Part B has been accepted, the State, county, and zip code of residence, and whether the enrollee is a participant in a group prepaid practice plan or health maintenance organization.

The remaining sections of the Medicare History Sample record contain charge, reimbursement, and utilization data for outpatient services supplied by an institutional provider, hospital inpatient stays, home health agency visits, SNF stays, physician services, and other services reimbursable under Medicare. The inpatient stay section of the Medicare History Sample provides information on principal diagnosis and surgical procedure. It is expected that the file will contain the expanded diagnosis and procedure information obtainable from the new Hospital Stay Record File (119).

HCFA's Bureau of Data Management and Strategy, which is responsible for developing and maintaining the Medicare History Sample file, is currently working on completion of the 1982 file. The Bureau anticipates that in the future the Medicare History Sample file will be completed 12 months after the end of the calendar year. The 1982 data, however, are taking at least twice the amount of time to complete. The latest available Medicare History Sample file is for 1981 and contains 1,900,000 records, an increase of approximately 100,000 records over the previous year (261).

Medicare Automated Data Retrieval System (MADRS)

Currently under development, the MADRS data file is intended to reorganize and merge Medicare's Part A and Part B claims files to facilitate research and make analysis less expensive. When it is completed, MADRS will sort the claims records in HCFA's files first by the year, then by the county in which the beneficiary resides, and finally by the beneficiary's health insurance number.

This presorted file will enable researchers to access the full array of Medicare claims made by all kinds of providers for a set of beneficiaries without sorting through an entire year's worth of Part A and Part B claims files.[8] MADRS will also contain an index to indicate the location of records for a particular county, beneficiary, or provider (other than individual physicians) on the automated data file, making access to particular records more convenient.

Because of a number of contract difficulties and resource limitations, as of May 1985 the file does not exist, and there is no indication of when it will be completed, although HCFA personnel indicate that there is a firm intention to do so.

---

[8]HCFA estimates that the cost of sorting through 1 year of the claims files to be about $15,000 (329).

Appendix F.—Sources of Data on Aggregate Measures of Technological Change

Research and Development Data

The level of ongoing research and development (R&D) activity can be measured in terms of research spending, number of research projects, or personnel involved. In the private sector, two sources of data on industrial R&D inputs are the National Science Foundation's (NSF) annual survey of industrial R&D and data on the size of venture capital investment in various areas. Unfortunately, the validity of either of these sources of data as an estimate of R&D on medical technology is limited.

Industrial R&D Data

For two reasons, it is difficult to identify and quantify industrial R&D activities specifically related to medical technologies. First, most basic and some applied research lays the scientific foundation for a wide range of future products and processes, without being specifically attributable to a single or even a class of medical technologies. Second, the R&D data that are published are usually too aggregated to be useful in identifying specific trends.

The most readily available source of health industry R&D estimates is the NSF's annual survey of industrial firms (308). Firms are categorized for the survey by primary manufacturing product, represented by Standard Industrial Classification (SIC) codes (see table F-1). However, many firms develop and manufacture a variety of different products, not necessarily all of the same type or even all relating to a single field such as health care. Because the NSF estimates are for company-wide R&D, they overestimate R&D in a specific product area when companies whose primary line of business is in that SIC category conduct R&D in other product categories. They underestimate it when R&D for that product is conducted by firms classified in other SIC codes (308). The balance of over- or underestimation probably varies depending on the type of technology. For instance, many medical devices firms are owned by large multiproduct firms; thus, the balance is likely to be toward underestimation of industrial R&D on medical devices.[1]

Venture Capital Investment Data

Venture capital has become a very important source of financing for many small and new firms and often funds investments in the development of new medical products (308). Analyzing data on the amount of venture capital invested in medical manufacturing firms is one way of assessing the level of private support for medical R&D. As a measure of innovation, however, such data are seriously flawed. The data themselves are limited in scope and specificity, and venture capital investments include investments in product commercialization and industrial expansion that do not necessarily contribute to R&D.

There are two sources of data on financial capital investment: 1) the Internal Revenue Service (IRS); and 2) private sources such as Venture Economics, Inc., a research and consulting division of Capital Publishing Corp. The IRS collects information on the sources of financial capital for firms in specific categories. (For example, IRS category 3698, "other electrical," includes X-ray and electromedical devices.) However, the IRS categories in which firms producing medical products are classified include a substantial number of firms not engaged in the production of drugs and devices, and the data pertain to the financing of all activities in these fields, not just the financing of R&D.

Venture Economics, Inc., maintains an extensive database on the U.S. venture capital industry (371). Information on manufacturers that have received venture capital financing can be retrieved according to product category, such as medical imaging or industrial products. Although the investments recorded do not account for all venture capital investments, they do include a high proportion of those in the last few

Table F-1.—Selected Four-Digit Standard Industrial Classification (SIC) Codes for Health Care Products

SIC code	Products
3693	X-ray and electromedical equipment
3841	Surgical and medical instruments
3842	Orthopedic, prosthetic, and surgical appliances and supplies
3843	Dental equipment and supplies
3851	Opthalmic goods
2831	Biological products, including vaccines and blood derivatives
2833	Medicinal chemicals and botanical products
2834	Pharmaceutical preparations

SOURCE: U.S. Executive Office of the President, Office of Management and Budget, *Standard Industrial Classification Manual*, Washington, DC, 1972.

---

[1] A further problem is that NSF's estimates of company-wide expenditures for applied R&D are subdivided into general product categories such as "professional and scientific instruments" and "other electrical machinery equipment and supplies." These categories are too broad to allow the extraction of applied R&D expenditures that pertain specifically to medical technologies. Basic research expenditures are collected for the company as a whole and are not broken down by product class (308).

years and offer a representative picture of venture capital investment activity.

Data on New Product Introductions

The most useful sources of data on new medical product introductions are the U.S. Patent and Trademark Office and the Food and Drug Administration (FDA). Like the data sources on R&D, they suffer from several problems. Data from the various sources tend to be incomparable, redundant, or incomplete; and they usually do not measure new techniques, small but important modifications, or new or unconventional ways of using old products.

Patent Data

The U.S. Patent and Trademark Office classifies patents into 400 to 500 functional categories. FDA has recategorized the patent classes according to its own definitions (308). Thus, data on patent applications can be compared with the FDA-designated categories to yield information on the annual numbers of patent applications for medical products.

Patent data are somewhat untimely, however, because the delay between the application for and issuance of a patent currently averages more than 2 years. In addition, patent data suffer as a measure of new product introduction because they do not distinguish between products that are marketed and those that are not. Furthermore, not all new products (or modifications of old products) are patented. Many firms depend on trade secrets and rapid changes in technology and design to protect their products and profits, rather than relying on the patent process (220).

Food and Drug Administration Data

No single FDA file can produce a listing of all new medical drugs and devices. Several separate databases can provide relevant information and might be merged to provide more useful and comprehensive information. The most applicable data files are the following:

- *510k Registry.*—Whenever a manufacturer wishes to market a new medical device, or an old device with new features or uses, it is required by section 510(k) of the 1976 Medical Device Amendments to notify FDA. If the device is found by FDA to be "substantially equivalent" to a preenactment device, it may be marketed without further proof of safety and efficacy. If not, further proof may be required, depending on whether FDA classifies the device as Class I, Class II, or Class III.[2]

FDA maintains a file of all active 510k applications to track their progress through the system. As a comprehensive measure of new devices, this database suffers some drawbacks. For instance, if a new device is accepted as "substantially equivalent" to a previous device, it may be listed under the product code of the old device even if it has some major technological differences. Thus, a listing of all new products in the database would not necessarily produce a comprehensive list of all new devices. More important, there is no way to distinguish between minor modifications and significant new products.

- *Premarket Approval Application* (PMAA) *Tracking File.*—Devices that are not found "substantially equivalent" and present a potentially high risk are categorized as Class III devices and require FDA approval before being marketed. Applications for premarket approval are submitted by manufacturers showing the results of clinical trials and other safety and efficacy information that FDA requires. A PMAA tracking file at FDA lists all devices in this category, but the file does not discriminate between devices actually marketed and those that are not. To obtain a list of Class III devices being marketed, the PMAA tracking file must be matched with the device registration file (see below).
- *Device Registration File.*—Each manufacturer of medical devices must report annually to FDA the devices being manufactured by that firm. This file contains all medical devices being manufactured in the United States, but it does not distinguish between new and old devices.
- *New Drug Evaluation Files.*—The FDA Office of Drugs' New Drug Evaluation database contains information on all new drugs that have been approved for marketing by FDA, both prescription and over-the-counter. Its analog, the Abbreviated New Drug Application file, contains information on "me-too" drugs that are not chemically new but have been approved for marketing by a new manufacturer. Neither file, however, records whether a drug is actually being marketed at present.
- *Drug Registration and Listing.*—This file contains information on the current marketing status of all prescription drugs, updated through an annual compliance report by manufacturers. New drugs listed by a manufacturer in this file can be cross-matched with the New Drug Evaluation file, but the process is a tedious one. There is an equivalent database for over-the-counter drugs, but it is not updated regularly and is currently about 2 years behind.

---

[2]Of more than 17,000 510(k) notifications of intent to market a new medical device that were received by FDA for fiscal years 1977-1981, only approximately 300 were found to be not substantially equivalent (308).

Appendix G.—PROs' Quality-of-Care Role in PPS[1]

The Utilization and Quality Control Peer Review Organization (PRO) program was established by the Tax Equity and Fiscal Responsibility Act of 1982 (Public Law 97-248) as a direct successor to the Professional Standards Review Organization (PSRO) program; it was modified the following year by the Social Security Amendments (Public Law 98-21) that inaugurated Medicare's prospective payment system (PPS) for inpatient hospital services.

PROs, which are administered by the Health Care Financing Administration (HCFA), have substantial responsibilities for containing costs by reviewing hospital behavior in response to PPS incentives; they are also expected to carry out quality-of-care review.

Expectations of and tasks assigned to PROs derive in part from the history of peer review efforts going back a generation to the development of Foundations for Medical Care and the Experimental Medical Care Review Organization program.

The PSRO program, established by 1972 legislation and charged with both containing costs and assuring quality in the Medicare and Medicaid programs (121, 272), set the stage for PROs. The members of PSROs were to ensure that institutional services provided through the Medicare and Medicaid programs were medically necessary, of a quality that met locally determined professional standards, and provided at the most economical level consistent with quality of care (304).

Ultimately, the PSRO program proved a disappointment. Results of several evaluations of its cost-effectiveness were ambiguous (11,128,293,294,296,314, 321). PSROs may have saved about as much money as the PSRO program cost to run, but they certainly did not meet expectations of Congress, the Administration, and others in the cost-containment area.

PSROs had demonstrably positive effects on quality of care, although these were difficult to assess in a cost-benefit framework. Quality assurance methods improved during the PSRO era. Changing attitudes of the medical community during the 1970s and early 1980s, which saw many more physicians willing to band together in the interests of assessing and improving the quality of medical care, were attributable in part to the spread and activity of the PSRO program.

Disenchantment with the PSRO program, especially because of its inability to curb costs, led two Administrations to try to abolish the program. Congress, on the other hand, recognized potential quality impacts and decided to establish the PRO program at the same time that it initiated major changes in the financing structure of the Medicare program. The PRO program differs from the PSRO program in many ways. For instance, individual PROs are awarded competitively bid contracts, not grants as with PSROs. Furthermore, in an extension of a process initiated in the last days of the PSRO program, PROs must negotiate with HCFA a wide variety of numerical objectives for curtailing the use of inpatient care and maintaining or improving quality of care; PROs are to be evaluated in part according to how well they meet or exceed those objectives.

Table G-1 lists the requirements of PROs. Most PRO activities focus on hospital admissions and the use of invasive procedures, largely for cost-containment purposes. Five objectives required of PROs relate to quality of care: 1) reducing unnecessary hospital readmissions due to previously substandard care; 2) assuring provision of medical services which, if not given, would have significant potential for causing serious patient complications; 3) "reducing the risk of mortality associated with selected procedures and/or conditions requiring hospitalization"[2]; 4) reducing unnecessary surgery; and 5) reducing avoidable postoperative or other complications.

Several required activities involving admissions review have stringent numerical objectives, as do all five quality-of-care areas. Over a 2-year period, to meet their stated admissions objectives the PROs must eliminate 1.25 million admissions, just under 5 percent of total Medicare admissions in 1982 (239). It is possible that under such stringent numerical objectives, quality of care and access to inpatient care could decline.

The required quality objectives for the first 2-year contract period, which are common to all PRO contracts, were defined by HCFA. Within them, however, PROs were given flexibility to identify local problems and devise local approaches to solve them. The actual quantitative objectives were developed during contract negotiations with HCFA. The presumed gain in accountability through contracting and specifying numerical objectives is regarded as an improvement in management capabilities for HCFA relative to what was possible in the PSRO program.

Specific examples of PRO objectives in each quality area are presented in box G-A. Several PROs have objectives concerning the same diagnoses, but they do not have the same numerical goals or procedures to

---

[1]This appendix is based on a contract paper prepared for OTA by K.N. Lohr, entitled "Peer Review Organizations (PROs): Quality Assurance in Medicare" (185). That paper is available from the National Technical Information Service.

[2]This objective has recently been changed by HCFA from the controversial phrase, "decreasing avoidable deaths."

Table G-1.—Major PRO Requirements

Hospital admission objectives:
- Reduce admissions for procedures that could be performed effectively and safely in an ambulatory surgical setting or on an outpatient basis.
- Reduce the number of inappropriate or unnecessary admissions or invasive procedures for specific DRGs.
- Reduce the number of inappropriate or unnecessary admissions or invasive procedures by specific practitioners or in specific hospitals.

Other hospital admission and utilization reviews:
- Review (before admission or before procedure) every elective case for 5 procedure-related DRGs (from a State-specific list of the top 20 procedures or procedure-specific DRGs for 1982).
- Review admissions occurring within 7 days of a discharge and deny all claims for inappropriate admissions.
- Review every permanent cardiac pacemaker implantation or reimplantation procedure and deny payment for all that are unnecessary.
- Review transfers from a PPS hospital to other hospitals or to specific PPS-exempt special unit or swing beds.
- Perform Admission Pattern Monitoring.
- Perform additional admission-related reviews in three distinct areas, including cases with specific principal diagnoses.
- Review admissions to and days of care in non-PPS hospitals or units.
- Carry out various other tasks relating to review and monitoring of hospital denials and notices of noncoverage.

Quality of care objectives:
- Reduce unnecessary hospital readmissions resulting from substandard care provided during the prior admission.
- Assure the provision of medical services which, when not performed, have "significant potential" (occurrence in 5 percent or more of cases) for causing "serious patient complications."
- Reduce the risk of mortality associated with selected procedures and/or conditions requiring hospitalization.[a]
- Reduce unnecessary surgery or other invasive procedures.
- Reduce avoidable postoperative or other complications.

Other reviews:
- DRG validation.
- Review every case involving day and/or cost outliers for necessity and appropriateness of admission and subsequent care.
- Carry out special sets of reviews on DRGs #462 and #468.
- Monitor denial notices that hospitals issue to Medicare beneficiaries to ensure that they do not mislead the patient (or family) or misstate the hospitals' authority or responsibility as to decisions to terminate care.
- Monitor hospitals' compliance with the physician attestation requirements.

[a]This objective was formerly "reduce avoidable deaths." It was changed by the Health Care Financing Administration in 1985.

SOURCE: K. N. Lohr, "Peer Review Organizations (PROs): Quality Assurance in Medicare," prepared for Office of Technology Assessment, U.S. Congress, Washington, DC, July 1, 1985.

---

meet those goals (380). Most quality objectives set by PROs for the first contract period concern problems that predated PPS and DRG-based payment. Whether the specific problems identified by the PROs persist in the PPS era or are supplanted by different problems, and whether the general areas of concern specified by HCFA are the crucial ones for PPS, remain open to question. One mark of the PROs' commitment to quality assurance, however, is that many took on more than just the five required objectives. The problems inherent in PRO quality activities have been noted by various observers, but PROs have a number of strengths as well. The more important limitations and strengths of quality assurance in the PRO program are listed in table G-2.

Some critics claim that the current quality objectives defined by HCFA are rather narrow and rigid. They

Table G-2.—Important Limitations and Strengths of Quality Assurance in the PRO Program

Limitations:
- Quality objectives are seen as rather rigid and narrow.
- Considerable ambiguity persists about program evaluation procedures and the weight to be given to quality assurance.
- If PPS has its intended effects on hospital use, questions about quality of care may arise for other providers (nursing homes, outpatient settings), but PROs do not have the mandate or the funding to carry out quality assurance activities in those areas.
- Many of the mandatory review tasks are also new activities (e.g., outlier review, DRG validation); getting them underway in a timely, effective manner may force PROs to skimp on quality review in the first year or so.
- Questions are raised that third-party payer organizations, such as fiscal intermediaries and insurers, are not as well equipped or disposed to emphasize quality concerns as are the PROs established by nonpayer organizations.
- Critics perceive the quality objectives (as well as objectives for admissions and invasive procedures) as quotas for limiting Medicare hospitalizations irrespective of whether the admission is appropriate or not.

Strengths:
- Several PROs formed by strong statewide PSROs (or amalgams of regional PSROs within a State) have a great deal of quality assurance experience.
- Many PROs are sufficiently committed to quality assurance efforts that they have taken on more than the required number (5) of quality objectives.
- All but 1 of the 54 PROs is a physician-sponsored (or physician-access) PRO; the 1 fiscal-intermediary PRO was organized by Blue Cross (of Idaho).
- Potential resources are broad: some PROs have substantial private review experience; some are independently developing analytic and research capabilities that might be applied to quality assurance.
- Medical record data are essential to comprehensive quality assurance. PROs are currently handling records from 30 to 40 percent of all Medicare admissions.

SOURCE: K.N. Lohr, "Peer Review Organizations (PROs): Quality Assurance in Medicare," prepared for Office of Technology Assessment, U.S. Congress, Washington, DC, July 1, 1985.

Box G-A — Specific Examples of PRO Objectives in Quality of Care

- **Reduce Unnecessary Readmissions Due to Substandard Care.** The South Carolina Medical Care Foundation detailed the following goals for this quality objective: "to reduce hospital readmissions resulting from substandard care provided during the prior admissions from 1,543 cases (17 percent) to 908 (10 percent)." The numerical goals for this objective were based on data for the first quarter of fiscal year 1984 (i.e., the first PPS year). Of a total of more than 33,000 Medicare discharges, about 2 percent resulted in readmissions; of these, about 17 percent were attributable to premature discharge. Similar findings were cited from Alabama. The South Carolina PRO concluded that, with its retrospective quality review and other procedures, it would be able to reduce the 17-percent figure to 10 percent.
- **Assure Provision of Necessary Medical Services.** The objective statement of the Utah PRO for this quality area was "to assure the provision of necessary medical services through improvement in measuring baseline renal function, calculating appropriate dosage, and monitoring serum concentration levels during the usage of aminoglycosides." Aminoglycosides are powerful antibiotics; their concomitant risks and a relatively narrow range between effective and possibly toxic levels require that dosage levels be calculated carefully and that use is monitored closely (see ref. 28). Although the PRO could not precisely specify numerical goals, it was able to estimate that about half of all Medicare patients receiving aminoglycosides during hospitalizations were inadequately monitored. It proposed, therefore, to cut the rate of noncompliance with explicit monitoring criteria by 50 percent in the first year of the contract and by another 40 percent in the second year.
- **Reduce Avoidable Deaths.*** The New York PRO will pursue the following goal in this area: "to reduce by 514 the number of avoidable deaths with the diagnosis of pneumococcal, aspiration, or bacterial pneumonia." Information from New York State and three PSRO-area studies from the 1982-84 period showed that about 20 percent of patients of Medicare age admitted with the principal diagnosis of pneumococcal, bacterial, or aspiration pneumonia died; about 25 percent of these deaths were found to be preventable. Assuming that about 1,028 patients admitted per year with these diagnoses would die, then about 257 deaths can be expected to be avoidable (0.25 × 1,028 deaths). Because the objective covers 2 years, the total number of avoidable deaths to be reduced is 514.
- **Reduce Unnecessary Surgery or Other Invasive Procedures.** In West Virginia, the PRO proposed to reduce by 528 cases the incidence of unnecessary surgery or other invasive procedures, with special reference to selected gastrointestinal procedures (esophagoscopy, gastroscopy, small bowel endoscopy, fiberoptic colonoscopy, large bowel endoscopy, and proctosigmoidoscopy). Factors that prompted this objective included a significant rise in gastrointestinal endoscopies, often in patients with at best minimal indications and frequently without prior X-ray studies that are usually considered critical diagnostic services. In perhaps as many as one-quarter of patients receiving such gastrointestinal procedures, the principal diagnoses were inappropriate or the procedure was otherwise apparently not indicated.
- **Reduce Avoidable Postoperative or Other Complications.** The Connecticut PRO proposed to reduce by 30 percent the number of postoperative urinary tract infections of indwelling catheters for patients receiving six procedures (abdominal hysterectomy, disc excision, total hip replacement, bowel resection, cholecystectomy, and repair of hip fracture). The estimated reduction of 237 infections is to be accomplished over 2 years. The goal was based on chart review in one of the State's PSRO areas which showed an 8.3-percent incidence of such infections. Data will be collected by retrospective chart review. Interventions range from written communications to physician sanctions.

---

*This objective is now "reduce the risk of mortality associated with selected procedures and/or conditions requiring hospitalization." It was changed by the Health Care Financing Administration in 1985.

SOURCE: U.S. Department of Health and Human Services, Health Care Financing Administration, Health Standards and Quality Bureau *Peer Review Organization Objectives: A Synopsis,* vol. 1, September 1984, cited in K.N., Lohr, "Peer Review Organizations (PROs): Quality Assurance in Medicare," prepared for Office of Technology Assessment, U.S. Congress, Washington, DC, July 1, 1985.

do not concern negative patient outcomes that fall short of death or major complications unless care was so poor that it necessitated a second admission, and they leave little room for modification if problems appear less serious than originally believed or if new problems surface.

Explicit criteria by which PROs' contract performance will be evaluated had not been issued (as of August 1985). HCFA has said that PROs' performance will be reviewed basically in terms of: 1) fulfilling numerical admissions and quality objectives, and 2) dollar benefits to the Federal Government (330). The relative weights to be given to meeting quality objectives, meeting admissions objectives, or adequately carrying out other tasks such as DRG validation or Admission Pattern Monitoring have not yet been made clear. Admissions objectives and other activities related directly to PPS could therefore take priority over quality objectives.[3]

PROs are not authorized by Medicare to review the quality of care delivered by nonhospital providers. Home health agencies and long-term-care facilities are of particular concern: If PPS has the expected effects on hospital use, caseloads for these long-term care providers will grow and patients will be on average sicker. The quality of some nursing home care has been questioned (158,373), and the methods to evaluate such care are still poorly developed (257,395).

Medicare beneficiaries have a great deal to lose if the quality of care in these settings is not monitored aggressively. The capacity for at least some PROs, especially those developed from strong PSROs, to take on such work is not in question. It seems unlikely that a second or complementary PRO program would be developed to take on such review, and it is not feasible for PROs to do so at their present funding and staffing levels.

PROs also do not have quality assurance responsibilities in nonacute or ambulatory care settings. As hospitals adapt to PPS by moving some services to the outpatient sector, a question that arises whether patients are more helped or harmed by the provision of care in such a wholly different way.[4] The validity of quality assurance efforts on behalf of Medicare beneficiaries can be questioned if the responsibility of the PROs stops at the hospital door. Again, at least a few PROs are probably capable at present of designing and implementing an effective ambulatory care review effort but not without additional resources and an explicit mandate to do so. HCFA is hoping to test quality review in nonacute and ambulatory settings by the start of fiscal year 1986 (78).

Whether PRO funding will prove adequate pervades the entire issue. PROs have a sizable budget—$339 million for the first 2-year cycle—but it is small in proportion to the $100+ *billions* that may be spent by Medicare just for hospital care in the equivalent 2 years. Furthermore, the portion of the PRO budgets directed to quality assurance may also be small because of the large number of other required functions and the uncertainty about the importance that will be placed on quality of care when contract performance is evaluated. If even as much as 25 percent of PRO budgets were spent for quality review, a miniscule proportion of the amount spent on inpatient care would be going for quality assurance. The interrelated effects of quality and admissions objectives further complicate the funding issue.

---

[3]On June 17, 1985, HCFA signed a contract with Systemetrics to be the "SuperPRO." The SuperPRO's three major responsibilities are to: 1) review PRO admission and DRG validation criteria; 2) replicate PRO reviews and compare them on a large sample of cases; and 3) identify quality issues not identified by the PROs. Results of the SuperPRO's monitoring activities will be available to HCFA for routine assistance to PROs and for contract purposes.

[4]The fact that the elderly will face increased out-of-pocket costs as a result of shifts in the site of care to the outpatient sector itself has quality-of-care ramifications, if Medicare patients do not obtain appropriate types or levels of care because of such financial barriers.

Appendix H.—Alternative Patient Classification Systems[1]

Introduction

In 1983, when Congress changed the basis for Medicare payment to the prospective payment system (PPS), the Diagnosis Related Groups (DRG) system was the best patient classification system available that could adjust for case-mix differences among hospitals. Other patient classification systems were not ready for use because data were unavailable or there were other administrative and technical problems. Although it is unlikely that the DRG system will be replaced in the near future, alternatives to and refinements of DRGs are under development.

This appendix describes and compares DRGs and five other existing systems for classifying hospital inpatients. Each patient classification system has been constructed from a set of principles and data sources that gives it advantages and disadvantages in various uses. The alternatives to DRGs described could be used as substitutes for or modifications of the DRG system. This appendix lays out criteria for evaluation the usefulness of any patient classification system in per-case hospital payment.

Even if they are not useful for payment, however, alternative patient classification systems could be valuable tools in evaluating the impacts of PPS. The effects of PPS on the quality of care can be measured with greater validity if patients with similar medical problems can be identified in both the pre-PPS and post-PPS periods. Patient classification systems that have very homogeneous groups of patients may help in this regard. Also, the underlying causes of changes in the distribution of hospital revenues and surpluses can be identified with greater precision using refined indexes of illness severity or patient resource needs to separate variations due to a hospital's relative efficiency from those due to intrinsic differences in patient needs.

Patient Classification Systems

A number of alternative patient classification systems have been considered for use in a prospective payment system for hospitals. Six such systems are described below:

- Diagnosis Related Groups (DRGs), 1980 Version;
- Disease Staging;
- Severity of Illness Index;
- Patient Management Categories;
- Medical Illness Severity Grouping System (MEDISGRPS); and
- Acute Physiology and Chronic Health Evaluation, Simplified Version (APACHE II).

Key attributes of each system are summarized in table H-1. More technical details are presented in the discussions of evaluation criteria. (Additional details can be found in refs. 142,305.)

Diagnosis-Related Groups (DRGs)[2]

Two sets of DRGs have been developed. The original set contained 383 categories, and the revised set on which Medicare's PPS is based contains 467 categories.[3] Both sets of DRGs were partially constructed from records of actual patient stays in a sample of hospitals. Creation of the DRGs relied both on statistical techniques to identify subgroups of patients with similar lengths of stay and on clinical judgment to confirm that patient subgroups also had compatible diagnoses. The second set was developed with greater reliance on the judgment of a panel of clinicians for the identification of clinically meaningful categories, although statistical analysis was still important in the development process.

Assignments of patients to DRGs are based on patient data available on patient discharge abstracts and, now, on Medicare's hospital bills. Principal diagnosis—i.e., the principal reason (after study) for a patient's hospitalization—was used to separate patients into 23 major diagnostic categories corresponding to organ systems. Other important variables are: 1) secondary diagnoses; 2) specific surgical procedures; 3) nature of coexisting conditions and complications; 4) discharge status (including death and "left hospital against medical advice"); 5) age; and 6) other factors for some categories. The data are commonly available in computerized form, and a computer algorithm (referred to as GROUPER) classifies each patient into the appropriate DRG. The diagnosis and procedure coding for DRGs is based on the International Classification of Diseases, 9th Revision, Clinical Modification (ICD-9-CM), which is an internationally recognized medical coding system developed for statistical monitoring of hospitalized patients.

---

[1]This appendix is based on S. Williams, G. Kominski, and G. Pickens, "The Evaluation of Alternative Patient Classification Systems," prepared for the Office of Technology Assessment, U.S. Congress, Washington, DC, December 1984.

[2]See also OTA's 1983 publication *Diagnosis-Related Groups and the Medicare Program: Implications for Medical Technology* (305).

[3]Medicare uses 470, but the 3 additional categories are ones in which "other" cases are placed before being paid for.

Table H-1.—Comparison of Six Case-Mix Measures

Characteristic	Diagnosis-Related Groups	Disease Staging	Severity of Illness Index	Patient Management Categories	MEDISGRPS	APACHE II
Number of classes	467 + 3	1,600 plus	4 plus	1,000 plus	Unique score for each patient	Unique score for each patient
Source data	Discharge abstract	Discharge abstract	Medical record	Discharge abstract	Medical record	Medical record
Type of classification	Objective	Objective	Combined subjective and objective	Objective	Objective	Objective
Classification variables	Principal diagnosis Secondary diagnosis Age Principal procedure Secondary procedure Sex Discharge disposition	Principal diagnosis Secondary diagnosis Sex Surgery Discharge disposition	Diagnoses History and physical Laboratory tests X-rays Progress and nursing notes	Principal diagnosis Secondary diagnosis Reason for chief problem Elective procedure	Reason for admission Significant history (associated problems) Illness severity (based on key clinical findings)	Principal diagnosis Laboratory tests History and physical
Comorbidity included?	Yes—specific diagnoses	Yes—secondary diagnosis as comorbidity and complications	Yes—any factor that affects length of stay	Yes—secondary diagnosis as comorbidity and complications	Yes	Yes—multiple system impacts
Deaths omitted?	No	No	No	No	No	Yes
Outliers omitted?	Yes	No	No	No	No	No
Affected by errors in diagnosis coding on abstracts?	Yes	Yes	No	Yes	No	No
Automated?	Yes	Yes	No	Yes	Yes	No
Mutually exclusive and exhaustive?	Yes	Yes	Yes	Yes	Yes	No
When applied?	After discharge	After discharge	After discharge	After discharge	Day 3 and day 10 after admission	24 hr. after admission

SOURCES: Based on a table in M. C. Hornbrook, "Techniques for Assessing Hospital Case Mix," *Ann. Rev. Public Health*, vol. 6, in press, 1985; and A. C. Brewster, B. G. Karlin, K. A. Hyde, et al., "Medical Illness Severity Grouping System (MEDISGRPs): A Clinically-Based Approach to Classifying Hospital Patients at Admission," mimeograph, 1984.

Disease Staging[4]

Disease Staging is the product of physicians' judgments about the biological progression of a given disease. Each disease is defined by four required elements: location of the problem, manifestations of the medical problem, cause of the problem, and the severity of the problem. Staging does not depend on observed utilization patterns or expected responses to therapy. Patients may be staged for each disease manifested.

A subset of 420 disease conditions was developed for two purposes: 1) to include the major diseases in each body system, and 2) to cover the majority of typical hospital admissions. Physician experts developed criteria for staging each disease. The criteria assigned patients to one of the following four major stages (substages were also developed for many diseases):

- Stage 1: Conditions with no complications or problems of minimal severity;
- Stage 2: Problems limited to an organ or system, significantly increased risk of complications over Stage 1;
- Stage 3: Multiple site involvement, generalized system involvement, poor prognosis; and
- Stage 4: Death.

Staging patients according to the medical criteria developed by the physician panelists originally required medical records review, but the system now in widespread use assigns patients to categories using information in the Uniform Hospital Discharge Data Set (UHDDS).[5] The computerized system may underestimate the severity in some cases; for example, when an ICD-9-CM code in the UHDDS applies to more than one stage of a disease, the lower stage is selected.

Severity of Illness Index[6]

The Severity of Illness Index reflects the overall severity of illness of the patient, not just the severity of each diagnosis. This index is based on seven dimensions, each of which is divided into four levels, based on criteria developed by researchers at Johns Hopkins University in conjunction with a panel of physicians and nurses. The seven dimensions deemed to be the best indicators of overall illness severity are as follows:

- stage of the principal diagnosis on admission;
- complications of the principal condition;
- concurrent, interacting conditions that affect the course of hospital treatment;
- dependency on the hospital staff;
- extent of non-operating-room life-support procedures;
- rate of response to therapy, or rate of recovery; and
- impairment remaining after therapy for the acute aspect of the hospitalization.

Relevant data from patients' medical records are abstracted manually by trained raters at the same time the hospital discharge abstract is prepared. Based on the combined patterns of severity levels within each dimension, the rater judges the overall index of severity of the patient's illness from 1 (least severe) to 4 (most severe). A computerized system is being developed that can be used with modified recordkeeping systems. Clinical data are to be used to modify the present 5-digit ICD-9-CM coding system to record severity considerations into discharge abstract data as a sixth digit for each disease condition.

Patient Management Categories[7]

Patient Management Categories were developed by panels of physician experts. The goal of this system was to specify patient attributes that identify patients with very similar needs for care. The categories are based on patient clinical characteristics and severity of the illness. The development of specific categories did not depend on empirical analysis of actual use of services, but the physician panelists did specify components of effective care in order to provide a basis for subsequently estimating the cost of providing care in each category. Components of care include diagnostic services, treatment procedures, and expected length of stay, which in the view of the physician panels are required for effective patient management (i.e., patient management paths).

Over 750 Patient Management Categories have been defined for patients in acute care hospitals. A computerized algorithm can be used to map cases into the categories from information on discharge abstracts.

---

[4]See also J.S. Gonnella, M.C. Hornbrook, and D.Z. Louis, "Staging of Disease: A Case-Mix Measurement," 1984 (120).

[5]The Uniform Hospital Discharge Data Set (UHDDS) is a minimum basic data set for acute care hospitals developed by a group of experts for the U.S. National Committee on Vital and Health Statistics, based on the work of a conference held in 1969 at Airlie House. The Secretary of the Department of Health, Education, and Welfare (now Health and Human Services) adopted the UHDDS in 1974, but Medicare and Medicaid have resisted using it. However, the Professional Standards Review Organization (now PRO—see ch. 6 and app. G) program adapted UHDDS for its PRO Hospital Discharge Data Set, which includes UHDDS information plus some PRO-specific information (214).

[6]For additional information and references, see OTA's 1983 publication *Diagnosis-Related Groups and the Medicare Program: Implications for Medical Technology* (305).

[7]See Blue Cross of Western Pennsylvania, *Hospital Case Mix: Development and Implementation*, 1983 (38).

The software criteria include combinations of diagnoses (ICD-9-CM codes) and specific surgical procedures when necessary. Sequencing of the codes on the abstract does not affect category assignment. Age and sex are used to categorize patients in only a few instances.

Medical Illness Severity Grouping System (MEDISGRPS)[8]

MEDISGRPS is a patient classification system that groups patients by severity levels on the basis of data acquired upon admission. Key clinical findings were selected by the group of researchers who developed the system. These key clinical findings include the results of laboratory, pathology, or radiology tests or physical examination findings that indicate illness. Test results, not their interpretations, are used. Each finding is assigned to one of the following severity groups:
- Severity group 0: No findings;
- Severity group 1: Minimal findings;
- Severity group 2: Severe or acute findings;
- Severity group 3: Severe and acute findings; and
- Severity group 4: Critical findings.

A computer program can be used to assign severity groups to each patient based on data from the medical record. The system is currently being tested in six sites.

Acute Physiology and Chronic Health Evaluation, Simplified Version (APACHE II)[9]

The APACHE classification system was developed to answer clinical questions about intensive care unit (ICU) patients. Data for the APACHE system are collected within 24 hours of ICU admission, rather than after hospital discharge as is typical of most other patient classification systems. The data used to assign patients are not available on discharge abstracts, and the extent of availability of the necessary data items from the medical records of non-ICU patients is unclear.

The original APACHE system consisted of an Acute Physiology Score based on 34 physiologic variables and a chronic health assessment, which is a four-category scale. The variables and the weights used to incorporate them into a total score for a specific patient were chosen by a group of ICU clinicians.

The simplified version, APACHE II, is based on 12 of the most commonly used physiologic measures of the original 34 variables. Again, clinicians chose the 12 measures based on their judgment of the validity

[8] See J.A. Brewster, C.M. Jacobs, and R.G. Bradbury, "Classifying Severity of Illness Using Clinical Findings," 1984 (43).

[9] See D.P. Wagner and E. Draper, "APACHE II and Medicare Reimbursement," 1984 (374).

and specificity of the measure, breadth of organ system coverage, and objectivity, reliability, and frequency of measurement. Most of these measurements are available for the majority of ICU patients shortly after hospital admission. The weighting scheme was also slightly modified for APACHE II. Data collection and analysis for payment purposes on large national samples of non-ICU patients have not been done.

Criteria for Evaluating the Usefulness of Patient Classification Systems in Prospective Payment

Six criteria that could be used to evaluate alternative patient classification systems for the purpose of paying hospitals for patient care are discussed below. For each criterion, the following information is presented: the rationale for its selection, how to conduct an evaluation using the criterion, a brief review of any evaluations that have been conducted, and speculations about how candidate patient classifications might perform when evaluated.

Criterion 1: How Well Does the Patient Classification System Account for Variations in Patient Needs for Hospital Services?

Prospective payment requires a method to adjust payment rates for differences among patients in their real need for resources. Without such an adjustment, hospitals would receive the same rate of payment for all patients, and strong incentives would exist for hospitals to treat only the less costly patients. Hospitals which, because of their mission, could not discriminate among patients in this way would suffer unfair financial burdens.

A patient classification system can comprise either a fixed number of discrete categories, each with a separate weight, or a scoring system which calculates a unique score for each patient from a formula based on individual patient characteristics. The objective of the patient classification system is to reduce as much as possible the difference between the amount paid for a given patient and the costs of needed care. If the price paid for a patient is based on the category weight or the patient's score, then the performance of the system depends upon the residual variation between patients' needs and the category weights. If there is high variation because patients with very different needs for care are contained in the same category (and therefore paid at the same rate), then the classification system can be said to perform poorly on this critical dimension. Thus, the primary criterion for evaluating the usefulness of any patient classification system for per-case prospective payment is the extent to which the system reduces the total variation in resource needs around the mean by forming subgroups, each of which has its own mean value.[10]

Identifying Patient Needs.—Unfortunately, a prescriptive measure of need for services is difficult or impossible to construct for most patients. Also, the complete separation of resource need from actual resource use in the construction of a patient classification system is probably infeasible.

There is an extensive literature on the objective measurement of health status or, conversely, medical needs. The basic measurement issue is the correlation between objective indexes of health status and clinical assessments of needed services. The capability of general health status instruments to measure patient needs is at best unclear. Some investigators have developed general health status measures for use in clinical settings (32,226,256). Although some studies have found general health status measures to be sensitive to the provision of medical care when there are dramatic changes in clinical status (247), other studies have failed to confirm such sensitivity in more common situations (81).

Recently, attention has been focused on specific patient groups, because resource needs are more likely to be measured successfully in patients who are similar. Intensive care patients form one such group, and APACHE II has been developed for them (374). The index based on APACHE II is significantly related to observed nursing resource use. Because APACHE II was developed only for patients who require intensive care, it is uncertain whether APACHE II will be useful as a general patient classification system. The MEDISGRPS classification system measures need using clinical laboratory, radiology, pathology, and physical examination findings. In these respects, MEDISGRPS attempts to generalize the approach used by the APACHE II system to nonintensive-care patients.

The developers of the six patient classification systems reviewed in this appendix recognized resource needs indirectly, often by attempting to define groups of patients with similar patterns of resource use. The developers of the DRG system, for example, used a combination of clinical judgment and data on variations among patients in length of stay (one measure of resource use) to develop the classification system. The Disease Staging system recognizes resource need indirectly by assuming that the severity of illness within a disease condition was correlated with need, but there was no direct reference either to the resource needs of patients or resource use in the construction of the system. Patient Management Categories were defined with clinically acceptable management patterns in mind. To the degree that the physicians who defined categories accurately specified appropriate services for each group, Patient Management Categories appear to be more strongly linked to patient resource need than other systems. The Severity of Illness Index attempts to measure resource need directly (such as the need for nursing services), but need is measured after examining resource use, and it is unclear how the Severity of Illness Index separates need from use.

Although desirable, it is not possible at present to identify a general measure of patient need for hospital resources that is sufficiently accurate. Furthermore, there is little expectation for substantial improvement in the near future. Until measures of patient need are developed, patient use of hospital resources, as measured by length of stay (LOS) and total cost, not the need for hospital resources, will continue to be used as the outcome variable in evaluation of this criterion.

The most commonly used measures of resource use are LOS, total charges, or estimated cost per admission. These measures appear to be highly correlated with one another. For example, the correlation between LOS and variable cost was high when estimated for a sample of patients in 77 New Jersey hospitals (168). The Pearson correlation coefficients were 0.84 for the total sample of patients and 0.78 for Medicare LOS inliers.

The methods used to estimate the cost of resources used can vary widely. Most studies have relied on cost allocation techniques used with hospital accounting data. Other approaches exist, but they require the collection of data that are not provided by routinely available data sources. For example, microcosting, which involves direct observation of resource use in a sample of patients, could be used to measure patient costs more accurately than estimates of per-case costs based on accounting data (397). Because they are more accurate, costs derived by microcosting techniques may be a useful alternative when classification systems are evaluated. Microcosting is, however, expensive and must be repeated periodically to reflect changes in hospital operations. Moreover, a high proportion of hospital costs are fixed and must be allocated to patients indirectly even with microcosting techniques. Despite these drawbacks, many hospitals are implementing microcosting techniques, and enough data might be available from them to be used in comparative evaluations of patient classification systems.

Statistical Issues.—For reasons enumerated above, the central question in comparative studies of patient classification systems has been: "How much reduction

---

[10]When the classification system calculates a unique score for each patient, the performance criterion is the extent of variance of the patient's true need for resources from the calculated score.

in the variance among patients in resource use is achieved by candidate patient classification systems?" Ideally, this comparison should occur on a nationally representative sample of discharges using the same dependent variables and the same statistical techniques. Few such studies have been conducted. For the most part, developers of each classification system have published studies that document the variance reduction capabilities of their own systems, or limited comparisons have been performed on local samples, often restricted to only a few patient categories. This is understandable, because most classification systems have been created recently and their developers must establish the reliability and validity of their products. The most extensively studied system has been the DRG system, in part because reduction in variation measures were used to create it (33,104,230).

Gonnella, Hornbrook, and Louis (120) have evaluated the performance of the Disease Staging system on a national stratified sample of patients who were discharged from 377 hospitals in 1977. In this study, attention was focused on LOS variation in diabetes mellitus cases. Mean LOS by stage, patient characteristics, and hospital characteristics were reported. The assessment was limited to pairwise LOS contrasts for patient and hospital subgroups by stage. No overall measure of variance reduction was provided. This patient classification system performed well in the limited situation in which it was tested.

Ament and colleagues (9) have reported comparative studies of the DRG and Disease Staging systems. Using a database for 50 hospitals from which extreme outlier cases had been removed, they found a 49-percent reduction in variance (measured as R^2)[11] for DRGs and a 35-percent reduction for Disease Stages.

Two studies (62,235) have reported a comparative evaluation of DRGs and Disease Staging in Maryland hospitals. Using a sample of DRGs, they found variance reduction values of about 15 percent for DRGs and 12 percent for Staged Disease Conditions and Disease Stages. Finally, an attempt to combine DRGs, Staged Disease Conditions and Disease Stages resulted in a reduction in variance of about 21.1 percent.

Computerized Patient Management Categories are only now being released, so there is little direct evidence about their variance reduction properties. The precursor to Patient Management Categories was studied by Horn, Sharkey, and Bertram (138) and found to have variance reduction values between 31 percent and 50 percent in a restricted sample.

[11]R^2 is the proportion of the total variance around the mean that is explained by a set of linear variables.

Horn, Sharkey, and Bertram (138) have compared reduction of variance measures for DRGs, the Severity of Illness Index, Disease Staging, and a precursor to Patient Management Categories in a sample of four hospitals and for limited groups of disease conditions. DRGs result in R^2 values in the 10- to 20-percent range for total charges in patients with gall bladder disease and congestive heart failure. The other classification systems are comparable, except that the Severity of Illness Index has higher R^2 values, especially when combined with the DRG system. Horn, Horn, and Sharkey (137) also have compared the performance of DRGs and the Severity of Illness Index in eight broad categories of disease in a sample of 14 hospitals using total charges. Percent reduction in variance for DRGs varied between 17 and 31 percent. The range for the Severity of Illness Index was 40 to 95 percent but was lower when outliers (i.e., cases with extremely high or low charges) were excluded (139).

In summary, although comparisons of variance reduction have been carried out for some of the classification systems, none of the evaluations has compared all the systems on a nationally representative sample of data. Thus, it is unknown at present how the alternative patient classification systems perform on this critical dimension.

Criterion 2: How Robust Is the Patient Classification System?

"Robustness" refers to the ability of the system to maintain its properties despite changes in the data used to create or operate the system. Roughly speaking, a system is robust if it preserves the same categories when different databases are used for its creation and if it preserves the same level of proportional reduction in variance when applied to different databases. Little is known about the robustness of most classification systems, but some speculation is possible.

Some of the classification systems relied on specific databases for their development. The DRG system is the best example. The procedure used to create the DRG system was partly based on reduction of variance in LOS, which is sensitive to the presence of outlier cases. Although regression techniques exist for the analysis of data containing outliers (149), these techniques were not used to develop the DRG system and apparently have not been used to develop any other system, probably because they are computer intensive and may not be suitable for large data sets. The expense and effort required probably prohibit a study that would examine DRG robustness by trying to reproduce the system with an alternative database (406).

Also, since DRGs were developed using expert advice, robustness of DRGs would need to be tested using a sample of expert panels.

Robustness also is an issue for systems that are created from expert judgment. For these systems, which include Disease Stages, the Severity of Illness Index, Patient Management Categories, and MEDISGRPS, robustness could be tested by determining if different expert panels would reproduce the original categories using the same principles. This evaluation also is probably unrealistic, considering the expense and effort that would be required.

Another aspect of robustness is the ability of a given system to classify patients reliably when different databases are used, for example, databases containing patients in different age groups or from different geographical regions. The study by Pettengill and Vertrees (230) suggests that the DRG system is sufficiently robust across geographic regions for it to be used in Medicare's PPS, but there are no published studies about the geographic robustness of the other patient classification systems.

Because of concerns about the DRG system's ability to classify children appropriately, most pediatric patients are excluded from Medicare's PPS. The National Association of Children's Hospitals and Related Institutions is conducting a study to determine if the DRG system is robust enough to be used for pediatric patients (217), and a special version of Disease Staging has been developed for pediatric patients.

One aspect of robustness that can be studied with existing data is the ability of alternative patient classification systems to preserve reduction in variance when applied to databases that include or exclude outliers, as defined by Medicare. The inclusion of outliers greatly increases overall variance. If outliers are to be paid outside the system, this means that alternative systems must be evaluated for their robustness for inliers only.

Criterion 3: How Reliable Are Patient Assignments to Category?

Previous studies have reported large random error rates in hospital abstracts (123), and there are many random errors in hospital charge data as well. These errors probably are less serious than they seem because data reporting will improve now that both hospitals and Medicare are monitoring reports to ensure accurate payments. Because of their tendency to cancel each other in relatively large data sets, random errors are less important than systematic errors (230), although selective correction of these errors could allow hospitals to report more of their patients in categories with high payment rates, which has been called "DRG creep" (267). Even if we assume that random errors are not a problem, however, data reporting could lead to problems of reliability and there could be important differences among the classification systems.

If patient assignments are reliable, each patient will be assigned to the same category when assignments are made more than once, even if assignments are made by different people under different circumstances. Reliability should be assessed at several levels.

One such level concerns the primary data. The more objective are the data used to assign patients to classifications, the more likely the assignments are to be reliable. For example, to the extent that a system, like MEDISGRPS, uses data directly from the clinical laboratory, it is more likely to be reliable than a system, like the Severity of Illness Index, that requires subjective judgments about the patient's illness. Some of the possible data elements are listed below in decreasing order of perceived objectivity (with few data available to establish exact order):

- sex, age, and the values for vital signs and laboratory test results;
- reports of imaging procedures, clinical laboratory examinations, and the findings at surgery and other procedures;
- primary or principal diagnoses;
- secondary diagnoses;
- symptoms reported by the patient and signs observed by clinicians; and
- judgments and interpretations, for example, about the relative severity of illness or the response to therapy.

Another level at which reliability should be assessed involves the integration of data into category assignment. Assignments based on specific criteria that can be incorporated into computer algorithms are more likely to be reliable than assignments that require subjective judgment.

Criterion 4: How Does the Patient Classification System Affect Economic Incentives Regarding Technology Use?

In general, patient classification systems can be separated into two types. The first type distinguishes between the clinical condition of the patient and the resources used to treat the condition by excluding all measures of resource use in the assignment of patients to categories. Disease Staging, MEDIGRPS, and APACHE II are three examples of this type. The second type combines measures of resource use with clinical information to assign patients to categories. DRGs and the Severity of Illness Index are examples of this type.

When the category to which a patient is assigned depends on whether or not a technology is used, hospital managers' and physicians' incentives for technology adoption and use can be very different from the incentives under systems in which assignment is unrelated to technology use. The DRG system, for example, classifies patients according to whether specific surgical procedures are performed. Depending on the relative payment rates associated with medical and surgical categories, the DRG system can encourage the use of some surgical procedures. Also, the DRG assignment of patients can change as new technologies are applied to patients. In patient classification systems in which assignment is neutral with respect to the kinds of technologies used, only technologies that reduce the cost per case are encouraged by the financial incentives of the system.

A more subtle example of technology-dependent assignment is the recent finding that the homogeneity of several surgical DRGs with respect to resource use could be substantially improved if they were differentiated on the basis of admission status (i.e., emergency vs. non-emergency). Because emergency admissions have significantly higher costs and lengths of stay, incorporating admission status into the definition of these DRGs would create an incentive for hospitals to classify as many patients as possible as emergency admissions. Unless more objective measures of emergency status can be found, improving the homogeneity with respect to resource use of the DRGs would encourage hospitals to label more admissions as emergency.

Criterion 5: To What Extent Is the Patient Classification System Meaningful to Clinicians?

In any classification system, patient categories should be consistent with generally accepted clinical practice. There are several reasons. Clinicians must understand the categories if they are to respond rationally to the inherent incentives of per-case payment. Clinical diagnoses (and levels of severity within diagnoses) dictate hospital management of resources. Clinical diagnoses supplemented with measures of prognosis and severity represent the most highly developed methods for determining a patient's need for hospital care. Finally, classification systems might affect clinical practice adversely if they do not recognize acceptable clinical practice in their category assignments. Being consistent with clinical practice, however, does not mean that the classification system must institutionalize current practice. When current practice and payment policy differ, users of the classification system should be able to relate the system's categories to the categories used for patient management.

Because alternative classification systems have been developed at different times over the last several years, and because development has relied on different physician experts whose qualifications for representing a national consensus often are unspecified, there likely is considerable variation in how well different systems reflect current clinical practice. The 1980 version of the DRG system and APACHE II, for example, reflected the consensus of panels of clinical experts drawn from national samples. The other systems relied on less representative authorities who may or may not have reflected the wide diversity in clinical practice that characterizes the nation's hospitals.

Criterion 6: How Feasible and Expensive Is the System To Use in Prospective Payment?

One effect of Medicare's PPS has been to accelerate hospital adoption of computer-processing capabilities. This widespread capability has made it feasible to consider classification systems that use more detailed data than do current ones. Therefore, differences in feasibility and expense among classification systems are probably limited to differences in the type of data required for category assignment and the process used for revision and recalibration, but not to differences in the number of categories in and of themselves. The required data elements should be available on existing hospital reporting systems. The following reporting systems can be used for category assignment, in descending order of availability, with availability determined largely by the extent to which these reports are managed with computer-based methods:

- the patient's itemized bill, perhaps modified by accepted accounting practices, such as Medicare's cost-to-charge ratio or more detailed microcosting methods;
- the Uniform Hospital Discharge Data Set (UHDDS);
- results of diagnostic tests, records of vital signs and other monitored indicators of clinical status, pathology reports, operative reports and other data that are processed by computer in some hospitals;
- the patient's medical record, which is available only on paper;
- patient characteristics that are not gathered as a routine part of the record, for example, the level of social support available to the patient after discharge; and
- the intensity and amount of hospital services that are not commonly measured in most hospitals, for example, nursing services.

Regardless of how data are collected, assignment of patients to categories should be capable of being done by computer to minimize cost and enhance feasibility.

Conclusions

The DRG system was not selected for use in Medicare's PPS by accident. It was (and remains at present) the classification system that most fully met two critical criteria: reduction in variation among patients in resource use, and feasibility. Though other systems may perform better by creating more homogeneous patient groups, they are not easily implemented or they lack objectivity in coding.

The relative cost and feasibility of alternative methods are changing as hospitals become more sophisticated in automated information processing. In the future, then, other systems that rely on more detailed data may become viable alternatives or refinements of DRGs.

References

References

1. Aaron, H.J., and Schwartz, W.B., *The Painful Prescription* (Washington, DC: The Brookings Institution, 1984).
2. Aday, L.A., Center for Health Administration Studies, University of Chicago, IL, personal communication, Sept. 4, 1985.
3. Aday, L.A., and Andersen, R.M., "The National Profile of Access to Medical Care: Where Do We Stand?" *Am. J. Public Health* 74(12):1331-1339, December 1984.
4. Aday, L.A., Andersen, R.M., and Fleming, G.V., *Health Care in the U.S.: Equitable for Whom?* (Beverly Hills, CA: Sage Publications, 1980).
5. Aday, L.A., Andersen, R.M., Loevy, S., et al., "Hospital-Sponsored Primary Care: II. Impact on Patient Access," *Am. J. Public Health* 74:792-798, 1984.
6. Alder, H.C., *Lithotripters: Noninvasive Devices for the Treatment of Kidney Stones*, AHA-012828 (Chicago, IL: American Hospital Association, 1985).
7. Allen, P.J., "The Effects of PPS on the Medical Supply Industry," *Hospitals* 58(13):64-68, July 1, 1984.
8. Alsofrom, J., "Hospitals Use TV in Battle for Patients," *American Medical News* 28(10):3-18, Mar. 8, 1985.
9. Ament, R.P., Dreachslin, J.L., Kobrinski, E.J., et al., "Three Case-Type Classifications: Suitability for Use in Reimbursing Hospitals," *Medical Care* 20:460-467, May 1982.
10. American Academy of Ophthalmology, "Cataract Surgery in the 1980's," prepared for Prospective Payment Assessment Commission, Washington, DC, January 1985.
11. American Association of Professional Standards Review Organizations Task Force, *PSRO Impact on Medical Care Serivces: 1980 Volumes I and II. A Report of the 1980 Ad Hoc Task Force on Impact* (Potomac, MD: AASPRO, 1981).
12. American Hospital Association, *Annual Survey of Hospitals, 1984 Edition* (Chicago, IL: AHA, 1984).
13. American Hospital Association, *Hospital Statistics, 1984 Edition* (Chicago, IL: AHA, 1984).
14. American Hospital Association, "Media Background Sheet," No. 5, Chicago, IL, Dec. 3, 1984.
15. American Hospital Association, "National Hospital Panel Survey," Chicago, IL, 1985.
16. American Hospital Association, Office of Public Policy Analysis, "Incorporating Capital Costs Into Medicare Prospective Prices," unpublished draft, Chicago, IL, July 1983.
17. American Medical Association "Physician Opinion on Health Care Issues: 1984," survey, Chicago, IL, September 1984.
18. American Medical Association, "AMA's DRG Monitoring Project and the Prospective Pricing System," in *AMA Report of the American Medical Association Board of Trustees* (Chicago, IL: AMA, December 1984).
19. American Medical Association, *Physicians' Current Procedural Terminology*, 4th ed. (Chicago, IL: AMA, 1985).
20. American Medical News, "More RNs, Fewer LPN's Finding Jobs at Hospitals-ANA Survey," *American Medical News* 28(15):24, Apr. 12, 1985.
21. American Medical News, "Hospital Industry's Margin Soared in '84," *American Medical News* 28(17):1, Apr. 26, 1985.
22. Anderson, G., and Lave, J., "State Rate-Setting Programs: Do They Reward Efficiency in Hospitals?" *Medical Care* 22(5):494-498, May 1984.
23. Anderson, G.F., and Steinberg, E.P., "To Buy or Not To Buy: Technology Acquisition Under Prospective Payment," *N. Eng. J. Med.* 311(3):182-185, July 19, 1984.
24. Anderson, G.F., and Steinberg, E.P., "Hospital Readmissions in the Medicare Population," *N. Eng. J. Med.* 311(21):1349-53, Nov. 22, 1984.
25. Arstein-Kerslake, C., "Hospital Personnel Reductions," *CHA Insight* 7(25):1, June 22, 1983.
26. Bacon, W., and Mullner, R., "National Health Care Surveys and Health Care Management," *J. Med. Systems* 7(6):469-479, 1983.
27. Banta, H.D., Ruby, G., and Burns, A.K., "Using Coverage Policy To Contain Medicare Costs," in *Proceedings of the Conference on the Future of Medicare*, Subcommittee on Health, Committee on Ways and Means, House of Representatives, U.S. Congress, Committee Print No. 23 (Washington DC: U.S. Government Printing Office, 1984).
28. Barr, J.T., "The Interaction of Therapeutic Drug Monitoring and DRG Payment Levels," prepared for Office of Technology Assessment, U.S. Congress, Washington, DC, Nov. 16, 1984.
29. Belin, C., Health Resources and Services Administration, U.S. Department of Health and Human Services, Rockville, MD, personal communication, March 1985.
30. Berenson, R.A., and Pawlson, L.G., "The Medicare Prospective Payment System and the Care of the Frail Elderly," *J. Am. Geriatr. Soc.* 32(11):843-8, November 1984.
31. Bergner, M., "Measurement of Health Status," *Medical Care* 23(5):696-705, May 1985.
32. Bergner M., Bobbitt R.A., Carter, W.B., et al.,

"The Sickness Impact Profile: Development and Final Revision of a Health Status Measure," *Medical Care* 19:787-805, August 1981.
33. Berki, S.E., Ashcraft, M.F., and Newbrander, W.C., "Length-of-Stay Variations Within ICDA-8 Diagnosis-Related Groups," *Medical Care* 22(2):126-142, 1984.
34. Bernstein, J., General Accounting Office, U.S. Congress, Washington, DC, personal communication, May 5, 1985.
35. Biles, B., Schramm, C.J., and Atkinson, J.G., "Hospital Cost Inflation Under State Rate-Setting Programs," *N. Eng. J. Med.* 303(12):664-668, Sept. 18, 1980.
36. Biomedical Business International, "Cost-Effective Surgical Devices," *Biomedical Business International* 8(9/10):102-103, May 28, 1985.
37. Blazer, D.G., and Pennybacker, M.R., "Epidemiology of Alcoholism in the Elderly," in *Alcoholism in the Elderly*, J.T. Hartford and T. Samorajski (eds.) (New York, NY: Raven Press, 1984).
38. Blue Cross of Western Pennsylvania, *Hospital Case Mix: Development and Implementation* (Pittsburgh, PA: Blue Cross of Western Pennsylvania, 1983).
39. The Blue Sheet, "Drug Clinical Research Costs Restraint Would Be Aided by FDA Acceptance of Home Bound and Hospitalized Patients as Equivalent," *The Blue Sheet* 28(20):7, May 15, 1985.
40. Bootman, J.L., et al., "Individualizing Gentamicin Dosage Regimens in Burn Patients With Gram Negative Septicemia: A Cost-Benefit Analysis," *J. Pharmac. Sci.* 68(3):267-72, 1979.
41. Boulding, K., "The Concept of Need for Health Services," *Milbank Mem. Fund Q.* 44:202-228, October 1966.
42. Breckenridge, R., "Pathology Practice Under TEFRA and DRGs," *Pathologist* 37(8):560-562, August 1983.
43. Brewster, A.C., Jacobs, C.M., and Bradbury, R.C., "Classifying Severity of Illness by Using Clinical Findings," *Health Care Financing Review* Annual Supplement:107-108, November 1984.
44. Brewster, J.A., Brown, R., Devaney, B., et al. (for Mathematica Policy Research, Inc.), "National Evaluation of the Medicare Competition Demonstrations: Final Evaluation Design Report," prepared for Health Care Financing Administration, U.S. Department of Health and Human Services, Baltimore, MD, June 15, 1984.
45. Broglie, W., Health Care Financing Administration, U.S. Department of Health and Human Services, Baltimore, MD, personal communication, Jan. 16, 1985.
46. Brook, R.H., and Lohr, K.N., "Efficacy, Effectiveness, Variations, and Quality: Boundary-Crossing Research," *Medical Care* 23(5):710-723, May 1985.
47. Brook, R.H., Ware, J.E., Jr., Rogers, W.H., et al., "Does Free Care Improve Adults Health?" *N. Eng. J. Med.* 309(23):1426-1434, Dec. 8, 1983.
48. Brown, P.W., "Slowdown in Equipment Innovation Tarnishes Domestic Imaging Market," *Diagnostic Imaging* 53(6):80-83, November 1984.
49. Buchanan, A., "The Right to a Decent Minimum of Health Care," in *Securing Access to Health Care, Volume Two: Appendices*, President's Commission for the Study of Ethical Problems in Medicine (Washington, DC: U.S. Government Printing Office, March 1983).
50. Burney, I., "Physician Reimbursment and Participation in Medicare," prepared for Health Care Financing Administration, U.S. Department of Health and Human Services, unpublished, Baltimore, MD, Sept. 29, 1984.
51. Business Week, "The Medicare Squeeze Pushes Hospitals Into the Information Age," *Business Week* 2847:87-90, June 18, 1984.
52. Butler, P.W., Bone, R.C., and Field, T., "Technology Under Medicare Diagnosis-Related Groups Prospective Payment: Implications for Medical Intensive Care," *Chest* 87(2):229-234, February 1985.
53. Caldwell, J.M., "Home Care: Utilizing Resources To Develop Home Care," *Hospitals* 56(21):68-72, Nov. 1, 1982.
54. Campbell, D.T., and Stanley, J.C., *Experimental and Quasi-Experimental Designs for Research* (Chicago, IL: Rand McNally College Publishing Co., 1973).
55. Carter, G.M., and Ginsburg, P.B. (for Rand Corp.), "The Medicare Case Mix Index Increase: Medical Practice Changes, Aging and DRG Creep," prepared for Health Care Financing Administration, U.S. Department of Health and Human Services, Pub. No. R-3292-HCFA, Baltimore, MD, June 1985.
56. Cerale, T., Alcohol, Drug Abuse, and Mental Health Administration, Public Health Service, U.S. Department of Health and Human Services, Washington, DC, personal communication, Aug. 30, 1985.
57. Chassin, M., *Variations in Hospital Length of Stay: Their Relationship to Health Outcomes* (Health Technology Case Study #24), prepared for Office of Technology Assessment, U.S. Congress, OTA-HCS-24 (Washington, DC: U.S. Government Printing Office, August 1983).
58. Chulis, G., Health Care Financing Administra-

tion, U.S. Department of Health and Human Services, Baltimore, MD, personal communication, Jan. 6, 1984.
59. Clopton, T., Office of Demonstrations and Evaluations, Health Care Financing Administration, U.S. Department of Health and Human Services, Baltimore, MD, personal communication, June 4, 1985.
60. Coelen, C., and Sullivan, D., "An Analysis of the Effects of Prospective Reimbursement Programs on Hospital Expenditures," *Health Care Financing Review* 2(3):1-40, Winter 1981.
61. Coffey, R.M., National Center for Health Services Research, Public Health Service, U.S. Department of Health and Human Services, Rockville, MD, personal communication, March 1985.
62. Coffey, R.M., and Goldfarb, M.G.,"DRGs and Disease Staging for Reimbursing Medicare Patients," prepublication draft, Rockville, MD, October 1984.
63. Cohn, D., "Medicare's New Money Game," *Washington Post*, Mar. 6, 1985.
64. Commission on Professional and Hospital Activities, "PAS Case Abstract" form, Ann Arbor, MI, 1984.
65. Converse, M., American Hospital Association, Chicago IL, personal communication, January 1985.
66. Copeland, R., "1984 Long-Term Care Survey Preliminary Report," U.S. Department of Commerce, memorandum, Washington, DC, Sept. 19, 1984.
67. Cornelius, B., Health Care Financing Administration, U.S. Department of Health and Human Services, Baltimore, MD, personal communication, May 1985.
68. Cornelius, B., Health Care Financing Administration, U.S. Department of Health and Human Services, Baltimore, MD, personal communication, May 1985.
69. Cromwell, J., and Ginsburg P., *Incentives and Decisions Underlying Hospitals' Adoption and Utilization of Major Capital Equipment* (Cambridge, MA: Abt Associates, 1975).
70. Cromwell, J., and Kanak, J., "The Effects of Prospective Reimbursement Programs on Hospital Adoption and Service Sharing," *Health Care Financing Review* 4(2):67, December 1982.
71. Crowley, S., Health Care Financing Administration, U.S. Department of Health and Human Services, Baltimore, MD, personal communication, August 1984.
72. Crowley, S., Health Care Financing Administration, U.S. Department of Health and Human Services, Baltimore, MD, personal communication, September 1984.
73. Curran, W.J., "Economic and Legal Considerations in Emergency Care," *N. Eng. J. Med.* 312(6):374-375, Feb. 7, 1985.
74. Dans, P.E., Charache, P., Fahey, M., et al., "Management of Pneumonia in the Prospective Payment Era. A Need for More Clinician and Support Service Interaction," *Arch. Int. Med.* 144(7):1392-7, July 1984.
75. Danzon, P., "Hospital Profits: The Effects of Reimbursement Policies," *J. Health Econ.* 1(1):29-52, 1982.
76. Davis, C.K., Administrator, Health Care Financing Administration, U.S. Department of Health and Human Services, testimony at hearing, *Proposed Prospective Reimbursement Rates for the End-Stage Renal Disease Program*, before the Subcommittee on Health of the Committee on Finance, U.S. Senate, U.S. Congress, Mar. 15, 1982 (Washington, DC: U.S. Government Printing Office, 1982).
77. Davis, C.K., "The Impact of Prospective Payment on Clinical Research" (editorial), *J.A.M.A.* 253(5):686-687, Feb. 1, 1985.
78. Davis, C.K., Administrator, Health Care Finance Administration, U.S. Department of Health and Human Services, "Statement Before the Subcommittee on Health, Committee on Finance, United States Senate," mimeo, Washington DC, Apr. 19, 1985.
79. Demkovich, L., "PPO-Three Letters That May Form One Answer to Runaway Health Costs," *National J.* 15(23):1176-1177, June 4, 1983.
80. Demkovich, L., "Verdict Is Still Out on Prototype of New Hospital Cost-Cutting Plan," *National J.* 15(50)1:2573-2576, Dec. 10, 1983.
81. Deyo R.A., and Inui, T.S., "Toward Clinical Applications of Health Status Measures: Sensitivity of Scales to Clinically Important Changes," *Health Services Research* 19(3):275-289, 1984.
82. District of Columbia Hospital Association, "The Inequity of Medicare Prospective Payment in Large Urban Areas," Washington, DC, September 1984.
83. Dobson, A., "Prospective Payment: Current Configuration and Future Direction," presented to the Prospective Payment Assessment Commission, Washington, DC, Feb. 2, 1984.
84. Dobson, A., Office of Research and Demonstrations, Health Care Financing Administration, U.S. Department of Health and Human Services, Baltimore, MD, personal communication, May 20, 1985.

85. Donabedian, A., "Evaluating the Quality of Medical Care," *Milbank Mem. Fund Q.* 44:166-203, July 1966.
86. Donabedian, A., *Explorations in Quality Assessment and Monitoring, Vol. I: The Definition of Quality and Approaches to its Assessment* (Ann Arbor, MI: Health Administration Press, 1980).
87. Donabedian, A., Wheeler, J.R., and Wyszewianski, L., "Quality, Cost and Health: An Integrative Model," *Medical Care* 20:975-992, October 1982.
88. Dowling W., "Prospective Reimbursement of Hospitals," *Inquiry* 11(3):163-180, September 1974.
89. Dowling, W.L., "Hospital Rate-Setting Programs: How, and How Well, Do They Work," *Topics in Health Care Financing/Rate Regulation* 6(1):15-23, Fall 1979.
90. Drummond, M.F., and Stoddart, G.L., "Economic Analysis and Clinical Trials," *Cont. Clin. Trials* 5:115-128, 1984.
91. Duff, R.S., and Hollingshead, A.B., *Sickness and Society* (New York, NY: Harper & Row, 1968).
92. Eastwood, M.R., *The Relation Between Physical and Mental Illness* (Toronto and Buffalo: Toronto Press, 1975).
93. Eckardt, M.H., Harford, T.C., Kaelber, C.T., et al., "Health Hazards Associated With Alcohol Consumption," *J.A.M.A.* 246(6):648, 1981.
94. The Economist, "Profitable American Hospitals," *The Economist* 295(7394):82-83, May 18, 1985.
95. Egdahl, R., "Ways for Surgeons To Increase the Efficiency of Their Use of Hospitals," *N. Eng. J. Med.* 309(19):1184-1187, Nov. 10, 1983.
96. Eggers, P.W., "Trends in Medicare Reimbursement for End-Stage Renal Disease: 1974-79," *Health Care Financing Review* 6(1):31-38, Fall 1984.
97. Enthoven, A.C., and Noll, R.G., "Prospective Payment: Will It Solve Medicare's Financial Problem?" *Issues in Science and Technology* 1:101-116, Fall 1984.
98. Equitable Life Assurance Society of the United States, "The Equitable Healthcare Survey: Options for Controlling Cost," conducted by Louis Harris & Associates, Inc., distributed by Information Resources International Inc., Tustin, CA, August 1983.
99. Farber, M.E., "DRG Payment and Medical Technology: DRG 39," prepared for the Office of Technology Assessment, U.S. Congress, Washington, DC, August 1985.
100. Feder, J.M., *Medicare: The Politics of Federal Hospital Insurance* (Lexington, MA: DC Heath & Co., 1977).
101. Feder, J.M., and Scanlon, W.M., "The Underused Benefit: Medicare's Coverage of Nursing Home Care," *Milbank Mem. Fund Q.* 60(4):604-632, 1982.
102. Fedorowicz, J., "Hospital Information Systems: Are We Ready for Case-Mix Applications?" *HCM Review* 8(4):33-41, Fall 1983.
103. Fein, R., "Medical Care Needs in the Coming Decade," *Bull. N.Y. Acad. Med.* 45:255-270, October 1969.
104. Fetter, R.B., Shin Y., Freema, J.L., et al., "Case Mix Definition by Diagnosis Related Groups," *Medical Care* 18(Supplement):1-53, 1980.
105. Feuerberg, M., "Hospital Data Systems and Their Adequacy for Evaluating PPS," prepared for the Office of Technology Assessment, U.S. Congress, Washington, DC, Mar. 14, 1985.
106. Flanagan, J.B., and Sourapas, K.J., "Preparing for Prospective Payment Part III: Information Systems," *Journal of AMRA* 55(1):11-15, January 1984.
107. Flood, A.B., Scott, W.R., and Eury, W., "Does Practice Make Perfect? Part 1: The Relation Between Hospital Volume and Outcomes for Selected Diagnostic Categories," *Medical Care* 22(2):98-114, February 1984.
108. Flood, A.B., Scott, W.R., and Eury, W., "Does Practice Make Perfect? Part 2: The Relation Between Volume and Outcomes and Other Hospital Characteristics," *Medical Care* 22(2):115-125, February 1984.
109. Florida Hospital Association, "Hospital Survey," Orlando, FL, Jan. 19, 1984.
110. Friedman, B., "Likely Effects of Medicare Prospective Payment System on the Veterans Administration Health Care System," prepared for the Office of Technology Assessment, U.S. Congress, Washington, DC, July 1985.
111. Friedman, B., Manheim, L., Davidson, S., et al., "A Decade of Medicaid Program Experience, 1973-1982," forthcoming in *Health Care Finance Administration Grant and Contract Reports*, 1984.
112. Frye, J., "Hospitals Offer Incentives To Attract Patients," *Medical World News* 25(19):70-71, Oct. 8, 1984.
113. Garnick, D.W., "The Impacts of Rate Regulation and Unionization on the Demand for Hospital Labor," prepared for Hospital Cost and Utilization Project, Division of Intramural Research, National Center for Health Services Research,

U.S. Department of Health and Human Services, Rockville, MD, January 1983.
114. Gent, M., Bureau of Data Management and Strategy, Health Care Financing Administration, U.S. Department of Health and Human Services, Baltimore, MD, personal communication, August 1984.
115. Gibson, D., and McMullan, M., "End-Stage Renal Disease: A Profile of Facilities Furnishing Treatment," *Health Care Financing Review* 6(2):87-90, Winter 1984.
116. Gitlow, S.E., "The Medical Aspects of Alcoholism," *Bull. N.Y. Acad. Med.* 59(2):167, March 1983.
117. Goldberg, D., Health Care Financing Administration, U.S. Department of Health and Human Services, Baltimore, MD, personal communication, May 1985.
118. Goldstein, I., Health Care Financing Administration, U.S. Department of Health and Human Services, Baltimore, MD, personal communication, September 1984.
119. Goldstein, I., Health Care Financing Administration, U.S. Department of Health and Human Services, Baltimore, MD, personal communication, May 1985.
120. Gonnella, J.S., Hornbrook, M.C., and Louis, D.Z., "Staging of Disease: A Case-Mix Measurement," *J.A.M.A.* 251(5):637-44, Feb. 3, 1984.
121. Goran, M.J., "The Evolution of the PSRO Hospital Review System," *Medical Care* 18(5):Supplement, 1979.
122. Gray, M.S., "Occupational Therapy Use Rises Under PPS," *Hospitals* 59:60-61, June 1, 1985.
123. Grimaldi, P.L., and Micheletti, J.A., *Diagnosis-Related Groups: A Practitioner's Guide* (Chicago, IL: Pluribus Press, 1983).
124. Gruentzig, A., "Percutaneous Transluminal Coronary Angioplasty: Six Years' Experience," *Am. Heart J.* 107:818, 1984.
125. Hadley, J., *More Medical Care, Better Health?* (Washington, DC: The Urban Institute Press, 1982).
126. Hadley, J., and Feder, J., "Hospital Cost Shifting: An Analysis of Hospitals' Markups and Financial Needs," Urban Institute Working Paper #3179-07, Washington, DC, The Urban Institute, 1984.
127. Hamilton, D., Walter, R., and Cromwell, J. (for Abt Associates, Inc.), "National Hospital Rate-Setting Study: A Comparative Review of Nine Prospective Rate-Setting Programs, First Annual Report," *Health Care Financing Grants and Contracts Report*, U.S. DHHS Pub. No. (HCFA) 80-03061 (Washington, DC: U.S. Government Printing Office, August 1980).
128. Health Care Management Systems, Inc., *Final Report: PSRO Ambulatory Care Quality Assurance Review* (La Jolla, CA: Health Care Management Systems, 1978).
129. Health Industry Manufacturers' Association, *Recalibration & Updating: A Means to Health Care Cost Control and Quality*, Report No. 84-4, Series No. 2 (Washington, DC: HIMA, 1984).
130. Health Research and Educational Trust of New Jersey, *DRG Evaluation: Volume IV-B Organizational Impact* (Princeton, NJ: HRET, January 1983).
131. Health Research and Educational Trust of New Jersey, *DRG Evaluation: Volume II Economic and Financial Analysis* (Princeton, NJ: HRET, February 1984).
132. Hellinger, F.J., "Recent Evidence on Case-Based Systems for Setting Hospital Rates," *Inquiry* 22:78-91, Spring 1985.
133. Himmelstein, D.V., Woolhandler, S., Harnly, M., et al., "Patient Transfers: Medical Practice as Social Triage," *Am. J. Public Health* 74(5):494-497, May 1984.
134. Hochman, A., "Effect of New Medicare Rules Disputed," *Washington Post*, p. B1, Apr. 28, 1985.
135. Home Health Line, "Changing Face of Medicare Home Health," *Home Health Line* 8:28, Feb. 4, 1983.
136. Home Health Line, "Region V Flatters Daily Care After Consulting HCFA; Says Patient Should Be in Skilled Nursing Facility if Cheaper," *Home Health Line* 7:167-168, Sept. 12, 1983.
137. Horn, S.D., Horn, R.A., and Sharkey, P.D., "The Severity of Illness as a Severity Adjustment to DRGs," prepublication draft, Baltimore, MD, 1984.
138. Horn S.D., Sharkey, P.D., and Bertram, D.A., "Measuring Severity of Illness: Homogeneous Case-Mix Groups," *Medical Care* 21(1):14-30, 1983.
139. Horn, S.D., Sharkey, P.D., Chambers, A.F., et al., "Severity of Illness Within DRGs," prepared for Health Care Financing Administration, U.S. Department of Health and Human Services, Baltimore, MD, December 1984.
140. Horn, S.D., Bulkley, G., Sharkey, P., et al., "Interhospital Differences in Severity of Illness," *N. Eng. J. Med.* 313(1):20-24, July 4, 1985.
141. Hornbrook, M.C., "Hospital Case Mix: Its Definition, Measurement and Use: Part II. Review of Alternative Measures," *Medical Care Review* 39:73, 1982.
142. Hornbrook, M.C., "Techniques for Assessing Hospital Case Mix," *Ann. Rev. Public Health*, vol. 6, in press, 1985.

143. Hornbrook, M.C., and Monheit, A.C., "Cost of Hospital Treatments: Volume, Case Mix, and Capacity," unpublished draft, Portland, OR, Jan. 4, 1985.
144. Hospital Affiliates International, "Hospital Care in America," survey conducted by Louis Harris & Associates, Inc., Nashville, TN, April 1978.
145. Hospital Research Association, "Certificate of Need Data," memorandum, Fairfield, NJ, December 1984.
146. Hospitals, "Admissions Fall But Margins Are Up in '84," *Hospitals* 59(9):70-72, May 1, 1985.
147. Hospitals, "Size of FEC Market a Matter of Opinion," *Hospitals* 59(10):43-44, May 16, 1985.
148. Hospitals, "Rise in LOS May Signal Case-Mix Changes," *Hospitals* 59(15):25-27, Aug. 1, 1985.
149. Huber, P., "Robust Statistics: A Review," *Annals of Mathematical Statistics* 43:1041-1067, 1972.
150. Hull, J.B., "Medicare Payment Plan Is Blamed for Hasty Release of Aged Patients," *Wall Street Journal*, June 25, 1985.
151. Hunt, K., "Government Cost Constraints Hindering R&D, Executive Claims," *Diagnostic Imaging* 7(3):25, March 1985.
152. Iezzoni, L.I., and Moskowitz, M.A., "The Clinical Impact of DRG-Based Physician Reimbursement," prepared with the support of the Office of Research, Health Care Financing Administration, under cooperative agreement No. 18-C-98526/1-01, to the Health Policy Research Consortium, Cooperative Research Center, Boston, MA, Dec. 31, 1984.
153. Jang, G., Block, P., Cowley, M., et al., "Relative Cost of Coronary Angioplasty and Bypass Surgery in a One-Vessel Disease Model," *Am. J. Cardiol.* 53:52C-55C, 1984.
154. Johnson, A.N., and Appel, G.L., "DRGs and Hospital Case Records: Implications for Medicare Case-Mix Accuracy," *Inquiry* 21:128-134, Summer 1984.
155. Joint Commission on Accreditation of Hospitals, *Accreditation Manual for Hospitals*, 1983 ed. (Chicago, IL: JCAH, 1982).
156. Jones, D.C., Chief, Statistical Methods Division, Bureau of the Census, U.S. Department of Commerce, "Statement of Objectives of the Long-Term Care (LTC) Survey Revisited (1984 LTC)," memorandum, Washington, DC, Mar. 22, 1984.
157. Joskow, P.L., *Controlling Hospital Costs: The Role of Government Regulation* (Cambridge, MA: The Massachusetts Institute of Technology Press, 1981).
158. Kane, R.L., Bell, R.M., Hosek, S.D., et al. (for Rand Corp.), "Outcome-Based Reimbursement for Nursing-Home Care," prepared for National Center for Health Services Research, Public Health Service, U.S. Department of Health and Human Services, Pub. No. R-3092-NCHSR, Rockville, MD, 1983.
159. Kappert, M., Acting Associate Administrator for Operations, Health Care Financing Administration, U.S. Department of Health and Human Services, "Statement Before the Select Committee on Aging and its Task Force on Rural Elderly, U.S. House of Representatives," mimeo, Washington, DC, Feb. 26, 1985.
160. Katterhagen, J.G., and Mortenson, L.E., "Clinical Research Patients Generate Significant Losses Under Diagnosis Related Groups (DRGs), *Semin. Oncol.* 11(3):xxxv-xxxvi, September 1984.
161. Keefe, J., Dube, P., and Jollie, W., "Managing DRGs: Knowing What To Cut and When," *Radio. Management* 5(4):2-6, 1983.
162. Keegan, A.J., "Hospitals Will Continue To Treat All DRGs To Snare Contribution Margin," *Modern Healthcare* 13(9):206-208, September 1983.
163. Kelsey, S., Mullin, S., Detre, K., et al., "Effect of Investigator Experience on Percutaneous Transluminal Coronary Angioplasty," *Am. J. Cardiol.* 53:54C-64C, 1984.
164. Kennedy, E., American Hospital Association, Chicago, IL, personal communication, Oct. 26, 1984.
165. Kennedy, J.W., Ritchie, J.L., Davis, K.B., et al., "The Western Washington Randomized Trial of Intracoronary Streptokinase in Acute Myocardial Infarction: A 12-Month Followup Report," *N. Eng. J. Med.* 312(17):1073-1078, Apr. 25, 1985.
166. Kidder, D., and Sullivan, D., "Hospital Payroll Costs, Productivity, and Employment Under Prospective Reimbursement," *Health Care Financing Review* 4(2):89-100, December 1982.
167. Kline, J., Congressional Research Service, U.S. Congress, Washington, DC, personal communication, Mar. 5, 1985.
168. Kominski, G.F., Williams, S.V., and Pickens, G.T., "A Comparison of DRGs and Disease Staging: Preliminary Report," draft of report to National Center for Health Services Research, Public Health Service, U.S. Department of Health and Human Services, Rockville, MD, 1985.
169. Kominski, G.F., Williams, S.V., Mays, R.B., et al., "Unrecognized Redistributions of Revenue in

DRG-Based Prospective Payment Systems," unpublished draft, Philadelphia, PA, July 1984.
170. Konoig, F., Health Care Financing Administration, U.S. Department of Health and Human Services, Baltimore, MD, personal communication, May 1985.
171. Kuntz, E., "Task Forces Scour Diagnosis, Therapy Methods for Cost-Cutting Procedures," *Modern Health Care* 14(3):138-142, Feb. 15, 1984.
172. Laffel, G.L., and Braunwald, E., "Thrombolytic Therapy: A New Strategy for the Treatment of Acute Myocardial Infarction," *N. Eng. J. Med.* 311(12):770-776, Sept. 20, 1984.
173. Langenbrunner, J.C., *The Safety, Efficacy, and Cost-Effectiveness of Therapeutic Apheresis* (Health Technology Case Study #23), prepared for the Office of Technology Assessment, U.S. Congress, OTA-HCS-23 (Washington DC: U.S. Government Printing Office, July 1984).
174. Lave, J.R., "Hospital Payment Under Medicare," in *Proceedings of the Conference on the Future of Medicare*, Subcommittee on Health, Committee on Ways and Means, House of Representatives, U.S. Congress, Feb. 1, 1984 (Washington, DC: U.S. Government Printing Office, 1984).
175. Lave, J.R., *The Medicare Adjustment for the Indirect Costs of Medical Education: Historical Development and Current Status* (Washington DC: Association of American Medical Colleges, January 1985).
176. Lee, H., "Coping With DRGs: Evanston Hospital, Evanston, Illinois," *Am. J. Hosp. Pharm.* 40(a):1508-9, September 1983.
177. Lefton, D., "Hospitals Score Record Profits Under DRGs," *American Medical News* 28(30):1, Aug. 9, 1985.
178. Levinson, R., National Institutes of Health, Public Health Service, U.S. Department of Health and Human Services, Bethesda MD, personal communication, October 1984.
179. Lewis, D.C., and Gordon, A.J., "Alcoholism and the General Hospital: The Roger Williams Intervention Program," *Bull. N.Y. Acad. Med.* 59(2):181-197, March 1983.
180. Lewis, S., "Speculations on the Impact of Prospective Pricing and DRGs," *West J. Med.* 140:638-644, April 1984.
181. Lichtenstein, P., Health Care Financing Administration, U.S. Department of Health and Human Services, Baltimore, MD, personal communication, August 1984.
182. Lintzeris, G., Bureau of Data Management and Strategy, Health Care Financing Administration, U.S. Department of Health and Human Services, Baltimore, MD, personal communication, Dec. 4, 1984.
183. Lintzeris, G., Bureau of Data Management and Strategy, Health Care Financing Administration, U.S. Department of Health and Human Services, Baltimore, MD, personal communication, Jan. 11, 1985.
184. Lipowski, Z.J., "The Need To Integrate Liaison Psychiatry and Geropsychiatry," *Am. J. Psychiatry* 140(8):1003, August 1983.
185. Lohr, K. N., "Peer Review Organizations (PROs): Quality Assurance in Medicare," prepared for the Office of Technology Assessment, U.S. Congress, Washington, DC, July 1, 1985.
186. Long, S.H., and Settle, R.F., "Medicare and the Disadvantaged Elderly: Objectives and Outcomes," *Milbank Mem. Fund Q.* 62(4):609-656, 1984.
187. Lubitz, J., "Different Data Systems, Different Conclusions? Comparing Hospital Use Data for the Aged From Four Data Systems," *Health Care Financing Review* 2:41-60, Spring 1981.
188. Lubitz, J., Health Care Financing Administration, U.S. Department of Health and Human Services, Baltimore, MD, personal communication, Mar. 13, 1985.
189. Luft, H.S., Bunker, J.P., and Enthoven, A.C., "Should Operations Be Regionalized? The Empirical Relation Between Surgical Volume and Mortality," *N. Eng. J. Med.* 301:1364, 1979.
190. Lundberg, C.J., "New Tax Bill Mandates Changes for HHAs," *Hospitals* 56(21):81-84, Nov. 1, 1982.
191. Martin, S.G., Frick, A.P., and Shwartz, M., "An Analysis of Hospital Case Mix, Cost, and Payment Differences for Medicare, Medicaid, and Blue Cross Plan Patients Using DRGs," *Inquiry* 21(4):369-379, Winter 1984.
192. May, J.J., and Wasserman, J., "Selected Results From an Evaluation of the New Jersey Diagnosis-Related Group System," *Health Serv. Res.* 19(5):547-559, December 1984.
193. McCarthy, E., National Center for Health Statistics, Public Health Service, U.S. Department of Health and Human Services, Hyattsville, MD, personal communication, Mar. 28, 1985.
194. McMenamin, P., "PPS Evaluation Issues With Respect to Health Care Costs," prepared for the Office of Technology Assessment, U.S. Congress, Washington, DC, Nov. 9, 1984.
195. McNamara, E., "Home Care: Hospitals Rediscover Comprehensive Home Care," *Hospitals* 56(21):60-66, Nov. 1, 1982.

196. McNeil, B., "Clinical Decisionmaking in an Era of DRG-Based Prospective Payment," paper presented at the Sixth Annual Meeting of the Medical Decision Making Society, Bethesda, MD, November 1984.
197. Means, K., Office of Assistant Secretary for Planning and Evaluation, U.S. Department of Health and Human Services, Washington, DC, personal communication, May 1985.
198. Medical Devices, Diagnostics, and Instrumentation, "Antitachycardia Devices: Conventional Pacing Energy," *M-D-D-I Reports* 11(26):3-5, July 1, 1985.
199. Mehta, C., Dana Farber Cancer Institute, Boston, MA, personal communication, Mar. 11, 1985.
200. Meier, B., and Gruentzig, A., "Learning Curve for Percutaneous Transluminal Coronary Angioplasty: Skill, Technology or Patient Selection," *Am. J. Cardiol.* 53:65C-66C, 1984.
201. Meiners, M.R., and Coffey, R.M., "Hospital DRGs and the Need for Long-Term Care Services: An Empirical Analysis," National Center for Health Services Research, U.S. Department of Health and Human Services, Rockville, MD, December 1984.
202. Meskin, S., "Possible Impacts of the Federal Prospective Payment System on the American Red Cross," prepared for American Red Cross, Washington, DC, August 1983.
203. Meyer, J., *Passing the Health Care Buck: Who Pays the Hidden Cost?* (Washington, DC: American Enterprise Institute, 1983).
204. Milstead, D., Health Care Financing Administration, U.S. Department of Health and Human Services, Baltimore, MD, personal communication, Mar. 28, 1985.
205. Moore, W.B., "CEOs Plan To Expand Home Health, Outpatient Services," *Hospitals* 59:74-77, Jan. 1, 1985.
206. Mortenson, L., Association of Community Cancer Centers, Washington, DC, personal communication, Mar. 11, 1985.
207. Moscowitz, M., Boston University Medical School, Boston, MA, personal communication, 1984.
208. Mosteller, F., and Tukey, J.W., *Data Analysis and Regression* (Boston MA: Addison-Wesley, 1977).
209. Mullner, R., "An Inventory of U.S. Health Care Data Bases," *A Review of Public Data Use* 2:85-192, June 1983.
210. Nathanson, M., "Labs Should Try To Cut Patients's Stay, Market Testing Services," *Modern Health Care* 14(3):146-148, Feb. 15, 1984.
211. Nathanson, P., Health Care Financing Administration, U.S. Department of Health and Human Services, Baltimore, MD, personal communication, April 1985.
212. National Academy of Sciences, Institute of Medicine, *Reliability of Hospital Discharge Abstracts*, Pub. No. IOM-77-01 (Washington, DC: NAS, February 1977).
213. National Academy of Sciences, Institute of Medicine, *Reliability of Medicare Hospital Discharge Records*, Pub. No. IOM-77-05 (Washington, DC: NAS, November 1977).
214. National Academy of Sciences, Institute of Medicine, *Reliability of National Hospital Discharge Survey Data* (Washington, DC: NAS, 1980).
215. National Academy of Sciences, Institute of Medicine, *Health Care in a Context of Civil Rights* (Washington, DC: NAS, 1981).
216. National Association for Ambulatory Care, "Statement Presented to the American Medical Association Committee on Medicolegal Problems," Dallas, TX, Mar. 10, 1985.
217. National Association of Childrens Hospitals and Related Institutions, "Request for Proposal: Children's Hospitals' Case-Mix Classification System Project," Alexandria, VA, 1984.
218. Neuhauser, D., and Pine, R., "DRGs and Elective Surgery: What's Best for the Provider? What's Best for the Patient?" *Medical Care* 23(2):183-188, February 1985.
219. Newhouse, J.P., "Two Prospective Difficulties With Prospective Payment of Hospitals," *J. Health Econ.* 2(3):269-274, 1983.
220. Obermayer, J., *The Role of Patents in the Commercialization of New Technology for Small Innovative Companies* (Cambridge, MA: Research & Planning, Inc., 1981).
221. Omenn, G.S., and Conrad, D.A., "Implications of DRGs for Clinicians," *N. Eng. J. Med.* 311(20):1314-1317, Nov. 15, 1984.
222. Packer, C.L., "Automation in the Medical Records Department," *Hospitals* 59(5):100-104, Mar. 1, 1985.
223. Palmer, R.H., "Components of Health Care Evaluations," in *Ambulatory Health Care Evaluation: Principles and Practice* (Chicago, IL: American Hospital Association, 1983).
224. Palmer, R.H., Harvard School of Public Health, Boston, MA, personal communication, Mar. 12, 1985.
225. Palmer, R.H., Strain, R., Maurer, J.V.W., et al., "Quality Assurance in Eight Adult Medicine Group Practices," *Medical Care* 22(7):632-643, July 1984.
226. Parkerson, G.R., Gehlbach, S.Y., Wagner, E.H.,

et al., "The Duke-UNC Health Profile: An Adult Health Status Instrument for Primary Care," *Medical Care* 19:806-828, August 1981.
227. Pattison, E.M., "The Selection of Treatment Modalities for the Alcoholic Patient," in *The Diagnosis and Treatment of Alcoholism*, H.H. Mendelson and N.K. Mello (eds.) (New York, NY: McGraw-Hill Book Co., 1979).
228. Perkins, J.B., "Streptokinase Treatment for Acute Myocardial Infarction and the DRG Payment System," prepared for the Office of Technology Assessment, U.S. Congress, Washington, DC, Dec. 14, 1984.
229. Pettengill, J., Congressional Research Service, U.S. Congress, Washington, DC, personal communication, August 1984.
230. Pettengill, J., and Vertrees, J., "Reliability and Validity in Hospital Case-Mix Measurement," *Health Care Financing Review* 4(2):101-127, December 1982.
231. Pincus, H.A., West, J., and Goldman, H., "DRG's and Clinical Research in Psychiatry," submitted to *Archives of General Psychiatry*, Mar. 27, 1985.
232. Porter, S., "How Ohio Hospitals Are Coping With DRGs," *Ohio State Med. J.* 80(4):263-5, April 1984.
233. Powe, N.R., "Percutaneous Transluminal Coronary Angioplasty: Efficacy, Cost and Effects of Prospective Payment," prepared for the Office of Technology Assessment, U.S. Congress, Washington, DC, July 1985.
234. President's Commission for the Study of Ethical Problems in Medicine and Biomedical and Behavioral Research, *Securing Access to Health Care: The Ethical Implications of Differences in the Availability of Health Services, Volume One: Report* (Washington, DC: U.S. Government Printing Office, March 1983).
235. Price, K.F., and Coffey, R.M., "Evaluating Patient Classification Systems for Hospital Reimbursement: The Case of Disease Staging," paper presented to the American Public Health Association meetings, Anaheim, CA, November 1984.
236. Pride Institute, "Symposium: The Potential Impact of Diagnosis-Related Groups on Long-Term Care," *Pride Inst. J. Home Health Care* 2(4):3-9, Fall 1983.
237. Prospective Payment Assessment Commission, *Report and Recommendations to the Secretary, U.S. Department of Health and Human Services*, vol. 1 (Washington, DC: U.S. Government Printing Office, Apr. 1, 1985).
238. Prospective Payment Assessment Commission, *Technical Appendixes to the Report and Recommendations to the Secretary, U.S. Department of Health and Human Services*, vol. 2 (Washington, DC: U.S. Government Printing Office, Apr. 1, 1985).
239. Pryga, E., American Hospital Association, Chicago, IL, personal communication, May 29, 1985.
240. Rabinowitz, R., "Alcoholism Consultation and Liaison in a General Hospital," *Bull. N.Y. Acad. Med.* 59(2):229, March 1983.
241. Rabkin, M.T., "Will the DRG Decimate Clinical Research?" (editorial), *Clin. Res.* 32(3):345-7, September 1984.
242. Reeder, G., Krishan, I., Nobrega, F., et al., "Is Percutaneous Coronary Angioplasty Less Expensive Than Bypass Surgery?" *N. Eng. J. Med.* 311:1157-1162, 1984.
243. Relman, A.S., "Economic Considerations in Emergency Care: What Are Hospitals For?" *N. Eng. J. Med.* 312(6):372-373, Feb. 7, 1985.
244. Rentrop, K.P., Feit, F., Blanke, H., et al., "Effects of Intracoronary Streptokinase and Intracoronary Nitroglycerin Infusion on Coronary Angiographic Patterns and Mortality in Patients With Acute Myocardial Infarction," *N. Eng. J. Med.* 311(23):1457-1463, Dec. 6, 1984.
245. Rettig, R.A., "The Politics of Health Cost Containment: End-Stage Renal Disease," *Bull. N.Y. Acad. Med.* 56:115-138, 1980.
246. Richards, G., "Layoff Wave Rolls Through Industry," *Hospitals* 58(16):76-82, Aug. 16, 1984.
247. Rockey P.H., and Griep, R.H., "Behavioral Dysfunction in Hyperthyroidism—Improvement With Treatment," *Arch. Intern. Med.* 140(9):1194-7, September 1980.
248. Romeo, A.A., *The Hemodialysis Equipment and Disposable Industry* (Health Technology Case Study #32), prepared for the Office of Technology Assessment, U.S. Congress, OTA-HCS-32 (Washington, DC: U.S. Government Printing Office, December 1984).
249. Romeo, A.A., Wagner, J., and Lee, R., "Prospective Hospital Reimbursement and the Diffusion of New Hospital Technologies," *J. Health Econ.* 3:1-24, 1984.
250. Rosko, M.D., "An Analysis of the Differential Impact of Hospital Rate Regulation on Routine Expenses Per Admission and Ancillary Expenses Per Admission," prepared for American Economic Association Annual Meeting, Washington, DC, Dec. 29, 1982.
251. Roth, M., "Surgery: Hospitals Trimming Budg-

ets in Medicare Billing Switch," *Pittsburgh Post-Gazette*, July 2, 1984.
252. Ruskin, P.E., "Geropsychiatric Consultation in a University Hospital: A Report on 67 Referrals," *Am. J. Psychiatry* 142(3):333-336, March 1985.
253. Russell, L.B., *Technology in Hospitals: Medical Advances and Their Diffusion* (Washington, DC: The Brookings Institution, 1979).
254. Rutstein, D.D., Berenberg, W., Chalmers, T.C., et al., "Measuring the Quality of Medical Care," *N. Eng. J. Med.* 294(11):582-588, Mar. 11, 1976.
255. SRI Research Center, "American Hospital Association National Opinion Study," Lincoln, NE, February 1983.
256. Sackett D.L., Chambers L.W., MacPherson A.S., et al., "The Development and Application of Indices of Health: General Methods and a Summary of Results," *Am. J. Public Health* 67(5):423-8, May 1977.
257. Sanazaro, P.J., "Quality Assessment and Quality Assurance in Medical Care," *Annual Review of Public Health* 1:37-68, 1980.
258. Saxe, L., Dougherty, D., Esty, K., et al., *The Effectiveness and Costs of Alcoholism Treatment* (Health Technology Case Study #22), prepared for the Office of Technology Assessment, U.S. Congress, OTA-HCS-22 (Washington DC: U.S. Government Printing Office, March 1983).
259. Scanlon, W.M., "A Theory of the Nursing Home Market," *Inquiry* 17:25-41, Spring 1980.
260. Schrage, M., "Spending Rules May Hurt Health Technology," *Washington Post*, p. G1, Oct. 28, 1984.
261. Schwartz, E., Bureau of Data Management and Strategy, Health Care Financing Administration, U.S. Department of Health and Human Services, Baltimore, MD, personal communication, September 1984.
262. Seymour, D., "What PPS Means for Hospital Marketing," *Hospitals* 58(12):70-2, June 16, 1984.
263. Sheingold, S., Congressional Budget Office, U.S. Congress, Washington, DC, personal communication, March 1985.
264. Sikora, D., Health Care Financing Administration, U.S. Department of Health and Human Services, Baltimore, MD, personal communication, Feb. 20, 1985.
265. Sickora, D., Health Care Financing Administration, U.S. Department of Health and Human Services, Baltimore, MD, personal communication, May 10, 1985.
266. Silverman, H., Health Care Financing Administration, U.S. Department of Health and Human Services, Baltimore, MD, personal communication, June 11, 1985.
267. Simborg, D.W., "DRG Creep: A New Hospital-Acquired Disease," *N. Eng. J. Med.* 304(26):1602-1604, 1981.
268. Sloan, F.A., "Regulation and the Rising Cost of Hospital Care," *The Review of Economics and Statistics* 63(4):479-487, November 1981.
269. Sloan, F.A., "Rate Regulation as a Strategy for Hospital Cost Control: Evidence From the Last Decade," *Milbank Mem. Fund Q.* 61(2):195-221, 1983.
270. Sloan, F.A., Valvona, J., Perrin, J.M., et al., "Diffusion of Surgical Technology: An Exploratory Study," unpublished manuscript, Nashville, TN, 1984.
271. Smith, S.E., "The Impact of DRGs on Educational Programs in Nursing," in *DRGs: Changes and Challenges*, F.A. Shaffer (ed.) (New York, NY: National League for Nursing, 1984).
272. Smits, H.L., "The PSRO in Perspective," *N. Eng. J. Med.* 305:253-289, 1981.
273. Smits, H.L., and Watson, R.E., "DRGs and the Future of Surgical Practice," *N. Eng. J. Med.* 311(24):1612-1615, Dec. 20, 1984.
274. Sobaski, W., Office of Research and Demonstrations, Health Care Financing Administration, U.S. Department of Health and Human Services, Baltimore, MD, personal communication, May 20, 1985.
275. Society for Medical Decision Making, "Panel: Clinical Decision Making in an Era of DRG-Based Prospective Payment," presented at Sixth Annual Meeting, Bethesda, MD, Nov. 28-30, 1984.
276. Spivey, B.E., "The Relation Between Hospital Management and Medical Staff Under a Prospective-Payment System," *N. Eng. J. Med.* 310(5):984-6, Apr. 12, 1984.
277. Stark, W.J., Terry, A.C., Worthen, D., et al., "Update of Intraocular Lenses Implanted in the United States," *Am. J. Ophthal.* 98:238-239, 1984.
278. Steel, K., Gertman, P., Crescenzi, C., et al., "Iatrogenic Illness on a General Medical Service at a University Hospital," *N. Eng. J. Med.* 304:638-642, Mar. 12, 1981.
279. Steinberg, E.P., and Cohen, A.B., *Nuclear Magnetic Resonance Imaging Technology: A Clinical, Industrial, and Policy Analysis* (Health Technology Case Study #27), prepared for the Office of Technology Assessment, U.S. Congress, OTA-HCS-27 (Washington, DC: U.S. Government Printing Office, September 1984).

280. Stern, R.S., and Epstein, A.M., "Institutional Responses to Prospective Payment Based on Diagnosis-Related Groups: Implications for Cost, Quality and Access," *N. Eng. J. Med.* 312:621-627, Mar. 7, 1985.
281. Stoiber, S., National Institutes of Health, Public Health Service, U.S. Department of Health and Human Services, Bethesda, MD, personal communication, May 1985.
282. Swartz, K., "Who Has Been Without Health Insurance? Changes Between 1963 and 1979," Urban Institute Working Paper, Washington, DC, April 1984.
283. Swartz, K. (Urban Institute), "The Changing Face of the Uninsured," paper prepared for presentation at the First Annual Meeting of the Association for Health Services Researchers, Panel on "Health Care for the Poor in an Era of Retrenchment," Washington, DC, June 11, 1984.
284. Tauke, T.J., "Rural Hospitals Suffer Prospective Payment Inequities," *Business and Health* 26:37-41, May 1985.
285. Teitelman, R., "Selective Surgery," *Forbes* 135(8):75-76, Apr. 22, 1985.
286. Technology Reimbursement Reports, "Medicare Lithotripter Coverage Includes Extracorporeal and Percutaneous Methods," *Technology Reimbursement Reports* 1(14):2, May 3, 1985.
287. Technology Reimbursement Reports, "Proposed Prospective Payment Freeze in FY 1986 Would 'Chill' Technological Innovation, HIMA Says," *Technology Reimbursement Reports* 1(24):4, July 12, 1985.
288. Technology Reimbursement Reports, "PROs Have 'Redflagged' 3,700 Inappropriate Discharges, More Enforcement Power Needed—Heinz," *Technology Reimbursement Reports* 1(77):7, Aug. 2, 1985.
289. Thompson, J.D., "The Measurement of Nursing Intensity," *Health Care Financing Review*, 1984 Annual Supplement:47-55, Winter 1984.
290. Thompson, M., and King, C., "Physician Perceptions of Medical Malpractice and Defensive Medicine," *Evaluation and Program Planning* 7:95-104, 1984.
291. Trafford, A., "Hospitals: A Sick Industry," *U.S. News and World Report* 98(10):39-45, Mar. 18, 1985.
292. Trauner, J., Luft, H., and Robinson, J., "Entrepreneurial Trends in Health Care Delivery: The Development of Retail Dentistry and Freestanding Ambulatory Services," prepared for Federal Trade Commission, Washington, DC, July 1982.
293. U.S. Congress, Congressional Budget Office, *The Effects of PSROs on Health Care Costs: Current Findings and Future Evaluations* (Washington, DC: U.S. Government Printing Office, 1979).
294. U.S. Congress, Congressional Budget Office, *The Impact of PSROs on Health Care Costs: Update of CBO's 1979 Evaluation* (Washington, DC: U.S. Government Printing Office, 1981).
295. U.S. Congress, Congressional Budget Office, "Impact of Medicare's Prospective Payment System," memorandum, Washington, DC, Nov. 31, 1984.
296. U.S. Congress, General Accounting Office, *Department of Health and Human Services Should Improve Monitoring of Professional Standards Review Organizations*, Report to the Subcommittee on Oversight, Committee on Ways and Means, House of Representatives, U.S. Congress, HRD-81-26 (Washington, DC: U.S. Government Printing Office, 1980).
297. U.S. Congress, General Accounting Office, "Information Requirements for Evaluating the Impacts of Medicare Prospective Payment on Post-Hospital Long-Term Care Services," Preliminary Report, GAO/PEMD-85-8, Washington, DC, Feb. 21, 1985.
298. U.S. Congress, General Accounting Office, Comptroller General of the United States, "Rising Hospital Costs Can Be Restrained by Regulating Payments and Improving Management," Report to Congress, HRD-80-72, Washington, DC, Sept. 19, 1980.
299. U.S. Congress, General Accounting Office, Comptroller General of the United States, "Use of Unaudited Hospital Cost Data Resulted in Overstatement of Medicare's Prospective Payment Rates," Report to Congress, GAO/HRD-85-74, Washington, DC, July 18, 1985.
300. U.S. Congress, General Accounting Office, Human Resources Division, "Reviewing the Medicare Prospective Reimbursement System for Hospitals," draft, Washington, DC, February 1984.
301. U.S. Congress, House of Representatives, Committee on Appropriations, *Committee Report Accompanying H.R. 6028* (Washington, DC: U.S. Government Printing Office, July 26, 1984).
302. U.S. Congress, House of Representatives, Select Committee on Aging, hearing on *Sustaining Quality Health Care Under Cost Containment*, H.R. 499, Feb. 26, 1985 (Washington, DC: U.S. Government Printing Office, 1985).
303. U.S. Congress, House of Representatives, Select Committee on Aging, Task Force on the Rural Elderly, "Results of Survey to State Nursing Home Ombudsmen," Washington, DC, February 1985.
304. U.S. Congress, Office of Technology Assess-

ment, *Strategies for Medical Technology Assessment* (Washington, DC: U.S. Government Printing Office, September 1982).
305. U.S. Congress, Office of Technology Assessment, *Diagnosis-Related Groups (DRGs) and the Medicare Program: Implications for Medical Technology*, OTA-TM-H-17 (Washington, DC: U.S. Government Printing Office, July 1983).
306. U.S. Congress, Office of Technology Assessment, *The Impact of Randomized Clinical Trials on Health Policy and Medical Practice*, OTA-BP-H-22 (Washington, DC: U.S. Government Printing Office, August 1983).
307. U.S. Congress, Office of Technology Assessment, *Medical Technology and Costs of the Medicare Program*, OTA-H-227 (Washington, DC: U.S. Government Printing Office, July 1984).
308. U.S. Congress, Office of Technology Assessment, *Federal Policies and the Medical Device Industry*, OTA-H-230 (Washington, DC: U.S. Government Printing Office, October 1984).
309. U.S. Congress, Office of Technology Assessment, "First Report on the Prospective Payment Assessment Commission (ProPAC) by the Office of Technology Assessment," Washington, DC, Mar. 25, 1985.
310. U.S. Congress, Senate, Committee on Finance, Subcommittee on Health, hearing on *Implementation of PRO's for Medicare*, Feb. 1, 1984 (Washington, DC: U.S. Government Printing Office, 1985).
311. U.S. Department of Commerce, Bureau of Census, *1976 Survey of Institutionalized Persons: Methods and Procedures* (Washington, DC: U.S. Government Printing Office, June 1978).
312. U.S. Department of Commerce, Bureau of Census, "Long-Term Care Survey," OMB No. 0990-0077, Form LTC-3, Washington, DC, April 1982.
313. U.S. Department of Defense, Office of Assistant Secretary for Defense, Health Affairs, Office of Quality Assurance, Washington, DC, personal communication, November 1984.
314. U.S. Department of Health, Education, and Welfare, Health Services Administration, Office of Planning, Evaluation, and Legislation, *An Evaluation of the Professional Standards Review Organization, Executive Summary*, DHEW Pub. No. (OPEL) 77-12, vol. 1 (Washington, DC: DHEW, 1977).
315. U.S. Department of Health, Education, and Welfare, Public Health Service, *Report of the President's Biomedical Research Panel*, DHEW Pub. No. (OS) 76-501 (Washington, DC: DHEW, Apr. 30, 1976).
316. U.S. Department of Health, Education, and Welfare, Public Health Service, National Center for Health Statistics, *Development of the Design of the NCHS Hospital Discharge Survey* (Washington, DC: U.S. Government Printing Office, September 1970).
317. U.S. Department of Health, Education, and Welfare, Public Health Service, National Center for Health Statistics, *Design and Methodology of the 1967 Master Facility Inventory Survey*, Series 1, No. 9 (Washington, DC: U.S. Government Printing Office, 1971).
318. U.S. Department of Health, Education, and Welfare, Public Health Service, National Center for Health Statistics, *Health Interview Survey Procedure*, DHEW Pub. No. (HRA) 75-1311 (Washington, DC: U.S. Government Printing Office, April 1975).
319. U.S. Department of Health, Education, and Welfare, Public Health Service, National Center for Health Statistics, *Plan and Operation of HANES 1 Augmentation*, DHEW Pub. No. (PHS) 78-1314 (Washington, DC: U.S. Government Printing Office, June 1978).
320. U.S. Department of Health, Education, and Welfare, Public Health Service, National Institutes of Health, *NIH Inventory of Clinical Trials: Fiscal Year 1975* (Bethesda, MD: NIH, 1975).
321. U.S. Department of Health and Human Services, Health Care Financing Administration, *Professional Standards Review Organization 1979 Program Evaluation*, HCFA Pub. No. 03041 (Baltimore, MD: HCFA, 1980).
322. U.S. Department of Health and Human Services, Health Care Financing Administration, *The International Classification of Diseases, 9th Revision, Clinical Modification*, vol. 1, 2d ed., DHHS Pub. No. (PHS) 80-1260 (Washington, DC: U.S. Government Printing Office, September 1980).
323. U.S. Department of Health and Human Services, Health Care Financing Administration, *The Medicare and Medicaid Data Book 1981* (Baltimore, MD: HCFA, April 1982).
324. U.S. Department of Health and Human Services, Health Care Financing Administration, *The Medicare and Medicaid Data Book 1982* (Baltimore, MD: HCFA, April 1983).
325. U.S. Department of Health and Human Services, Health Care Financing Administration, *Medicare Statistical Files Manual* (Baltimore, MD: HCFA, September 1983).
326. U.S. Department of Health and Human Services, Health Care Financing Administration, *The

Medicare and Medicaid Data Book 1983, HCFA Pub. No. 03156 (Baltimore, MD: HCFA, December 1983).

327. U.S. Department of Health and Human Services, Health Care Financing Administration, "PRO Hospital Discharge Data Set Tape Layout," Baltimore, MD, 1984.

328. U.S. Department of Health and Human Services, Health Care Financing Administration, "Selected Activities for Short-Term and Long-Term Agenda," unpublished, Baltimore, MD, 1984.

329. U.S. Department of Health and Human Services, Health Care Financing Administration, "MADRS Summary," draft, Baltimore, MD, February 1984.

330. U.S. Department of Health and Human Services, Health Care Financing Administration, "Request for Proposal: Operation of Utilization and Quality Control Peer Review Organizations," RFP No. HCFA-84-015, Baltimore, MD, Feb. 29, 1984.

331. U.S. Department of Health and Human Services, Health Care Financing Administration, *HCFA Coverage Manual* (Baltimore, MD: HCFA, September 1984).

332. U.S. Department of Health and Human Services, Health Care Financing Administration, "Background Paper," Baltimore, MD, December 1984.

333. U.S. Department of Health and Human Services, Health Care Financing Administration, "Background Paper," Baltimore, MD, January 1985.

334. U.S. Department of Health and Human Services, Health Care Financing Administration, "Background Materials for Technical Advisory Panel Meeting," unpublished, Baltimore, MD, Mar. 12, 1985.

335. U.S. Department of Health and Human Services, Health Care Financing Administration, "Research, Demonstration, and Evaluation Spending Plan," Baltimore, MD, draft, April 1985.

336. U.S. Department of Health and Human Services, Health Care Financing Administration, *Status Report*, HCFA Pub. No. 03185 (Washington, DC: U.S. Government Printing Office, April 1985).

337. U.S. Department of Health and Human Services, Health Care Financing Administration, "Background Paper," Baltimore, MD, July 1985.

338. U.S. Department of Health and Human Services, Health Care Financing Administration, Bureau of Data Management and Strategy, "Medicare Data," Baltimore, MD, 1985.

339. U.S. Department of Health and Human Services, Health Care Financing Administration, Health Standards and Quality Bureau, *Peer Review Organization Objectives: A Synopsis*, vol. 1, September 1984, cited in K.N. Lohr, "Peer Review Organization (PROs): Quality Assurance in Medicare," prepared for the Office of Technology Assessment, U.S Congress, Washington, DC, Nov. 9, 1984.

340. U.S. Department of Health and Human Services, Health Care Financing Administration, Office of Research and Development, "Annual Impact Report," draft, Baltimore, MD, September 1984.

341. U.S. Department of Health and Human Services, Health Care Financing Administration, Office of Statistics and Data Management, "Health Care Financing Trends," *Health Care Financing Review* 6(1):91-93, Fall 1984.

342. U.S. Department of Health and Human Services, Office of Inspector General, "Long-Term Care: Service Delivery Assessment, Report to the Secretary," Washington, DC, 1981.

343. U.S. Department of Health and Human Services, Office of Inspector General, "The Prospective Payment System and the Office of Inspector General," Washington, DC, Mar. 8, 1984.

344. U.S. Department of Health and Human Services, Public Health Service, Food and Drug Administration, "Summary of Safety and Effectiveness Data: Dornier Lithotripter, Model HM3," unpublished manuscript, Washington, DC, December 1984.

345. U.S. Department of Health and Human Services, Public Health Service, Health Resources and Services Administration, *Area Resource File (ARF) System*, DHHS Pub. No. HRS-P-OD-84-6 (Rockville, MD: HRSA, May 1984).

346. U.S. Department of Health and Human Services, Public Health Service, Health Resources and Services Administration, *Report to the President and Congress on the Status of Health Personnel in the United States*, DHHS Pub. No. HRS-P-OD 84-4 (Rockville, MD: HRSA, May 1984).

347. U.S. Department of Health and Human Services, Public Health Service, Health Resources and Services Administration, *Status Report on State Certificate of Need Programs* (Rockville, MD: HRSA, 1985).

348. U.S. Department of Health and Human Services, Public Health Service, National Center for Health Services Research, *NMCES Household Interview Instruments*, DHHS Pub. No. (PHS) 81-3280 (Hyattsville, MD: NCHSR, April 1981).

349. U.S. Department of Health and Human Services, Public Health Service, National Center for Health Services Research, *Project Overview: Hospital Cost and Utilization Project Research Note 1*, DHHS Pub. No. (PHS) 83-3343 (Rockville, MD: NCHSR, June 1983).

350. U.S. Department of Health and Human Services,

Public Health Service, National Center for Health Services Research, "Project Description and Justification: Impacts of the Prospective Payment System on Clinical Cancer Research," unpublished, Rockville, MD, Aug. 3, 1984.
351. U.S. Department of Health and Human Services, Public Health Service, National Center for Health Services Research and Health Care Technology Assessment, "Public Health Service Prospective Payment Activity as of April 30, 1985," Rockville, MD, April 1985.
352. U.S. Department of Health and Human Services, Public Health Service, National Center for Health Statistics, *Current Estimates Health Interview Survey*, DHHS Pub. No. (PHS) 80-1551 (Washington, DC: U.S. Government Printing Office, 1979).
353. U.S. Department of Health and Human Services, Public Health Service, National Center for Health Statistics, *Data Systems of the National Center for Health Statistics*, Series 1, No. 16, DHHS Pub. No. (PHS) 82-1318 (Washington, DC: U.S. Government Printing Office, 1981).
354. U.S. Department of Health and Human Services, Public Health Service, National Center for Health Statistics, *Public Use Data Tape Documentation, National Ambulatory Medical Care Survey* (Washington, DC: U.S. Government Printing Office, April 1981).
355. U.S. Department of Health and Human Services, Public Health Service, National Center for Health Statistics, *Highlights From Wave 1 of the National Survey of Personal Health Practices and Consequences, U.S. 1979*, DHHS Pub. No. (PHS) 81-1162 (Washington, DC: U.S. Government Printing Office, June 1981).
356. U.S. Department of Health and Human Services, Public Health Service, National Center for Health Statistics, *Plan and Operation of the Second National Health and Nutrition Examination Survey: 1976-80*, DHHS Pub. No. (PHS) 81-1317 (Washington, DC: U.S. Government Printing Office, July 1981).
357. U.S. Department of Health and Human Services, Public Health Service, National Center for Health Statistics, *Procedures and Questionnaires of the National Medical Care Utilization and Expenditure Survey*, DHHS Pub. No. 83-20001 (Washington, DC: U.S. Government Printing Office, March 1983).
358. U.S. Department of Health and Human Services, Public Health Service, National Center for Health Statistics, *Nursing and Related Care Homes*, DHHS Pub. No. (PHS) 84-1824 (Washington, DC: U.S. Government Printing Office, December 1983).
359. U.S. Department of Health and Human Services, Public Health Service, National Center for Health Statistics, "Discussion Paper: Planning for a Survey of Health Care Utilization and Expenditures," unpublished, Hyattsville, MD, Mar. 1, 1984.
360. U.S. Department of Health and Human Services, Public Health Service, National Center for Health Statistics, unpublished data, Hyattsville, MD, 1985.
361. U.S. Department of Health and Human Services, Public Health Service, National Institutes of Health, *General Clinical Research Centers*, NIH Pub. No. 83-1433 (Bethesda, MD: NIH, February 1983).
362. U.S. Department of Health and Human Services, Public Health Service, National Institutes of Health, *NIH Data Book 1984*, NIH Pub. No. 84-1261 (Bethesda, MD: NIH, June 1984).
363. U.S. Department of Health and Human Services, Public Health Service, National Institutes of Health, National Cancer Advisory Board, letter to the Secretary of Health and Human Services, Bethesda, MD, Sept. 25, 1984.
364. U.S. Department of Health and Human Services, Public Health Service, National Institutes of Health, National Cancer Institute, "Fact Sheet—Community Clinical Oncology Program," Bethesda, MD, November 1983.
365. U.S. Department of Health and Human Services, Public Health Service, Office of Health Technology Assessment, "Public Health Service Assessment of Streptokinase Infusion for Acute Myocardial Infarction," Report No. NCHSR 84-232, Rockville, MD, 1984.
366. U.S. Department of Health and Human Services, Social Security Administration, Office of Policy, *1978 Survey of Disability and Work*, SSA Pub. No. 13-11745 (Washington, DC: SSA, January 1982).
367. U.S. Executive Office of the President, Office of Management and Budget, *Standard Industrial Classification Manual* (Washington DC: U.S. Government Printing Office, 1972).
368. U.S. National Science Foundation, *Federal Funds for Research and Development: Fiscal Years 1980, 1981, and 1982*, NSF 81-325 (Washington DC: NSF, 1981).
369. Vaida, M., "The Financial Impact of Prospective Payment on Hospitals," *Health Affairs* 3(1):112-119, Spring 1984.
370. Vaida, M., California Hospital Association,

Sacramento, CA, personal communication, Sept. 27, 1984.
371. Venture Economics (Wellesley Hills, MA), "Venture Capital Investment in the Medical Health Care Field," prepared for the Office of Technology Assessment, U.S. Congress, Washington, DC, August 1983.
372. Verstraete, M., Bory, M., Collen, D., et al., "Randomised Trial of Intravenous Recombinant Tissue-Type Plasminogen Activator Versus Intravenous Streptokinase in Acute Myocardial Infarction," *Lancet* 1:842-847, Apr. 13, 1985.
373. Vladeck, B., *Unloving Care: The Nursing Home Tragedy* (New York, NY: Basic Books, 1980).
374. Wagner, D.P., and Draper, E., "APACHE II and Medicare Reimbursement," *Health Care Financing Review* Annual Supplement:91-105, November 1984.
375. Wagner, J.L., and Krieger, M.J., *The Implications of Cost-Effectiveness Analysis of Medical Technology, Background Paper #5: Four Common X-Ray Procedures: Problems and Prospects for Economic Evaluation,* prepared for Office of Technology Assessment, U.S. Congress, OTA-BP-H-14 (Washington, DC: U.S. Government Printing Office, April 1982).
376. Waldhauser, C., Health Care Financing Administration, U.S. Department of Health and Human Services, Baltimore, MD, personal communication, March 1985.
377. Waldron, C., Health Care Financing Administration, U.S. Department of Health and Human Services, Baltimore, MD, personal communication, May 1985.
378. Ware, J.E., Jr., Brook, R.H., Davies, A.R., et al., "Choosing Measures of Health Status for Individuals in General Populations," *Am. J. Public Health* 71(6):620-625, June 1981.
379. Washington Report on Medicine and Health, "DRGs, LOS, and FTEs," *Washington Report on Medicine and Health* 35(38):(Perspectives), Oct. 1, 1984.
380. Washington Report on Medicine and Health, "PROs Set To Go," *Washington Report on Medicine and Health* 38(45):(Perspectives), Nov. 19, 1984.
381. Washington Report on Medicine and Health, "DRGs and Quality of Care," *Washington Report on Medicine and Health* 39(1):(Perspectives), Jan. 7, 1985.
382. Washington Report on Medicine and Health, "DRGs Spur Hospital Interest in Long-Term Care," *Washington Report on Medicine and Health* 39(4):(Perspectives), Jan. 28, 1985.
383. Washington Report on Medicine and Health, "Public Hospitals Have Higher Costs, HHS Says," *Washington Report on Medicine and Health* 39(11):1, Mar. 18, 1985.
384. Washington Report on Medicine and Health, "Can Rural Hospitals Survive?" *Washington Report on Medicine and Health* 39(18):(Perspectives), May 6, 1985.
385. Watts, C.A., and Baker, F.D., "Hospital Cost Inflation Under State Rate-Setting: Some Additional Evidence," draft, Seattle, WA, 1981.
386. Webster's *Third New International Dictionary* (Unabridged) (Springfield, MA: G. & C. Merriam Co., 1981).
387. Wennberg, J.E., "Dealing With Medical Practice Variations: A Proposal for Action," *Health Affairs* 3(2):6-32, Summer 1984.
388. Wennberg, J.E., "Small Area Variations in Hospitalized Case-Mix," Final Report, Department of Community and Family Medicine, Dartmouth Medical School, Hanover, NH, Oct. 31, 1984.
389. Wennberg, J.E., and Gettlesohn, A., "Variations in Medical Care Among Small Areas," *Sci. Am.* 246(4):120-34, April 1982.
390. Wennberg, J.E., McPherson, K., and Caper, P., "Will Payment Based on Diagnosis-Related Groups Control Hospital Costs?" *N. Eng. J. Med.* 311(5):295-300, Aug. 2, 1984.
391. Werner, M., Southerland, E.W., and Abramson, F.P., "Concepts for the Rational Selection of Assays To Be Used in Monitoring Therapeutic Drugs," *Clin. Chem.* 21:1368-1371, September 1975.
392. West, H., Marcus, L., McMenamin, P., et al. (for Mandex, Inc.), prepared for Health Care Financing Administration, U.S. Department of Health and Human Services, *Physician and Hospital Reimbursement Study* (Vienna, VA: Mandex, Inc., Jan. 31, 1985).
393. Williams, A., "Need—An Economic Exegesis," in *Economic Aspects of Health Services,* A.J. Culyer and K.G. Wright (eds.) (London: Robertson & Co., 1978).
394. Williams, A., Carter, G., Melnick, G., et al., "Medicare Part A Data: A Prospective Payment Systems Perspective," prepared for the Office of the Secretary for Planning and Evaluation, U.S. Department of Health and Human Services, WD 2173-HHS, draft, Washington, DC, 1984.
395. Williams, K.N., and Brook, R.H., "Quality Measurement and Assurance: A Review of the Recent Literature," *Health and Medical Care Services Review* 1(3):1-15, May/June 1978.
396. Williams, S., Kominski, G., and Pickens, G.,

"The Evaluation of Alternative Patient Classification Systems," prepared for the Office of Technology Assessment, U.S. Congress, Washington, DC, Mar. 26, 1985.
397. Williams, S.V., Finkler, S.A., Murphy, C.M., et al., "Improved Cost Allocation in Case-Mix Accounting," *Medical Care* 20(5):450-59, May 1982.
398. Wisconsin Hospital Association News, "Hospital Layoffs May Hit 4,000 by End of Year," *Wisconsin Hospital Association News*, Apr. 23, 1984.
399. Wood, D., Bureau of Data Management and Strategy, Health Care Financing Administration, U.S. Department of Health and Human Services, Baltimore, MD, personal communication, August 1985.
400. World Health Organization, "Constitution of the World Health Organization," in *Basic Documents* (Geneva, Switzerland: WHO, 1948).
401. Worthington, N.L., and Piro, P.A., "The Effects of Hospital Rate-Setting Programs on Volumes of Hospital Services: A Preliminary Analysis," *Health Care Financing Review* 4(2):47-61, December 1982.
402. Wrenn, K., "No Insurance, No Admission," *N. Eng. J. Med.* 312(6):373-374, Feb. 7, 1985.
403. Yaffe, R., Office of Demonstrations, Health Care Financing Administration, U.S. Department of Health and Human Services, Baltimore, MD, personal communication, Aug. 7, 1984.
404. Yarbro, J.W., and Mortenson, L.E., "The Need for Diagnosis-Related Group 471," *J.A.M.A.* 253(5):684-685, Feb. 1, 1985.
405. Yavner, S., Yavner, D., and Finklestein, S.M., "Medical Technology and DRGs: The Case of the Implantable Infusion Pump," prepared for the Office of Technology Assessment, U.S. Congress, Washington, DC, December 1984.
406. Young, W.W., Swinkola, R.B., and Hutton, M.A., "Assessment of the AUTOGRP Patient Classification System," *Medical Care* 18(2):228-244, 1980.
407. Zuckerman, S., Becker, E., Adams, K, et al., "Physician Practice Patterns Under Hospital Rate-Setting Programs," *J.A.M.A.* 252(18):2589-2592, Nov. 9, 1984.

springer publishing company

The Encyclopedia of Aging

George L. Maddox, Editor-in-Chief
Robert C. Atchley, Leonard W. Poon,
George S. Roth, Ilene C. Siegler,
Raymond J. Steinberg, Associate Editors
Raymond J. Corsini, Managing Editor

This major new reference work will provide concise, authoritative explanations for hundreds of terms and concepts relating to the aging process. Up-to-date and comprehensive, the Encyclopedia includes information on research and practice, as well as on the rapidly growing range of programs and professional services to the elderly. The level of presentation makes this volume readily accessible to students, and professionals from many fields, with particular attention to the needs of information-seeking nonspecialists.

This Encyclopedia is the only one of its kind in the world, and it offers a total state-of-the-art perspective on aging.

Ca. 500 Entries   Approx. 1,000 pp.   One Volume   Double Column

November, 1986

Among the 225 distinguished contributors are:

Reubin Andres, M.D.
Robert Binstock, Ph.D.
Bonnie Bullough, R.N., Ph.D.
Robert N. Butler, M.D.
Gene D. Cohen, M.D.
Carl Eisdorfer, M.D., Ph.D.
Carroll L. Estes, Ph.D.
Barry J. Gurland, M.D.
Leonard Hayflick, Ph.D.

Carol C. Hogue, Ph.D.
Robert Kastenbaum, Ph.D.
Richard Lazarus, Ph.D.
Zhores Medvedev, Ph.D.
Erdman B. Palmore, Ph.D.
Joan Quinn, R.N., M.S.N.
Matilda W. Riley, D.Sc.
Nathan Shock, Ph.D.
Barbara M. Silverstone, D.S.W.
Philip Weiler, M.D.

Order from your bookdealer or directly from publisher.
Springer Publishing Co. 536 Broadway, New York, NY 10012

springer publishing company

The Journal of Compliance in Health Care
Raymond A. Ulmer, Editor-in-Chief

Here is the only periodical to focus exclusively on patient noncompliance problems, bringing together information on research, practice, education, and training, from the entire range of health-related disciplines. Two issues a year beginning in Spring, 1986. Subscription rates: Individual $25 ($45/2 yrs) Institutions $44 ($78/2 yrs)

Health Care Delivery in the United States
3rd Edition
Steven Jonas, Editor

This comprehensive resource has become the standard work of its kind. Now completely updated. "An extremely well-documented description... non-technical, very interesting, and well integrated." —*Medical Care.* 512pp / 1986

Basic Nursing Home Administration
James Allen

This comprehensive volume covers the nine core areas of knowledge required by the federal government for state licensure as a nursing home administrator. Its clear, easy to follow format also makes it a valuable text for college courses as well as an essential professional reference. 512 pp / 1986

Cancer Treatment and Research in Humanistic Perspective
Steve Gross and **Solomon Garb,** Editors

A forum of views on the pressing humanistic concerns that accompany the onset and treatment of cancer. Discusses drug experimentation, ineffective therapies, pain treatment, psychosocial problems, needs of cancer-care professionals, and more. 256pp / 1985

Vitalizing Long-Term Care
The Teaching Nursing Home and Other Perspectives
Stuart Spicker and **Stanley Ingman,** Editors

This interdisciplinary volume contributes to the efforts to reverse the status of America's nursing homes as isolated custodial institutions—and to fostering a new spirit in long-term care emphasizing service, teaching, and research.   256pp / 1984

Geriatrics and the Law
Patient Rights and Professional Responsibilities
Marshall Kapp and **Arthur Bigot**

Examines every aspect of geriatrics practice from a legal viewpoint: health-care financing, involuntary commitment, guardianship, powers of attorney, informed consent, and more. Explains complex medicolegal issues in clear, easy-to-understand language. 272pp / 1984

Assessing Clinical Competence
Neufeld, Norman, Spaulding, Editors

Here is a comprehensive overview of the concept of competence as it relates both to practicing physicians and medical students.   384pp / 1985

Social Work in the Emergency Room
Carole Soskis

Addresses issues ranging from treating psychiatric emergencies and drug abuse cases to setting up a social work service and anticipating legal needs. 240pp / 1984

Order from your bookdealer or directly from publisher.
Springer Publishing Co. 536 Broadway, New York, NY 10012